Spontaneous Abortion

Advances in Reproductive Health Care

LHRH and Its Analogs: Contraception and Therapeutic Applications
H. Vickery, J. J. Nestor, Jr., E. S. E. Hafez (editors)

Spontaneous Abortion
E. S. E. Hafez (editor)

Voluntary Termination of Pregnancy
E. S. E. Hafez (editor)

Biomedical Aspects of IUDs
H. Hasson, W. A. A. van Os, E. S. E. Hafez (editors)

Prostaglandins and Fertility Regulation
M. Toppozada, M. Bygdeman, E. S. E. Hafez (editors)

Male Fertility and Its Regulation
T. Lobl, E. S. E. Hafez (editors)

Advances in Reproductive Health Care

Spontaneous Abortion

Editor

E. S. E. Hafez

Executive Director,
Reproductive Health Center (USA)
& IVF/Andrology International

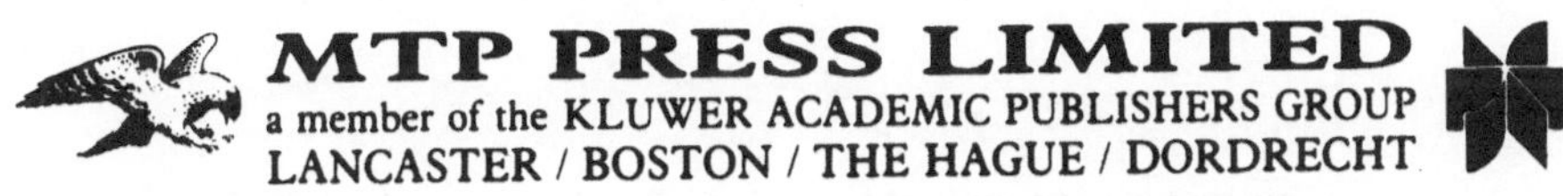

Published in the UK and Europe by
MTP Press Limited
Falcon House
Lancaster, England

British Library Cataloguing in Publication Data

Spontaneous abortion.—(Advances in reproductive health care)
1. Miscarriage
I. Hafez, E. S. E. II. Series
618.3'92 RG648

ISBN 978-94-010-9791-8 ISBN 978-94-010-9789-5 (eBook)
DOI 10.1007/978-94-010-9789-5

Published in the USA by
MTP Press
A division of Kluwer Boston Inc
190 Old Derby Street
Hingham, MA 02043, USA

Library of Congress Cataloging in Publication Data

Main entry under title:

Spontaneous abortion.

(Advances in reproductive health care)
Bibliography: p.
Includes index.
1. Miscarriage. 2. Miscarriage—Etiology.
I. Hafez, E. S. E., 1922- . II. Series.
(DNLM: 1. Abortion—congresses. WQ 225 S7633 1982)
RG648.S68 1984 618.3'3 84-7840
ISBN 978-94-010-9791-8

Softcover reprint of the hardcover 1st edition 1984

Typeset by Macmillan India Ltd, Bangalore.

Dedication

To our teacher

Tommy Nicholas Evans

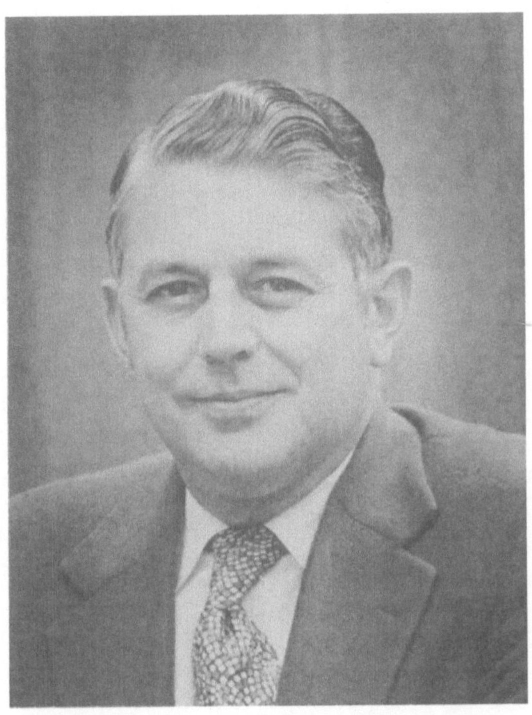

The Editor most appropriately has dedicated this series on *Advances in Reproductive Health Care* to Dr Tommy N. Evans, a true giant and pioneer in the field of human reproduction. Dr Evans' lifelong contributions to this important field of medicine are unmatched and encompass teaching, research, national and international organizational leadership, and most importantly, genuine concern for patients, physicians, and other researchers.

I feel honored and privileged to have been given this opportunity to recognize Dr Tommy N. Evans, a true colleague, teacher and friend.

Amir H. Ansari
Director, Department of OB/GYN
Georgia Baptist Medical Center
Atlanta, Georgia 30312

Contents

List of Contributors

J. J. AMY
Department of Obstetrics/Gynecology,
Free University of Brussels,
Academisch Ziekenhuis, Laarbeeklaan,
101,
B-1090 Brussels, BELGIUM

A. J. M. AUDEBERT
40 Cours de Verdun,
33000 Bordeaux, FRANCE

D. BARSOUM
El Batal Ahmed, Abd El Aziz At.,
Bab El Louk, Cairo,
EGYPT

R. E. BATT
Department of Gynecology–Obstetrics,
State University of New York at
Buffalo,
1000 Youngs Road, Williamsville,
N.Y. 14221, USA

F. R. BATZER
Pennsylvania Hospital, Department of
Obstetrics and Gynecology,
330 S. 9th Street,
Philadelphia, PA 19107–6096, USA

G. S. BERGER
Obstetrics and Gynecology
Department,
Chapel Hill Fertility Services,
109 Conner Drive, Suite 2104,
Chapel Hill,
North Carolina, USA

R. S. BERKOWITZ
Department of Obstetrics/Gynecology,
Harvard Medical School,
New England Trophoblastic Disease
Center,
Brigham and Women's Hospital,
75 Francis Street, Boston,
Massachusetts 02115, USA

M. BULIĆ
Department of Obstetrics and
Gynecology, Dr 'Ozren Novosel'
Hospital, 41000
Zagreb, Zajceva 19, YUGOSLAVIA

J. B. CALIXTO
Divisao De Farmacologia,
Universidade Federal De Santa
Catarina, Campus Universitario–
Trindate, 88000 Florianópolis, SC
BRAZIL

E. CITTADINI
Clinica Obstetrica e Ginecologica (R)
dell'Universita' di Palermo, Palermo,
ITALY

M. COGNAT
Department of Obstetrics/Gynecology,
Hospital St. Joseph, Lyon, FRANCE

S. L. CORSON
Department of Obstetrics and
Gynecology,
Pennsylvania Hospital, 330 S-9th
Street, Philadelphia, PA 19107–6096
USA

N. J. COSSLER
Department of Obstetrics/Gynecology,
Wayne State University School of
Medicine,
4707 St. Antoine, Detroit, Michigan
48201, USA

B. COUTIFARIS
Department of Obstetrics/Gynecology,
University of Athens, Aretaison
Hospital,
76 Vasilissis Sophias Avenue, Athens,
611 GREECE

C. COUTIFARIS
Department of Obstetrics/Gynecology, Hospital of the University of Pennsylvania,
3400 Spruce Street, Philadelphia, PA, 19104, USA

B. DAHLBERG
University of Lund, Department of Obstetrics/Gynecology, S-21401 Malmo, SWEDEN

P. DE BRUCKER
Department of Obstetrics/Gynecology, Free University of Brussels,
Academisch Ziekenhuis, Laarbeeklan, 101,
B-1090 Brussels, BELGIUM

I. DELKE
Department of Obstetrics/Gynecology, State University of N.Y. Downstate Medical Center, Obstetrics and Gynecology,
450 Clarkson Ave, Box 24, Brooklyn, N.Y. 11203, USA

Y. S. DE MEDEIROS
Laboratory of Pharmacology,
Health Sciences Center, Universidade Federal de Santa Catarina, 88000 Florianopolis, SC BRAZIL

K. I. EL-LAMIE
Department of Obstetrics/Gynecology, Faculty of Medicine, Ein-Shams University, Cairo, EGYPT

T. EL-MEKKAWI
Department of Obstetrics/Gynecology, Al Azhar University, Faculty of Medicine,
56 Giza Street,#17, Giza, Cairo, EGYPT

Z. EL-SHEIKHA
Department of Obstetrics/Gynecology, Al Azhar University, Faculty of Medicine,
56 Giza Street,#17, Giza, Cairo, EGYPT

I. FIGÁ-TALAMANCA
Institute of Physiology,
University of Rome,
Piazzo Aldo Moro,
00100 Rome, ITALY

W. FOULON
Department of Obstetrics/Gynecology & Adrology
Academisch Ziekenhuis, Vrije Universiteit Brussel, Laarbeeklaan 101, B.1090 Brussels, BELGIUM

I. GERHARD
Klinikum Universität Heidelberg, Frauenklinik Gynäkologische Endokrinologie,
Voßstr. 9, D-6900 Heidelberg, WEST GERMANY

D. P. GOLDSTEIN
Department of Obstetrics/Gynecology, New England Trophoblastic Disease Center,
Harvard Medical School, Brigham and Women's Hospital,
75 Francis Street, Boston, Massachusetts 02115, USA

E. S. E. HAFEZ
Reproductive Health Center
IVF/Andrology International
78 Switsong, Kiawah Island, SC 29455, USA

M. HAYES
Department of Obstetrics/Gynecology, Wayne State University School of Medicine,
275 East Hancock Avenue, Detroit, Michigan 48201, USA

J. B. HERTZ
Department of Obstetrics and Gynecology,
Gentofte Hospital, University of Copenhagen,
DK-2900 Hellerup, DENMARK

B. HO YUEN
Department of Obstetrics and Gynaecology, University of British Columbia, 4490 Oak Street, Grace Hospital, Vancouver, B.C., CANADA V6H 3V5

P. HUSSLEIN
Department of Obstetrics/Gynecology, Vienna University,
Spitalgasse 23, A-1090 Vienna, AUSTRIA

O. KANDIL
Department of Obstetrics/Gynecology, Al Azhar University, Faculty of Medicine,
56 Giza Street, 17, Giza, Cairo, EGYPT

L. G. KEITH
Department of Obstetrics/Gynecology, Prentice Women's Hospital and Maternity Clinic, Northwestern University,
333 E. Superior Street, 465 Chicago, Illinois 60611, USA

J. KLEINHOUT
Department of Obstetrics/Gynecology
St. Elizabeth of Groote Gasthuis, Postbus 417, 2000 AK Haarlem, The NETHERLANDS

K. MADAN
Institute of Human Genetics,
Faculty of Medicine, Free University,
Postbus 7161, 1007 MC Amsterdam, The NETHERLANDS

D. M. MAGYAR
Department of Obstetrics/Gynecology, Wayne State University School of Medicine,
275 East Hancock Avenue, Detroit, Michigan 48201, USA

M. MERCKX
Department of Obstetrics/Gynecology, Free University of Brussels,
Academisch Ziekenhuis, Laarbeeklan, 101, B-1090 Brussels, BELGIUM

M. W. METHOD
Department of Obstetrics & Gynecology,
Northwestern University Medical School and Prentice Women's Hospital,
333 E. Superior Street, Chicago, Illinois 60611, USA

M. MIZUNO
Department of Obstetrics/Gynecology, Faculty of Medicine,
University of Tokyo 7-3-1, Hongo, Bunkyo-Ku, Tokyo 113, JAPAN

M. MOUSA
Department of Obstetrics/Gynecology, Al Azhar University, Faculty of Medicine, 56 Giza Street, 17 Giza, Cairo, EGYPT

A. NAESSENS
Department of Microbiology, Academisch Ziekenhuis, Vrije Universiteit Brussel, Laarbeeklaan 101, B. 1090 Brussels, BELGIUM

J. D. NAPLES
Department of Gynecology–Obstetrics, State University of New York at Buffalo,
1000 Youngs Road, Williamsville, N.Y. 14221, USA

H. NISHIMURA
Central Institute for Experimental Animals, 1430 Nogawa, Miyamae, Kawasaki 213, JAPAN

M. PAJNTAR
Hospital of Obstetrics and Gynecology, Kidričeva 38a, 64000 Kranj, YUGOSLAVIA

B. J. POLAND
Department of Obstetrics/Gynecology, Vancouver General Hospital, 4490 Oak Street, Grace Hospital,
The University of British Columbia, Vancouver, British Columbia, CANADA V6H 3V5

S. M. PRIDE
Department of Obstetrics/Gynecology, Vancouver General Hospital, University of British Columbia, 4490 Oak Street, Grace Hospital, Vancouver, British Columbia, CANADA V6H 3V5

G. A. RAE
Laboratory of Pharmacology, Health Sciences Center,
Universidade Federal de Santa Catarina, 88000
Florianopolis, SC BRAZIL

J. ROJSEK
Department of Clinical Psychology, Polyclinic for mental health and neurology, Gosposvetska lo,
64000 Kranj, YUGOSLAVIA

B. RUNNEBAUM
Department of Gynecological Endocrinology, University of Heidelberg, Voßstr. 9, D-6900, Heidelberg, WEST GERMANY

S. SAKAMOTO
Department of Obstetrics/Gynecology,
Faculty of Medicine,
University of Tokyo 7-3-1, Hongo,
Bunkyo–Ku, Tokyo 113, JAPAN

K. SATO
Department of Obstetrics/Gynecology,
Faculty of Medicine,
University of Tokyo 7-3-1, Hongo,
Bunkyo–Ku, Tokyo 113 JAPAN

W. SCHNEDL
Department of Histology and
Embryology,
University of Vienna,
Schwarzspanierstr. 17, A–1090,
Vienna, AUSTRIA

L. SETTIMI
Institute of Physiology,
University of Rome,
Piazza Aldo Moro,
00100 ROME, ITALY

K. SHIOTA
Congenital Anomaly Research Center,
Faculty of Medicine, Kyoto University,
Yoshida Koneo-cho, Sakyo-Ku, Kyoto
606, JAPAN

N. J. SPIRTOS
Department of Obstetrics/Gynecology,
Wayne State University School of
Medicine,
275 East Hancock Avenue, Detroit,
Michigan 48201, USA

M. TAKADA
Department of Obstetrics/Gynecology,
Juntendo University, School of
Medicine 2-1-1, Hongo Bunkyo-ku,
Tokyo 113, JAPAN

M. L. TANCER
Department of Obstetrics/Gynecology,
Brookdale Medical Center,
Brookdale Plaza and Linden Boulevard
Brooklyn, N.Y. 11212, USA

K. TSUJI
Department of Obstetrics/Gynecology,
Wakayama Medical College,
1 Shichibancho, Wakayama 640,
JAPAN

N. P. VERIDIANO
Department of Obstetrics/Gynecology,
Brookdale Medical Center,
Brookdale Plaza and Linden Boulevard
Brooklyn, N.Y. 11212, USA.

P. WAGENBICHLER
Department of Gynecology/Obstetrics,
University of Vienna, Spitalqasse 23,
A–1090, Vienna, AUSTRIA

S. WEINER
Section of Perinatology, Department of
Obstetrics and Gynecology,
Pennsylvania Hospital, 8th and Spruce
Sts, Philadelphia, Pennsylvania 19107–
6096, USA

J. W. WLADIMIROFF
Department of Obstetrics/Gynecology,
Academic Hospital Rotterdam-Dijkzigt,
Erasmus University Rotterdam,
Dr Molewaterplein 40, 3015 GD
Rotterdam, The NETHERLANDS

Foreword

This series of volumes dealing with reproductive health care has as its primary objective the improvement of the quality of human reproduction. The explosion of knowledge and new technology give us opportunities as never before to accomplish this end.

The Editor has brought together contributors who are outstanding scientists from around the world. A number of the authors have personally made significant contributions to our body of knowledge in reproductive medicine. Bringing all this information together in an easily readable format is a great service. This is essential reading for all concerned with the control and improvement of human reproduction and the correction of its many deficits.

TN Evans

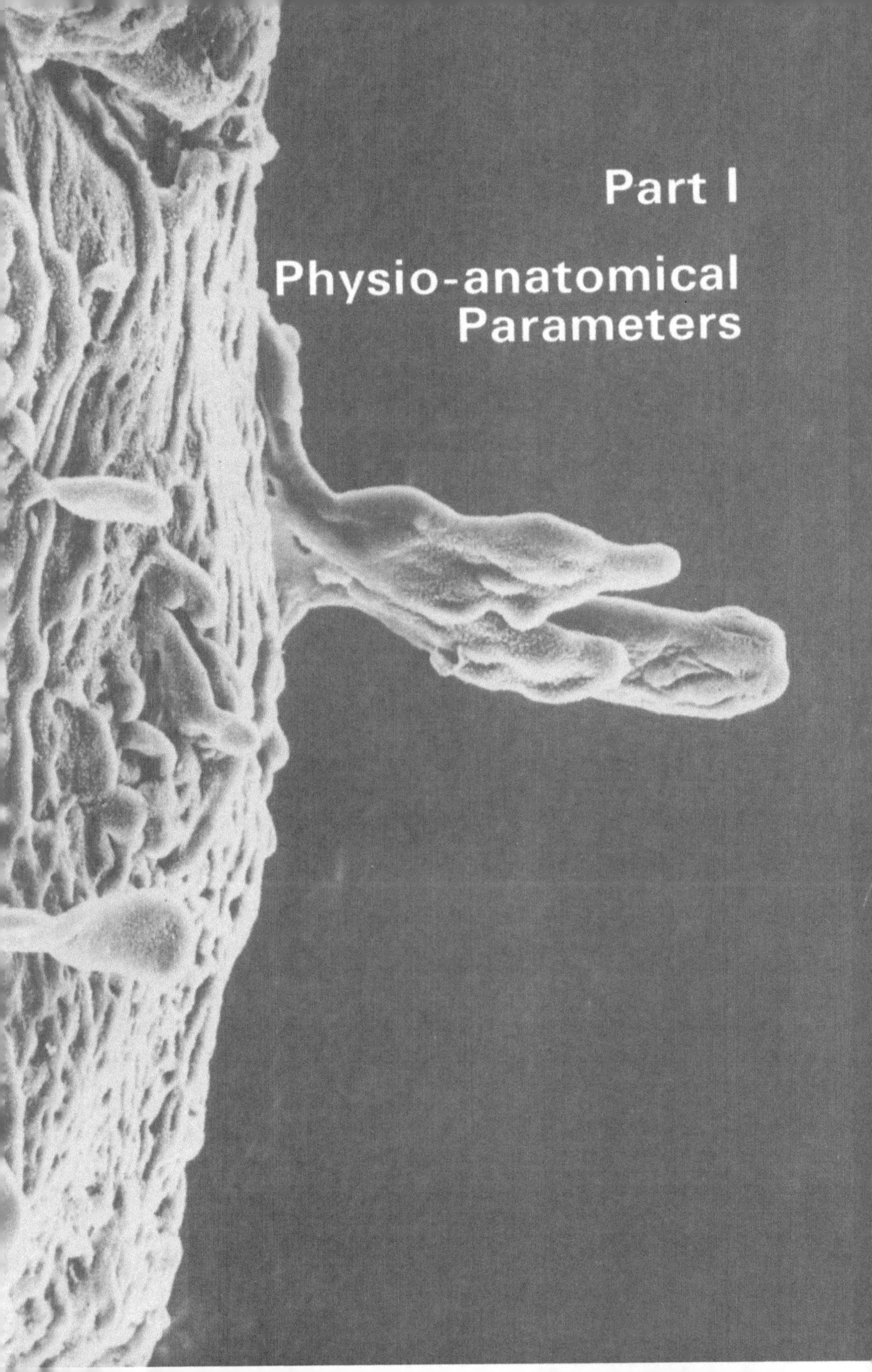

Part I

Physio-anatomical Parameters

1 Uterine microvasculature and spontaneous abortion

M. TAKADA

In the implantation and subsequent development of a fertilized ovum, its integrity is most significant. However, with maternal local factors, i.e., unsatisfactory uterine conditions, implantation may not succeed even if the integrity of the fertilized ovum is excellent; if implantation is made, the maturation of the fetoplacental unit following implantation is disturbed, which leads to abnormalities in fetal development or to miscarriage. Thus, the uteroplacental unit, as well as the fetoplacental unit, plays an important role in the establishment and maintenance of pregnancy.

Among the mechanisms of the uteroplacental unit, most significant is the physiological mechanism of the uterine microvasculature and its correspondence to gestation. In particular, homeostasis of simultaneous cooperative development of the uterine wall and the placenta is most important.

The simultaneous cooperative homeostasis and the mechanism of abortion resulting from the impairment of the microvasculature is explained with the findings of the microvasculature of the pregnant uterus with myoma uteri.

SPECIFICITY OF UTERINE MICROVASCULATURE IN MAINTENANCE OF PREGNANCY

The human uteroplacental unit, from the aspect of microvasculature, shows specific and staged changes which are essential for the maintenance of pregnancy.

(1) 1*st stage.* Dilatation and extension of the uterine microvasculature by steroid hormones secreted from the corpus luteum in pregnancy and opening of the a. spiralis to the intervillous space resulting from competition between the gestational decidua and the trophoblast occur.

(2) 2*nd stage.* More rapid dilatation, extension, and shunt formation of the uterine microvasculature by steroid hormones supplied from the placenta via the intervillous space take place.

(3) *3rd stage.* A rapid increase in blood supply and its pooling, accompanying gestational changes in the uterine microvasculature and consequent hyperpermeability of the vascular wall; an increase in the response dose of steroid hormones derived from the placenta; hypertrophy and extension of the uterine muscular cells due to prolonged acting time; softening, stretching, and expansion of the uterine cavity due to edema in interstitial tissues.

Interdependent homeostasis in the uterine wall and the placenta, established under the conditions in which these alterations affect one another, is an important factor required for maintenance of pregnancy (Figure 1.1).

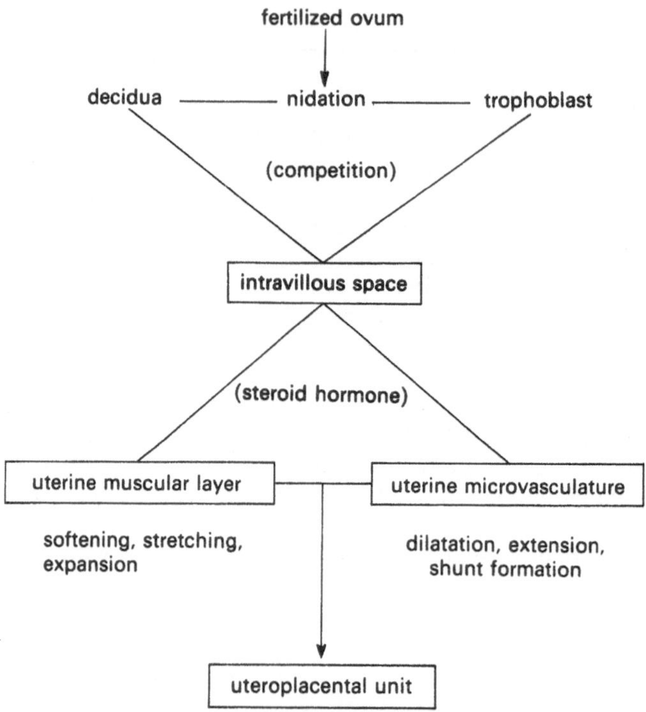

Figure 1.1 Development of the uteroplacental unit.

Each of the stages is explained by the findings of the uterine microvasculature required for maintenance of pregnancy in microangiographical examinations on the extirpated pregnant uterus, histological examinations with serial sections and examinations of the plastoid cast.

Changes in uterine microvasculature during gestation

A. spiralis, which have a significant role in the implantation of a fertilized ovum and the formation of the intervillous space in the uterus, number about sixty in the direction of the uterine cavity on the entire circumference in transversal sections of 5–10 mm in thickness. In the non-gestational uterus, the distribution of a. spiralis is relatively dense at an interval of 1.2 mm on the anterior and posterior walls and the bilateral walls up to the height of the hysterosalpingo angle from the orificium uteri internum. However, its distribution is

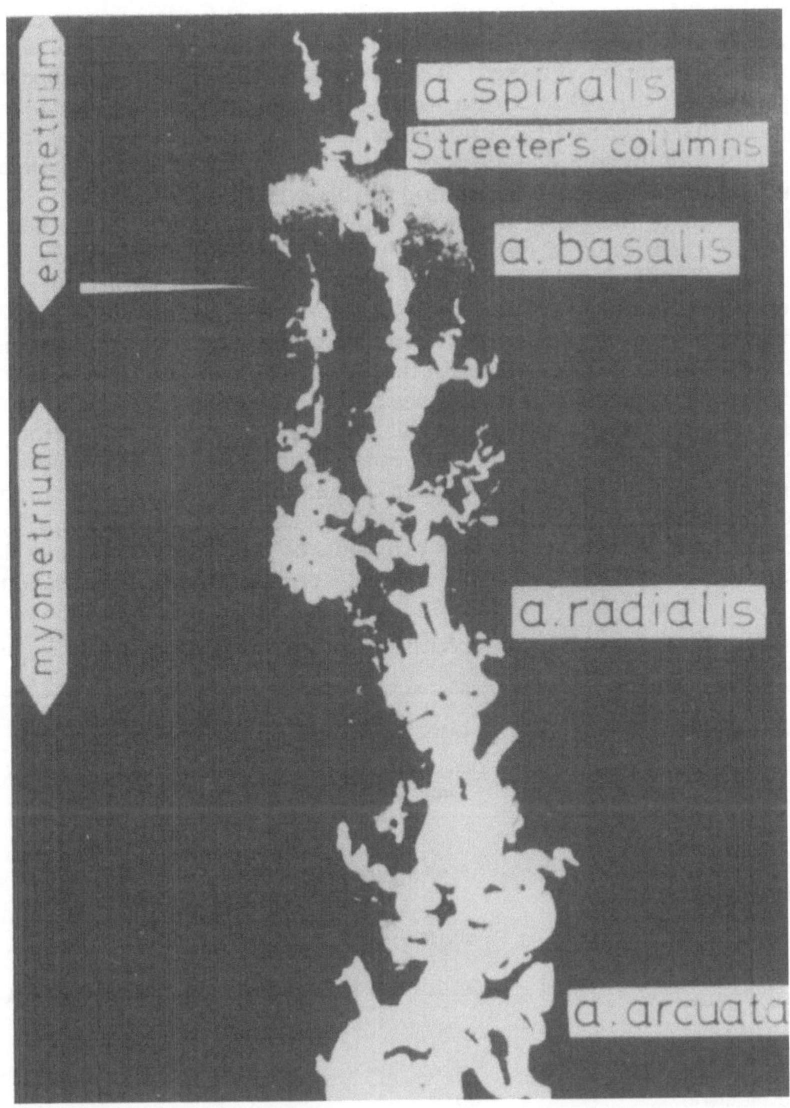

Figure 1.2 Microangiogram of the uterine spiral arterial system. The figure was prepared by connecting and integrating each of the pictures obtained in the epidiamicroscopic observation and photographing of the uterine microvasculature in the serial sections of the extirpated human uterus for which microangiography was performed.

sparse in the endometrium of the fundus, which is a disadvantageous condition for the establishment of the implantation of a fertilized ovum and prognosis of the implanted ovum. The cyclic structure of a. arcuata and marked coiling of the uterine spiral arterial system in the non-gestational uterus are organo-specificity-prepared for the increased transversal and longitudinal diameters and the kinetics of blood circulation (Takada *et al.*, 1974).

The arteriole system in the uterine wall consists of a. arcuata, a. radialis, a. basalis, and a. spiralis. Such formation of the uterine arteriole is affected greatly by gestation (Figure 1.2). It is rapidly dilated and extended after implantation of a fertilized ovum, with the diameters of a. radialis increasing to 1.5 times that of the non-gestational time at 2 months of gestation and to twice that at 4 months; the diameters of a. spiralis, to 2.5 times and 3 times at 2 months and 4 months of gestation (Table 1.1).

Extension of the coiled artery (a. radialis and a. spiralis) is marked; the a. radialis, especially, is conspicuously extended. The coiled artery of the uterine wall with the placenta *in situ* in the 7 months gestational uterus has extended to about eight times that in the non-implantation site (Figure 1.3). When the degree of extension of the uterine wall is judged from the extension of the coiled artery, the extension of the uterine wall with the placenta *in situ* is considered to amount to several times that of the non-implantation site. The coiled artery is displaced across the muscular fibers of the uterine wall accompanying dilatation of the uterine cavity and extension of the uterine wall (Figure 1.4a). Dilatation and extension of the venule and shunt formation are also conspicuous (Figure 1.4b).

Such changes as dilatation and extension of the coiled artery and shunt formation, being attributed to the effect of steroid hormones produced in the

Table 1.1 Measurement of the degree of dilatation of the a. radialis and a. spiralis accompanying pregnancy

	A. spiralis		*A. radialis*	
	Diameter (μm)	*Ratio*	*Diameter* (μm)	*Ratio*
Plastoid cast				
non-pregnant uterus	21.07	1	222.54	1
pregnant uterus				
2 month	33.29	1.56 (× 1.5)	522.96	2.35 (× 2)
4 month	45.08	2.14 (× 2)	694.32	3.12 (× 3)
7 month	668.20	31.71 (× 30)	1218.80	5.4 (× 6)
Microangiogram				
non-pregnant uterus	20.76	1	185.25	1
pregnant uterus				
2 month	30.93	1.49 (× 1.5)	494.61	2.67 (× 2)
4 month	42.14	2.03 (× 2)	563.16	3.04 (× 3)
7 month	615.10	29.63 (× 30)	1254.20	6.77 (× 6.0)

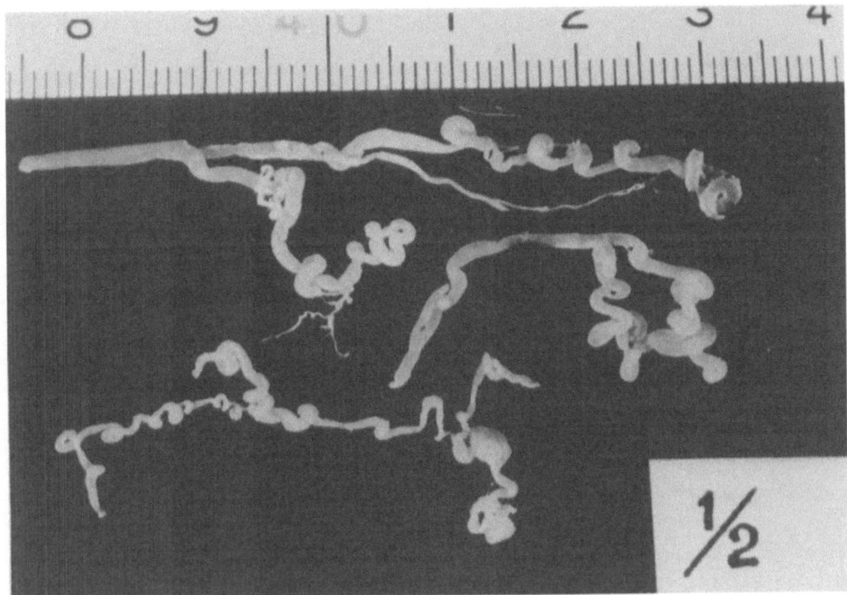

Figure 1.3 Plastoid cast of the coiled artery in the uterine wall with the placenta *in situ* at 27 weeks of gestation.

placenta, are structural changes easily associated with retention of blood flow in the venule as well as increased reflux blood flow via the arteriole. They are suitable correspondence for an increase in response dose of steroid hormones on the myometrium and extension of response time.

The uterine microvasculature is highly sensitive to the effect of steroid hormones. In rats (Takada, 1977), estrogen has the action of extending the uterine microvasculature while progesterone dilates it results in shunt formation (Takada, 1978) (Figure 1.5). Steroid hormones produced in the placenta enter the circulation system and spread directly into the uterine wall via the intervillous space in larger amounts than those in which they act on the uterine wall via the uteroartery (Barnes, 1962; Mitsui *et al.*, 1965). Concentration of progesterone on the myometrium is higher than that in the antiplacental site. Gestational changes in microvasculature in the uterine wall with placenta *in situ* are more remarkable than those in the non-implantation site because of the direct infiltration of placental steroid hormones into the uterine wall.

Open outlets of the a. spiralis to the intervillous space

The number of open outlets of the a. spiralis formed by penetrating trophoblast cells or endothelial cells (Marais, 1968; Aladjem, 1970; Knoth and Larsen, 1972; Enders, 1976) varies, with 102–156 at 3–4 months of gestation, 180–320 at the last stage of gestation (Boyd, 1956), 300–400 in placental-maternal colposcopic examinations in monkeys (Haller, 1968), and in

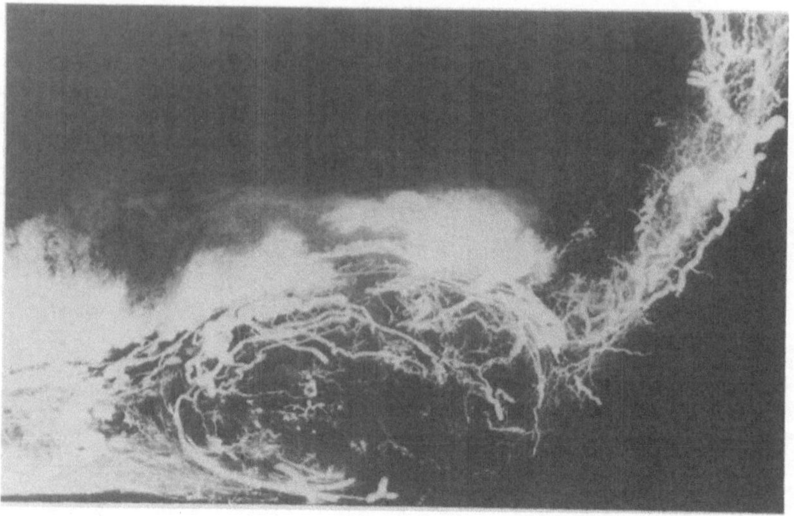

a

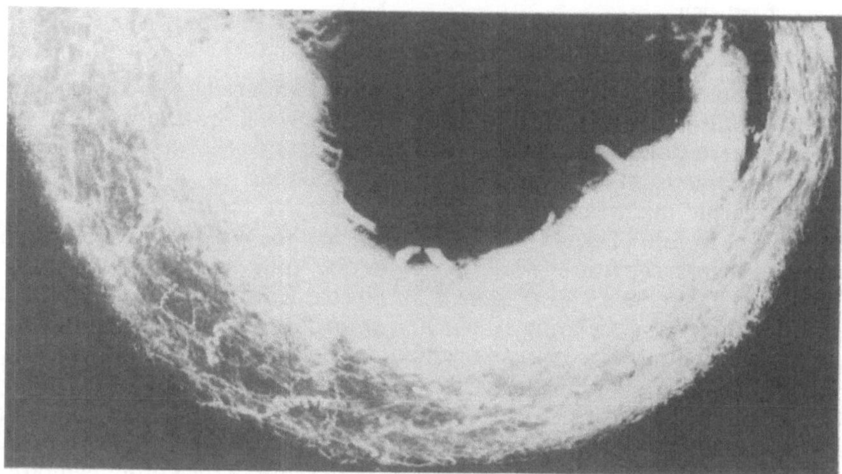

b

Figure 1.4 Microangiogram of the uterine microvasculature at 12 weeks of gestation, **a**, Arteriola. Uteroplacental microvasculature (arteriole) in the case where implantation was made into the endometrium with a myoma nodule. A. radialis is markedly dilated, extended, and circumvented avoiding myoma nodules, transferring to a. spiralis. A. spiralis is intensely coiled and dilated just short of opening. **b**, Veniplex. Veniplex in the uterine wall with the placenta *in situ* is markedly dilated when compared with that at non-gestational time and shunt formation was observed. It has a structure to facilitate the reflux blood flow via the arteriole to be pooled.

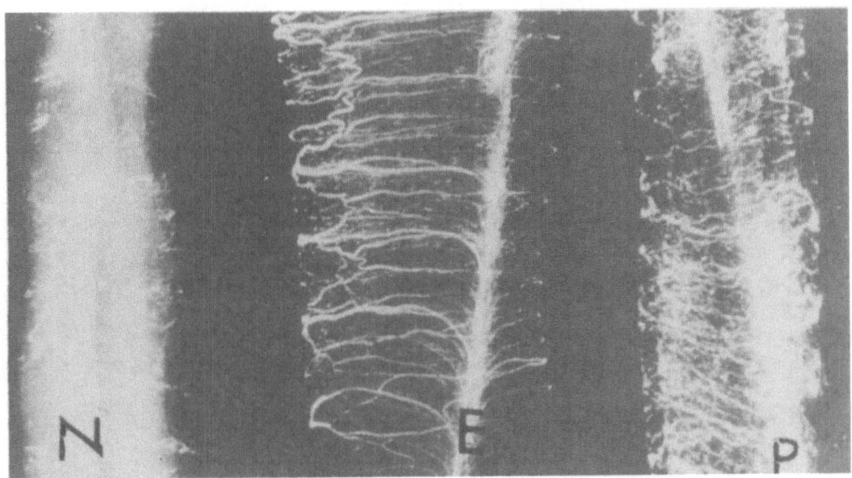

Figure 1.5 The effect of estrogen and progesterone on the uterine microvasculature. N = 250 g female rat, control. E = 250 g female rat (spayed); estrogen 2 mg/day, i.m. for 7 days. P = 250 g female rat (spayed); progesterone 10 mg/day, i.m. for 7 days.

25 arteriographical examinations (Borell *et al.*, 1965; Ramsey, 1962). Microangiographical examinations with serial sections of the pregnant uterus and examinations on the whole placenta with simultaneous infusion of plastoid into the umbilical vein and bilateral uteroartery reveal the number of open outlets of the a. spiralis to the intervillous space to be 32 at 12 weeks of gestation, 27 at 24 weeks, and 27 at 32 weeks, decreasing with an increase in the number of months of gestation. Thus, the number of open outlets of the a. spiralis is settled by the end of the third month of gestation.

Open outlets of the a. spiralis are classified into two types. In type I, marked replacement of the villi was observed in the outlets with large diameters and marked coiling (Figure 1.6a). In type II, rare replacement of the villi with small diameters and meandering without coiling was noted (Figure 1.6b). There is another type of open outlets of the a. spiralis which may be called type III, i.e., those which close just short of the opening due to hyalin degeneration (Kamemori, 1976; Takada, 1977).

The whole plastoid cast in the uteroplacental unit shows that there is a relation of 'one cotyledon, one opening' in principle between the location of the opening of the a. spiralis to the intervillous space and cotyledon (Freese, 1968; Martin and Ramsey, 1970; Gruenwald, 1973; Arts, 1974; Kamemori, 1976). The number of cotyledons in the placenta is defined by the number of open outlets of the a. spiralis to the intervillous space. Since the number of open outlets of the a. spiralis is settled by the end of the third month of gestation, the number of cotyledons in the placenta is nearly settled by the third month (Takada, 1977). Therefore, not only are the number of openings of the a. spiralis to the intervillous space and open outlets greatly involved in the morphological and functional formation of the placenta, which is an

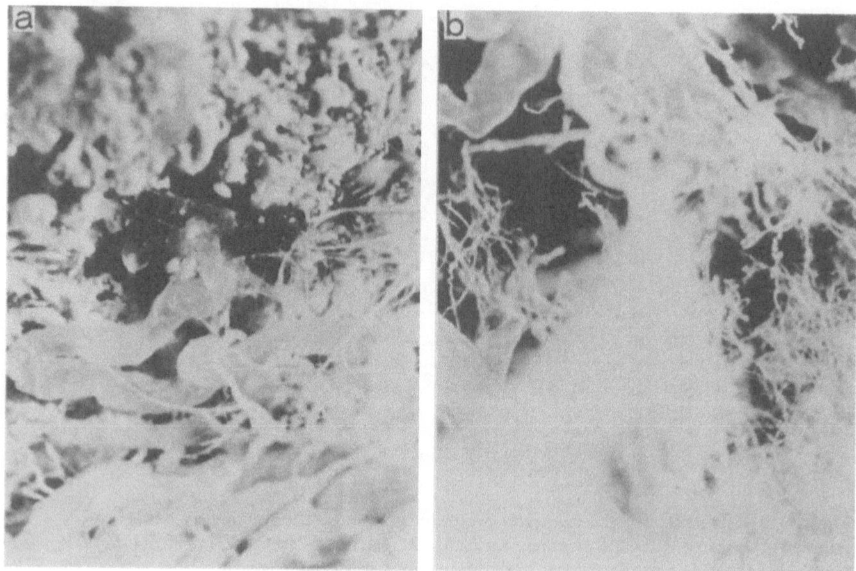

Figure 1.6 Open outlets of the a. spiralis to the intravillus space at 27 weeks by plastoid cast.

aggregate of cotyledons, but in the subsequent placental development, simultaneous cooperative development of the uterine wall, i.e., an area of the placenta *in situ*, must show nearly as much dilatation as a placental-maternal area does. There is no possibility that the a. spiralis is newly opened to the intervillous space and cotyledons are newly formed in and after the third months of gestation. In most primates, the base of placental attachment to the endometrium does not expand greatly beyond the original implantation site, and no new a. spiralis is opened there-after.

ABORTION DUE TO IMPAIRMENT OF GESTATIONAL SYNCHRONY OF THE UTERINE MICROVASCULATURE

If gestational synchrony of the uterine microvasculature which is required for the simultaneous cooperative development of the uterine wall and placenta is impaired, slip and separation are caused at the junction of the two, and signs of abortion may appear.

If the a. spiralis opened to the intervillous space is disturbed or shunt formation in the microvasculature is decreased, uteroplacental blood flow is decreased and thereby the life of a fetus is threatened or fetal development is suppressed (Caldeyro-Barcia, 1957).

Experiments in rhesus monkeys with the uteroartery ligated show fewer cases of livebirth at term and more cases of stillbirth (Misenhimer *et al.*, 1970). In recent years, techniques in which thrombosis is induced in the a. spiralis employing radioactive microspheres, and uteroplacental blood flow is allowed to decrease, have been attempted to observe the outcome of pregnancy (James *et al.*, 1974; Panigel *et al.*, 1975). However, these techniques cannot be applied to the human uterus. Thus, abortion based on such a mechanism has not been verified in the human pregnant uterus. Relations between threatened abortion which is observed in cases of pregnancy in the uterus with myoma nodules and uterine microvasculature are herein explained.

Implantation of a fertilized ovum into an area of the endometrium in the vicinity of a myoma nodule is comparatively rare, and in many cases implantation is made into an area without a myoma nodule. Among 32 cases of extirpation of the pregnant uterus with a uterine myoma nodule, six cases (18.7%) showed implantation into an area of the endometrium in the vicinity of the uterine myoma nodule, any of which are cases of myoma multiplex. It is possible to distinguish the location of chorion frondosum from that of myoma nodule by means of ultrasonography, i.e., no contact between myoma and placenta, margin of placenta in contact with myoma and partial or complete overlapping, if the case is in the 7th week of gestation or more (Muram *et al.*, 1980).

When comparing gestational cases (Group 1) in which implantation was made into an area of the endometrium without a myoma nodule with gestational cases (Group 2) in which implantation was made into an area of the endometrium with a myoma nodule, Group 2 shows smaller diameters of the a. radialis and the a. spiralis with smaller numbers of open outlets. The rate of open outlets including type II and type III is overtly higher in Group 2. In addition, Group 2 shows poor branching of the a. radialis in the myometrium, extended circumvention of the coiled artery avoiding myoma nodules, and disordered local circulation. Gestational changes in the uterine muscle are also unsatisfactory in Group 2 (Table 1.2). Such impairment of the uterine microvasculature is a direct cause of slip and separation between the decidua basalis and the chorion frondosum, and it is an indirect cause of development disturbance and regressive degeneration of the chorion frondosum.

Table 1.2 Microvasculature in site complicated by uterine myoma. Comparative results of uterine microvasculature between the pregnant group in which implantation was in an area without uterine myoma nodules (Group 1) and the pregnant group in which implantation was in an area with uterine myoma nodules (Group 2)

	*Group 1**	*Group 2**
A. spiralis diameter (mean)	36.2 μm	24.2 μm
A. radialis diameter (mean)	602.5 μm	590.3 μm
A. spiralis opening	27 ~ 32	21 ~ 25
A. spiralis open outlets (II, III combined types)	7 ~ 9%	18 ~ 22%
Abnormal displacement of coiled artery	no	yes
Shunt formation in the microvasculature	marked	reduced
Softening and stretching of the uterine muscular layer	favorable	poor

* Results from three cases, 12 weeks pregnant Type I: marked replacement of villi, coiling, thick; Type II: few replacement of villi, meandering, thin; Type III: none opening, meandering

Abortion is induced by the influences of myoma nodules alone in a few cases only. According to the report by Muram *et al.* (1980), the rate of abortion is not increased owing to myoma. In many of the abortion cases in pregnancies with myoma uteri, not only myoma but also other tolerant factors are responsible for abortion. Contraction of the uterine muscles around the myoma or uterine contraction induced by psychosomatic stress and high implants (implants into the uterine fundus) are one of the tolerant factors.

We compared 55 cases of normal term pregnancies and 32 cases of miscarriage using ultrasonography in order to study relations between implantation sites in the uterine cavity and the outcome of pregnancies (Takeuchi, 1973). The frequency of high implants (implants into the uterine fundus) was found to be 14.9% in normal pregnancies and 50.0% in miscarriages, and the sparse distribution of the microvasculature in the uterine fundus (Takada *et al.*, 1974) seems to be related closely to miscarriages.

References

Aladjem, S. (1970). Studies in placental circulation. Vascular area of the terminal villus in normal and abnormal pregnancies. *Am. J. Obstet. Gynecol.*, **107,** 88

Arts, N. F. and Lohman, A. H. M. (1974). An injection-corrosion study of the fetal and maternal vascular systems in the placenta of the rhesus monkey. *Eur. J. Obstet. Gynecol. Reprod. Biol.*, **4/4,** 133

Barnes, A. G., Kumar, D. and Goodno, J. A. (1962). Studies in human myometrium during pregnancy. *Am. J. Obstet. Gynecol.*, **84,** 1207

Borell, U., Fernström, I., Ohlson, L. and Wiqvist, N. (1965). Influence of uterine contractions on the uteroplacental blood flow at term. *Am. J. Obstet. Gynecol.*, **90,** 44

Boyd, J. D. (1956). Morphology and physiology of the uteroplacental circulation. In Ville, C. A. (ed.) *Gestation*, pp. 132–194. (New York: Macy)

Brown, G. F. and Beilby, J. O. W. (1970). Microvasculature of the uterus – an injection method of study. *Obstet. Gynecol.*, **35,** 21

Bryce, T. H. and Teacher, J. H. (1908). *An Early Ovum Imbedded in the Decidua. Contributions to the Study of the Early Development and Imbedding of the Human Ovum.* (Glasgow: University of Glasgow Press)

Caldeyro-Barcia, R. (1957). In Larman, J. T. (ed.) *Physiology of Prematurity*, pp. 20–25, 128–135. (New York: Macy)

Dalgaard, J. B. (1946). The blood vessels of the human endometrium. *Acta Obstet. Gynecol. Scand.*, **26,** 342

Farrer-Brown, G., Beilby, J. O. W. and Tarbit, M. H. (1970). The vascular patterns in myomatous uteri. *J. Obstet. Gynecol. Br. Commonw.*, **77,** 967

Freese, U. E. (1968). The uteroplacental vascular relationship in the human. *Am. J. Obstet. Gynecol.*, **101,** 8

Gruenwald, P. (1973). Lobular structure of hemochorial primate placentas and its relation to maternal vessels. *Am. J. Anat.*, **136,** 133

Haller, U. (1968). Beitrag zur Morphologie der Utero-Placentargefäße. *Arch. Gynäk.*, **205,** 185

James, A. E., Siegel, M. E., Ramsey, E. M., Panigel, M., Misenhimer, H. R. and Donner, M. W. (1974). Imaging with radioactive microspheres to demonstrate maternal circulation in the placenta of rhesus monkey. *Invest Radiol.*, **9,** 65

Kamemori, H. (1976). The histological, microangiographic and plastoid cast studies on the fine vascular construction of the nonpregnant and pregnant human uterus. *Acta Obstet. Gynecol. Jpn.*, **28,** 635

Knoth, M. and Larsen, J. F. (1972). Ultrastructure of human implantation site. *Acta Obstet. Gynecol. Scand.*, **51,** 385

Marais, W. D. (1968). Human decidual spiral arteries – ultrastructure of the intima in normal vessels. *J. Obstet. Gynecol. Br. Commonw.*, **75,** 552

Martin, C. B. Jr. and Ramsey, E. M. (1970). Gross anatomy of the placenta of rhesus monkeys. *Am. J. Obstet. Gynecol.*, **36,** 167

Misenhimer, H. R., Ramsey, E. M., Martin, C. B. Jr., Donner, M. W. and Margulies, S. I. (1970). Chronically impaired uterine artery blood flow. Effect on uteroplacental circulation and pregnancy outcome. *Obstet. Gynecol.*, **36,** 415

Mitsui, T., Ogata, E., Saito, M., Fujita, T., Akamine, K. and Kikuchi, S. (1965). Progesterone determination in myometrial tissue using Gas-Liquid Chromatography. *J. Jpn. Obstet. Gynecol. Soc.*, 107

Muram, D., Gillieson, M. and Walters, J. H. (1980). Myomas of the uterus in pregnancy. ultrasonographic follow-up. *Am. J. Obstet. Gynecol.*, **138,** 16

Panigel, M., James, A. E. Jr., Siegel, M. and Donner, M. W. (1975). Radionuclide and angiographic studies of placental circulation in man and rhesus monkeys. *Eur. J. Obstet. Gynecol. Reprod. Biol.*, **5/5,** 251

Ramsay, E. M. (1962). Circulation in the intravillus space of the primate placenta. *Am. J. Obstet. Gynecol.*, **84,** 1646

Takada, M. (1977). Influence of maternal factors upon fetal development. *Acta Obstet. Gynecol. Jpn.*, **29,** 1275

Takada, M., Matsumoto, K. and Kamemori, T. (1974). Studies on human uterine microvasculature. *Clin. Gynecol. Obstet.*, **28,** 341

Takeuchi, H. (1973). Ultrasound placentography in early pregnancy. *Excerpta Medica Int. Congr. Ser.*, **227,** 25

2
Repeated abortions and uterine malformations

A. J. M. AUDEBERT, E. CITTADINI, and M. COGNAT

Uterine malformations have long been considered as a cause of repeated abortions (Mauriceau, 1865). Recent progress in the field of human reproduction has not led to any major change in the concepts on this subject. After reviewing the basic principal elements of uterine abnormalities, this report will place emphasis on certain aspects of congenital Mullerian anomalies.

FREQUENCY OF UTERINE MALFORMATION

The frequency of uterine malformations is difficult to determine with precision and varies greatly according to populations studied and the diagnostic means utilized. Many forms are asymptomatic and never discovered. The frequency of anomalies related to developmental defects of the Mullerian ducts is between 0.05 and 2%. In infertile women, the frequency varies from 1 to 5% (Tulandi *et al.*, 1980; Siegler, 1967). In a series of 1053 laparoscopies performed for infertility, a uterine anomaly was present on 31 studies (3%) (Audebert, 1980). The rate of anomaly increases from 15% to as high as 25% in women with a history of several spontaneous abortions (Musset, 1973). The frequency also varies according to the type of Mullerian anomaly (Buttram, 1983).

CLASSIFICATION OF MALFORMATIONS

Various classifications of malformations have been proposed and include the following: anatomic and embryological (Jarcho, 1946), embryological (Semmens, 1962), functional (Jones, 1957) or morphological (Musset, 1967). There is no classification which is universally accepted. The most recent classification is based on the embryological, morphological and functional concept (Buttram and Gibbons, 1979). The latest classification distinguishes malformations in women who were exposed to diethylstilbestrol (Kaufman *et al.*, 1977; Barnes *et al.*, 1983; Stillman, 1982) and uses therapeutic and prognostic concepts.

PHYSIOPATHOGENIC MECHANISM

Of the various uterine causes of repeated abortion (Table 2.1), the group represented by malformations (approximately 8.5%) is the most widely accepted. The physiopathogenic mechanism is not always perfectly clear. Some of these are as follows.

(1) A defect in expansion of the uterine cavity with increase in intrauterine pressure and increase in prostaglandin synthesis may play a part.

(2) Endometrial anomalies reduce the chances of implantation of the blastocyst (Moyer, 1968; Muller, 1977). These functional alterations are secondary to either a disturbance of steroid receptors or a decrease in vascularization (Salvatierra, 1976).
    These anomalies occur mostly in the septate uterus, but also in the horns of bicornuate uteri with the difference according to the side on some occasions.

(3) Other anomalies often associated with the malformation (hypoplasia, cervical incompetence, endometriosis, traumatic synechia occurring after repeated curettages, polyps) may be the real cause of the abortion.

According to the mechanism, the occurrence of late abortions can be understood. There is not complete agreement on the possible correlations between the type of malformation and the risk of an accident. Bicornuate uteri had been considered to represent the group with the greatest risk (Jones and Wheeless, 1969). Today it appears that the risk may be greater for septate uteri (Musset, 1973; Palmer, 1981; Buttram, 1983). Surgical correction of uterine anomalies, because of repeated abortions, include many septate uteri and very few bicornuate, arcuate or didelphic uteri (Audebert *et al.*, 1983; Kusuda, 1982).

The explanation of the mechanism of primary infertility linked with malformation is uncertain. Alterations of gamete transport (defects in cervical function or by increase in uterine contraction) have not yet been demonstrated. These mechanisms are alluring but become troublesome when a pregnancy evolves normally in a malformed uterus. This clinical finding has been observed in all types of malformations. The livebirth rate, without surgical correction, is 55% for uterus didelphys, 57% for bicornuate uteri and 28% for septate uteri (Buttram, 1983). The rate of abortions is respectively 43%, 35% and 67% in the same series.

DIAGNOSIS

Uterine malformation is sometimes confirmed by inspection during a simple clinical examination, for example, the presence of two cervices with or without vaginal septum. A complete workup specifies the type and degree of malformation (Musset, 1973).

Hysterography is the fundamental examination for determining the exact morphology of the uterine cavity as well as fallopian tube permeability and

Table 2.1 Repeated abortions: causes and treatment due to uterine abnormality

Uterine causes of repeated abortion	*Treatment for repeated abortions due to uterine abnormality*	*Additional procedures performed during metroplasty by laparoscopy*
Endometrial – hormonal infectious immunologic synechiae *Myometrial* – myoma adenomyosis *Malformation* – hypoplasia	1. Medical 2. Surgical (a) bicornuate uterus: Strassman metroplasty (laparotomy) (b) septum: – laparotomy Jones (resection) } metroplasties Bret-Palmer } metroplasties Tompkins } metroplasties – hysteroscopic resection	Adhesiolysis Salpingoplasty Douglassectomy – ligamentopexy Myomectomy Cystectomy (ovarian) Wedge resection of ovary Fulguration or resection of endometriotic implants

Table 2.2 Results of some published series of metroplasties

	No.	*Living child*	*Abortion*	*Ectopic*	*Failures*	*Lost for follow-up*
Musich and Behrman (1978)	21	9(45%)	2	—	7	3
Buttram (1979)	46	23	1	1	—	—
Palmer (1981)	100	67	4	—	7	22
Seffert (1981)	38	29	2	—	4	3
Candiani (1981)	68	31	2	—	5	30
Audebert (1983)	54	29 +2	3	—	2	8
Total —	327	190 = (60%)	14	1	—	20

other associated lesions (synechia). Certain images could correspond to several types of anomalies. A detailed analysis permits the distinction (Siegler, 1967). Despite appropriate technique and interpretation of the films, hysterography cannot accurately differentiate a bicornuate from a septate uterus. Hysteroscopy supplemented by laparoscopy is required to establish the final diagnosis (Siegler, 1983). Hysteroscopy can appreciate the morphology of the uterine cavity, the importance of a septum and the symmetry of the uterine cavity in case of a double uterus. Synechia can be discovered and treated by this same method. It can also be used in postoperative procedures to evaluate healing and to eliminate synechia.

A laparoscopy is necessary to differentiate between a bicornuate and a septate uterus. It also specifies the condition of the pelvis, revealing endometriotic lesions or periadnexal adhesions. In the case of a unicornuate uterus, a contralateral rudimentary horn will be seen on some occasions.

Ultrasonography permits a precise diagnosis in certain cases. A frontal section visualizes the septum, evaluates the number of uterine cavities (producing the same image as an hysterogram) and the thickness of the myometrium. This provides an essential element in the diagnosis of an associated hypoplasia (Leroy *et al.*, 1981).

Ultrasonography can also evaluate the ovaries, discover a rudimentary horn and avoid an intravenous pyelogram. This is carried out in diagnosing a solitary kidney associated with solitary unicornuate uterus and in 10–20 % of cases with a uterus didelphys. Ultrasonography is useful in pregnancy to locate the conceptus after successful surgical correction.

Hysterophlebography is used to evaluate hypoplasia and to estimate vascularization of the myometrium (Viala, 1981).

TREATMENT

Medical treatment

Before surgical correction of a possible uterine malformation, various medical treatments may be tried, especially if hypoplasia plays a part. Essentially, estrogen and sympathomimetic drugs are used, which improve the vascularization of the myometrium and facilitate hyperplasia and the multiplication of muscle fibers. Pregnancy produces the same results.

Surgical treatment

Various surgical techniques are used to correct uterine anomalies since the reconstruction of a solitary uterine cavity from a bicornuate uterus by Strassman in 1907.

Abdominal route

The abdominal route is the most widely used method.

(1) Bicornuate uterus is preferably corrected by the Strassman metroplasty.

(2) Two types of techniques are used to treat the septate uterus, according to excision or conservation of the septum and adjacent myometrium.

A wedge resection of the septum and part of the uterine wall can be performed to remove the abnormal tissue (Jones, 1957), but the resulting uterine cavity, which is carefully reconstructed in two planes, has a size dependent upon the amount of resection required. A simple incision up to the level of the two cavities, in a frontal plane (Strassman, 1957) or in a sagittal plane (Tompkins, 1962; Bret and Guillet, 1959; Palmer, 1981) permits the reconstruction of a solitary uterine cavity. The frontal incision should stop before the interstitial portion of the fallopian tubes, in order to avoid the risk of tubal occlusion after suturing the myometrium. This type of operation with a sagittal incision is performed whenever possible. An infiltration of the myometrium with lidocaine (Xylocaine), epinephrine or PORE 8 limits bleeding. A tourniquet can also be used. An intrauterine device, like the 'Duck Foot' type of Massouras, can be placed in the uterine cavity and left for several weeks in order to prevent synechiae; the use of IUDs, however, has been abandoned.

The extramucosal suture should be strong whereas the serosal suture should be meticulously performed with fine absorbable or non-absorbable materials (with the exception of catgut which should never be used) in order to avoid secondary adhesions. Omental or peritoneal grafts are sometimes placed on the serosal suture.

Humidification of the operative field should be constant and a careful rinsing should precede closing. Corticosteroids, estrogens and progestins are also used postoperatively.

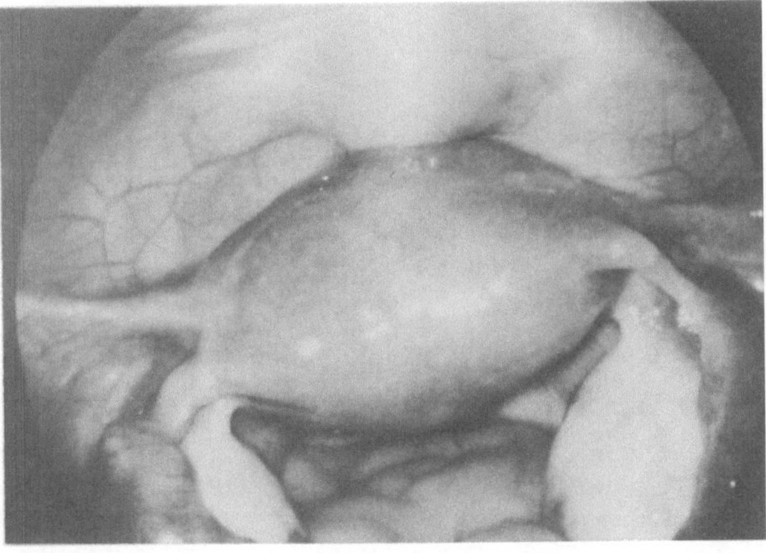

Figure 2.1 Laparoscopic view of a septate uterus. Note the transverse elongation of the fundus.

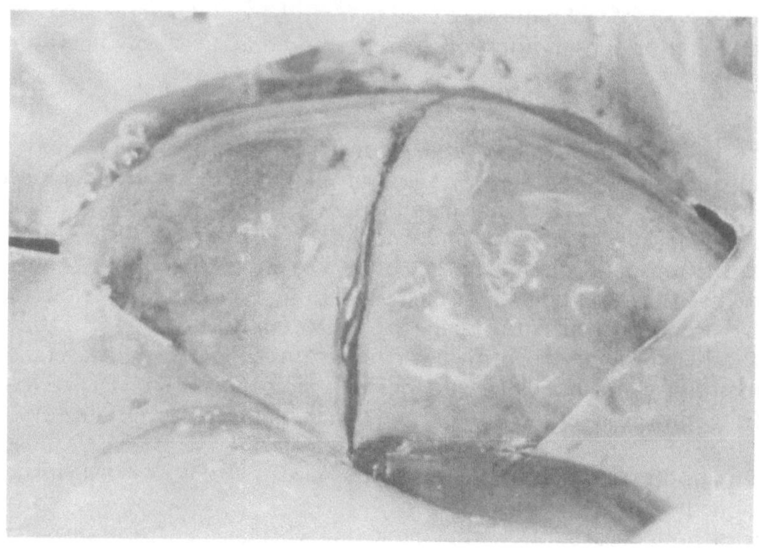

Figure 2.2 Sagittal serosal incision on a septate uterus.

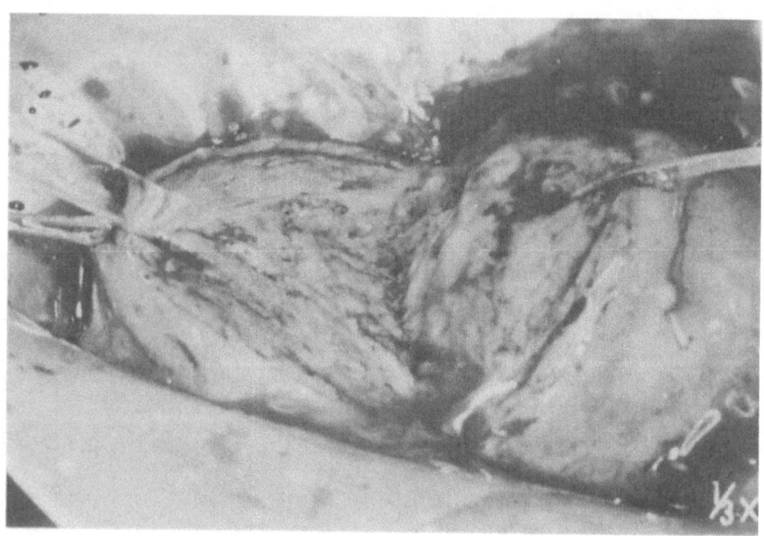

Figure 2.3 Exposure of the septum.

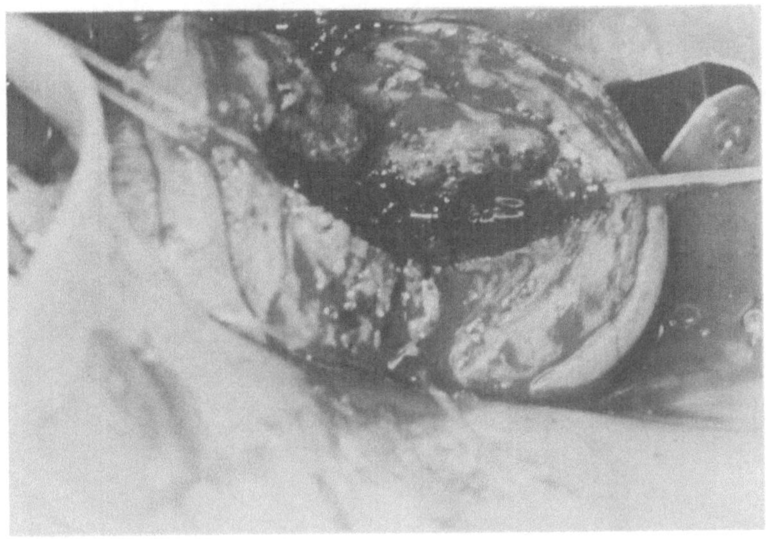

Figure 2.4 Incision of the septum showing the endometrium colored in blue by the dye.

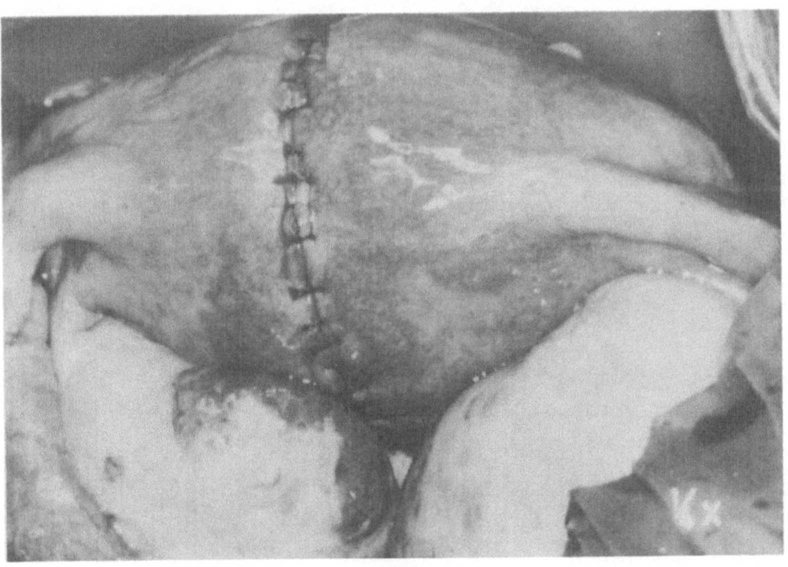

Figure 2.5 Careful serosal suture.

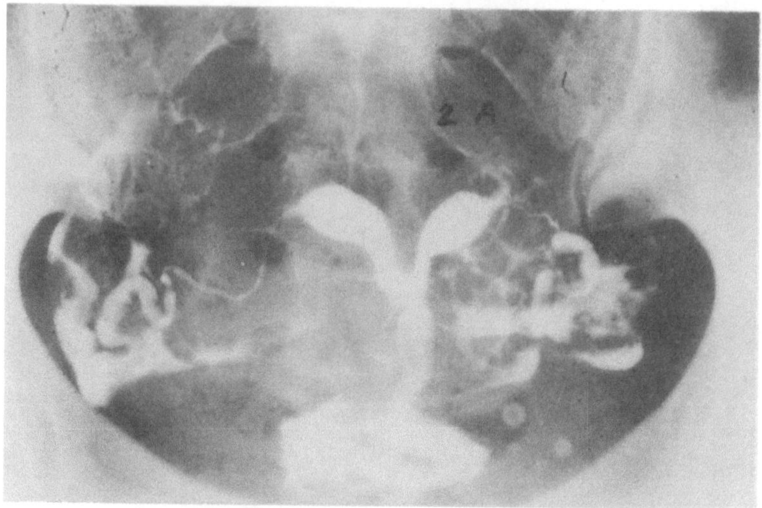

a

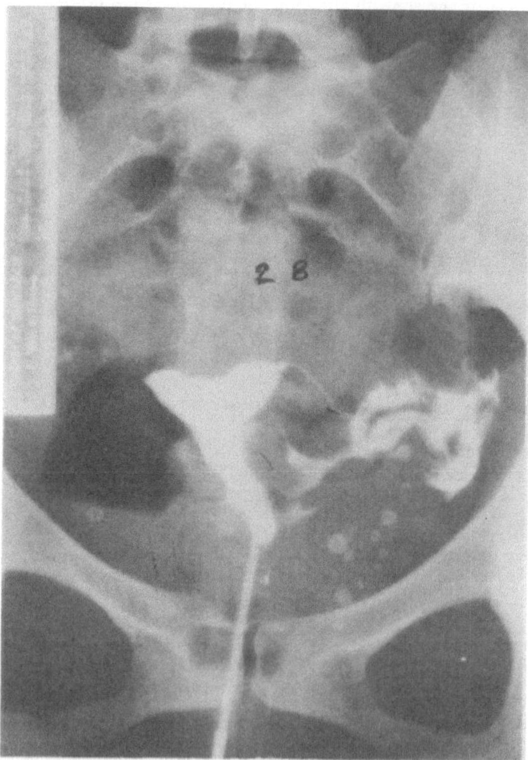

b

Figure 2.6 Hysterographic views before (**a**) and after (**b**) surgical correction of a septate uterus.

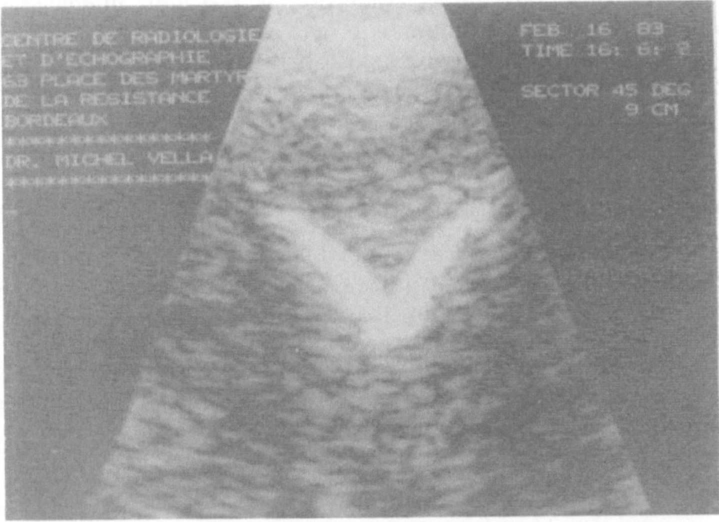

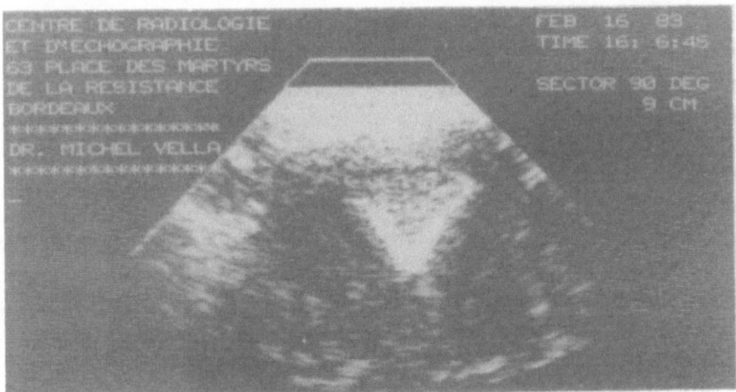

Figure 2.7 Ultrasonography: frontal view of a septate uterus.

Numerous additional procedures may be carried out according to each case (Table 2.1).

Vaginal route

In minor or moderate cases, an opertion using the vaginal technique is employed with success. A section of the septum is 'blindly' dissected out with scissors (use of endoscopic scissors avoids undue cervical dilatation). The procedure can be performed under radioscopic or hysteroscopic control (Edstrom, 1974; Chervenak and Neuwirth, 1981). The vaginal technique can complete the abdominal operation in case of persistence of the lower portion of the septum or in case of a vaginal septum.

In the case of septate uterus, hysteroscopic resection, under laparoscopic control, is performed. In addition to its operative and postoperative simplicity, the vaginal route does not cause postoperative adhesions and also avoids cesarean section (Daly *et al.*, 1983*a*, *b*).

Results of surgical treatment

There are not many metroplasty studies and comparisons are difficult because classifications vary according to author. However, there are some recognizable studies (Table 2.2). Statistics show that the results of the metroplasty are better as the indication becomes more selective. The results obtained by hysteroscopic metroplasty (Daly *et al.*, 1983*a*, *b*) are very encouraging but need further confirmation by other authors. Although the role of metroplasty is well established, there are no controlled series.

Surgical indication

Indications for operation is the most delicate and disputed aspect. The occurrence of miscarriages after corrective surgery would indicate the involvement of the uterine tissues and, in certain cases, the volume of the endometrial cavity being a secondary factor.

The morbidity of the surgical procedure and its consequences (risk of adhesions, scarred uterus) should also be considered. A surgical indication is considered only after a serious study of past history and a complete workup.

In dealing with repeated abortions it is customary to consider surgery after two miscarriages, after failure of the medical treatment and if laparoscopy reveals other pelvic factors. In treating a bicornuate uterus metroplasty is only undertaken as a last resort. The indication is rare in reality.

The simplicity of the hysteroscopic metroplasty performed at the time of a laparoscopy without enhancing morbidity of the procedure may modify our attitude in the future, when faced with a uterine septate.

CONCLUDING REMARKS

Uterine malformations represent one of the oldest recognized causes of repeated abortions. The progress observed in human reproduction during this past decade has not modified the physiopathogenic or therapeutic concepts. Ultrasonographic examination is the most important diagnostic advancement. Surgical intervention should only be considered after meticulous analysis of all determining elements and after conservative treatment. The simplification of the surgical correction obtained by hysteroscopic metroplasty may also represent a major advance, if the favorable results published are confirmed.

References

Audebert, A. J. M., Larue-Charlus, S. and Emperaire, J. C. (1980). Coelioscopie et infertilité: évaluation des indications. A propos d' une série de 1053 cases. *Rev. Fr. Gynecol. Obstet.*, **75**, 419

Audebert, A. J. M., Deniano, M. A., Cittadini, E. and Cognat, M. (1983). Risultati di uno studo multicrentico nelle metroplastidie. *Contraccez. Fertil. Sessualita*, **10**, 21

Barnes, A. B., Colton, T., Gundersen, J., Noller, K. L., Tilley, B. C., Strama, T., Townsend, D. E., Hatab, P. and O'Brien, P. C. (1983). Fertility and outcome of pregnancy in women exposed in utero to diethylstilbestrol. *N. Engl. J. Med.*, **302**, 609

Bret, A. J. and Guillet, B. (1959). Hystéroplastie reconstitutive sans résection musculaire, dans les malformations utérines causes d'avortements à repetition. *Presse Med.*, **67**, 394

Buttram, V. C. (1983). Mullerian anomalies and their management. *Fertil. Steril.*, **40**, 159

Buttram, V. C., Zanotti, L., Acosta, A. A., Banderheyden, J. S., Besch, P. K. and Franklin, R. R. (1974). Surgical correction of the septate uterus. *Fertil. Steril.*, **25**, 373

Buttram, V. C. and Gibbons, W. C. (1979). Mullerian anomalies: a proposed classification (an analysis of 144 cases). *Fertil. Steril.*, **32**, 40

Candiani, G. B. and Fedele, L. (1981) Clinical management of uterine anomalies. *Acta Eur. Fertil.*, **12**, 83

Chevenak, F. A. and Neuwirth, R. S. (1981). Hysteroscopic resection of the uterine septum. *Am. J. Obstet. Gynecol.*, **141**, 351

Daly, D. C., Tohan, N., Walters, C. and Riddick, D. H. (1983*a*). Hysteroscopic resection of the uterine septum in the presence of a septate cervix. *Fertil. Steril.*, **39**, 560

Daly, D. C., Walters, C. A., Soto-Albors, C. E. and Riddick, D. H. (1983*b*). Hysteroscopic metroplasty: surgical technique and obstetric outcome. *Fertil. Steril.*, **39**, 623

Edstrom, K. G. B. (1974). Intrauterine surgical procedures during hysteroscopy. *Endoscopy*, **6**, 175

Jarcho, J. (1946). Malformations of the uterus. *Am. J. Surg.*, **71**, 106

Jones, H. W. (1957). Obstetric significance of female genital anomalies. *Obstet. Gynecol.*, **10**, 113

Jones, H. W. and Wheeless, C. R. (1969). Salvage of the reproductive potential of women with anomalous development of Mullerian ducts: 1868–1968–2068. *Am. J. Obstet. Gynecol.*, **104**, 348

Kaufman, R. H., Binder, G. L., Gray, P. J. Jr. and Adam, E. (1977). Upper genital tract changes associated with exposure in utero to diethylstilbestrol. *Am. J. Obstet. Gynecol.*, **128**, 51

Kusuda, M. (1982). Infertility and metroplasty. *Acta Obstet. Gynecol. Scand.*, **61**, 407

Leroy, B., Bessis, R. and Jeny, R. (1981). L'échotomographie. In Boury-Heyler, C., Mauléon, P. and Rochet, Y. (eds.) *Utérus et fécondité*, pp. 201–203. (Paris: Masson)

Mauriceau, F. (1865). *Traité des maladies des femmes grosses*. (Paris)

Moyer, D. L. (1968). Endometrial diseases in infertility. In Behrman, S. J. and Kistner, R. W. (eds.) *Progress in Infertility*, p. 91. (Boston: Little, Brown)

Muller, P. (1977). Endomètre et malformation utérine. *"L'Endomètre"*, p. 245. (Paris: Masson)

Musset, R. (1967). Classification globale des malformations utérines. *Gynecol. Obstet.*, **66**, 145

Musset, R. (1973). Les explorations nécessaires à l'identification des anomalies congénitales du vagin et de l'uterus. *Gaz. Med. Fr.*, **80**, 4997

Palmer, R. (1981). Anomalies utérines congénitales. In Boury-Heyler, C., Mauléon, P. and Rochet, Y. (eds.) *Utérus et fécondité*. (Paris: Masson)

Rock, J. A. and Zacur, H. A. (1983). The clinical management of repeated early pregnancy wastage. *Fertil. Steril.*, **32**, 123

Salvatierra, V., Comino, R., Beltran, E. Y. and Florida, J. (1976). Desarollo glandular y vascularisation del endometrio en las malformaciones uterinas. VIII World Congress of Gynecology and Obstetrics. Excerpta. Medica – Mexico – DF, n° **672**, 320

Seffert, P. and Rochet, Y. (1981). A propos de 41 hystéroplasties pour bifidité utérine. In Boury-Heyler, C., Mauléon, P. and Rochet, Y. *Uterus et fécondité*, p. 225. (Paris: Masson)

Semmens, J. P. (1962). Congenital anomalies of the genital tract. *Obstet. Gynecol.*, **19**, 328

Siegler, A. M. (1967). *Hysterosalpingography*. (New York: Harper & Row, Hoeber Medical Division)

Siegler, A. M. (1983). Hysterosalpingography. *Fertil. Steril.*, **40**, 139

Stillman, R. J. (1982). In utero exposure to diethylstilbestrol: adverse effects on the reproductive tract and reproductive performance in male and female offspring. *Am. J. Obstet. Gynecol.*, **142**, 905

Strassman, P. (1907). Die operative Vereinigung eines Doppelten Uterus-Zentralbe. *Gynekol.*, **43**, 1322

Tompkins, P. (1962). Comments on the bicornuate uterus and twinning. *Surg. Clin. North Am.*, **42**, 1049

Tulandi, T., Arronet, G. H. and McInnes, R. A. (1980). Arcuate and bicornuate uterine anomalies in infertility. *Fertil. Steril.*, **34**, 362

Viala, J. L. (1981). Hypoplasie utérine. In Boury-Heyler, C., Mauléon, P. and Rochet, Y. (eds.) *Uterus et fécondité*, pp. 119–123. (Paris: Masson)

3
Control of uterine activity in pregnancy

J. J. AMY, P. DE BRUCKER and M. MERCKX

The pregnant uterus, as a viscus, behaves in a peculiar way, in that it accommodates for a considerable length of time a large foreign body in its cavity. During the greater part of gestation, myometrial contractions are infrequent and of low intensity. Possibly, the slow and very gradual distension of the muscle wall by the growing conceptus prevents up to a point the appearance of trains of contractions leading to expulsion of the latter. Much more likely, however, the quiescence of the normal pregnant uterus is achieved by an extrinsic mechanism of neuroendocrine nature.

Evacuation of uterine contents is effected either by suppression of myometrial inhibition, or by an increase in efficacy of one or more stimuli, or by a combination of both factors. As a result, contractions become more frequent and more intense, ultimately giving rise to a regular rhythmic contractile pattern.

PROPERTIES OF MYOMETRIUM

Structure of the myometrium

The smooth muscle cells of the myometrium are elongated and spindle-shaped, about 300 μm long and 10 μm in diameter. The nucleus is eccentrically placed in the thickest part of the cell. The cytoplasm contains *myofilaments*, mitochondria, and the sarcoplasmic reticulum that surrounds the myofilaments. In the smooth muscle cell, these latter are of three kinds: in addition to the 15 nm *myosin* (thick) filaments and the 6 nm *actin* (thin) filaments, the cell contains 10 nm *intermediate filaments*. Intermediate filaments are attached to the so-called *dense bodies* which are randomly distributed in the cell membrane and in the cytoplasm (Huszar, 1981).

The myosin molecule is about 160 nm long. It is composed of two *heavy chains* (molecular weight: 200 000) and, in smooth muscle, of two additional *light chains* (molecular weight: 15 000 and 20 000, respectively). Actin, the other major muscle protein, has a molecular weight of 45 000 (Huszar, 1981).

The cells are arranged in a network of intricately interwoven bundles which follow a spiral course; some of these end up in the cervix. The smooth muscle elements are separated by thin sheets of connective tissue composed of collagen, elastic fibers, fibroblasts and mast cells. The connective tissue supports the muscle fibers and also serves to transmit the tension developed by contraction of the latter.

Uterine enlargement during pregnancy is mainly due to stretching and hypertrophy of existing muscle cells, the appearance of new muscle cells being much less important. Concomitantly, there is an accumulation of fibroelastic tissue, especially in the external muscular layer (Pritchard and MacDonald, 1980).

Coordination of myometrial activity

Functionally, the smooth muscle elements of the myometrium behave like a syncytium wherein excitation, which causes depolarization and a decrease in the resting potential of the cell membrane, is spread from cell to cell by myogenic conduction. Generalized spread of these trains of action potentials to the entire myometrium is a prerequisite for the coordinated uterine activity of labor or abortion. This is made possible by the appearance of increasing numbers of *gap junctions* between adjacent muscle cells. Gap junctions are thought to be sites of low impedance to the flow of current between cells. Before labor, the scarcity of these contacts very likely limits the spread of current, thereby preventing any activity generated in one area to propagate to other parts of the myometrium. With the onset of labor, the appearance of gap junctions may permit the spread of action potentials and synchronize muscle contractility (Garfield and Hayashi, 1981). A contraction generalized to the entire myometrium can thus be obtained within 10–20 seconds in response to a localized stimulus. During coordinated uterine activity, such as that seen during labor, contractions usually originate in the fundal area, close to one of the cornua.

Biochemistry of myometrial contraction

The action potential generated upon electrical stimulation of the cell membrane is transferred inside the cell by means of the transverse tubular system of the sarcoplasmic reticulum. The latter, which together with the mitochondria constitutes a storage system for part of the intracellular calcium, releases calcium ions into the cytoplasm. Calcium activates *myosin light-chain kinase* (also called *myosin-ATP-ase*) and, by means of the latter, catalyses hydrolysis of ATP to ADP and phosphorylation of the 20000 molecular weight myosin light chains. This brings about actin–myosin interaction, and the muscle cell contracts: the actin filaments slide past the myosin filaments, without either changing in length (Figure 3.1). Relaxation occurs when another enzyme, *myosin light-chain phosphatase*, removes the phosphate group from the myosin molecule. During relaxation, Ca^{2+} is bound and stored again in the vesicles of the sarcoplasmic reticulum and in the mitochondria, and ATP is resynthesized, with consumption of oxygen (Carsten, 1976; Huszar, 1981).

The activity of myosin light-chain kinase appears to be regulated by at least three factors. Activation requires the presence of *calmodulin* (a calcium-

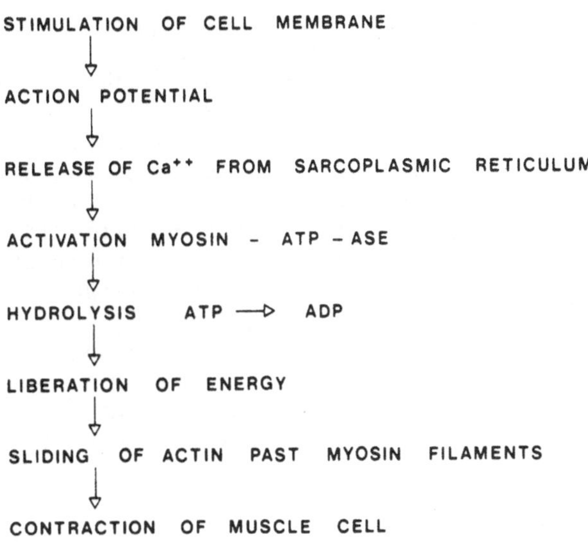

Figure 3.1 Sequence of biochemical events leading to contraction of the muscle cell. The stimulus (e.g. binding of the oxytocic substance to its receptor on the outer cell membrane) effects in succession: (1) an increase in the concentration of activator calcium in the cytoplasm, (2) the activation of myosin light-chain kinase (myosin ATP-ase) and phosphorylation of the myosin light chain and (3) the sliding of the actin past the myosin filament.

dependent regulatory protein) and an intracellular free Ca^{2+} concentration of 10^{-7}–10^{-6} mol/l. On the contrary, its activity is inhibited by cyclic AMP (cAMP)-dependent protein kinase (Huszar, 1981).

Beside the sarcoplasmic reticulum and the mitochondria, which constitute intracellular storage sites for the ion, the cytoplasmic concentration of free Ca^{2+} is also dependent on its passage through specific channels in the outer cell membrane. Progesterone appears to enhance sequestration of calcium in the mitochondria and the sarcoplasmic reticulum, thus increasing the threshold necessary for stimulation. On the contrary, both oxytocin and prostaglandins E_2 and $F_2\alpha$ promote the influx of calcium from the membranes towards the myofilaments. Prostaglandin $F_1\beta$, that does not modify uterine contractility, has no such effect (Carsten, 1976, 1979). Calcium antagonists (e.g. verapamil, nifedipine) which interfere with transmembranal passage of Ca^{2+} display a definite tocolytic effect both in patients with premature uterine contractions and in those undergoing termination of pregnancy with intra-amniotic prostaglandin $F_2\alpha$ (Forman *et al.*, 1981). The uterorelaxant effect of Mg^{2+} is probably mediated by means of an intracellular displacement of Ca^{2+}.

Thus, movements of activator calcium within the cell control the contractile activity of the myometrium. Activator calcium is the final common pathway by which all substances active on the myometrium exert their effect. The role played by the cyclic nucleotide cAMP is more difficult to grasp. Changes in the levels of cAMP are observed in response to several pharmacologic agents, but there is no consistency in this respect. β-Agonists (e.g. isoproterenol, epinephrine) appear to have as sole mechanism of action the stimulation of membrane-associated adenylate cyclase, resulting in the rise of the intracellular concentration of cAMP and relaxation of the myofilaments.

Beside β-agonist stimulation, myometrial relaxation also follows treatment with cAMP, dibutyryl cAMP and phosphodiesterase inhibitors such as theophylline, all of which raise the intracellular content of cAMP (Figure 3.2). Cyclic AMP-dependent protein kinase causes calcium to be taken up by the sarcoplasmic reticulum and it lowers the activity of myosin light-chain kinase (Krall *et al.*, 1977; Huszar, 1981). Prostaglandins E_1 and E_2 also activate adenylate cyclase and thereby elevate the intracellular level of cAMP, although they are potent oxytocics. Therefore, there is no strict relation between the intracellular content of cAMP and the degree of activity of the myometrium. Prostaglandins $F_1\alpha$ and $F_2\alpha$ and oxytocin have no effect on the basal levels of

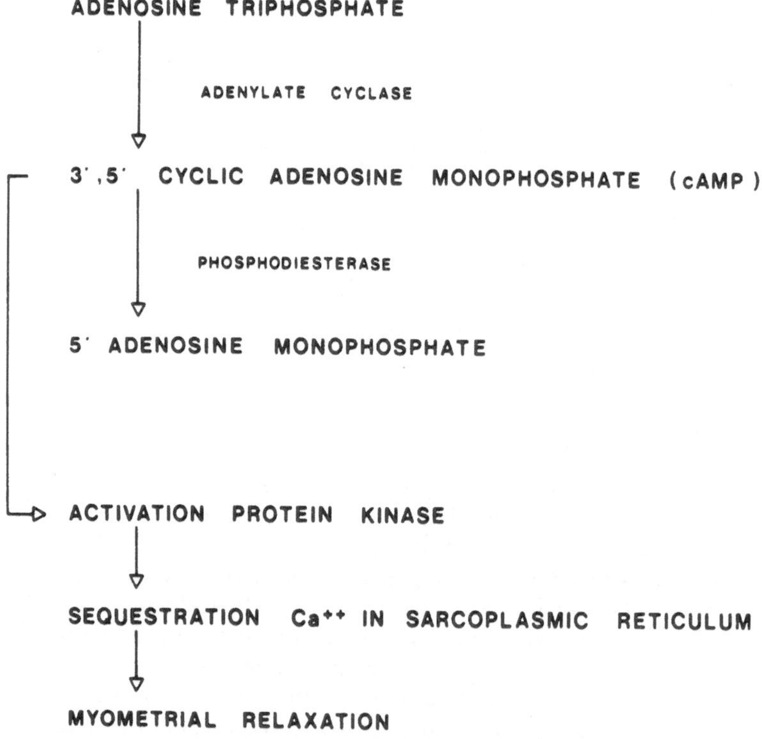

Figure 3.2 Stimulation of adenylate cyclase (e.g. β-adrenergic agonists) leads to an increase in the intracellular concentration in cAMP. The latter substance, by means of activation of cAMP-dependent protein kinase, causes Ca^{2+} to be stored in the sarcoplasmic reticulum and in the mitochondria. This results in relaxation of the myometrial cell. Cyclic AMP is metabolized under control of the enzyme phosphodiesterase. Inhibitors of phosphodiesterase (e.g. theophylline) cause myometrial relaxation.

cAMP but inhibit isoproterenol-induced increases in concentration of the cyclic nucleotide. Prostaglandin antagonists such as polyphloretin phosphate and 7-oxa-13-prostynoic acid block prostaglandin E- and F-induced contractions, without modifying the ability of prostaglandin E to raise cAMP levels (Krall *et al.*, 1977; Harbon *et al.*, 1979).

PROPERTIES OF UTERINE CERVIX

Structure of cervical stroma

The lower uterine segment and the cervix contain relatively much more connective and elastic tissue and less muscle than the corpus. Collagen makes up 80% of the protein in the cervical stroma. Its fibers are arranged in a regular matrix of bundles with few intervening cellular elements. A ground substance, the main constituents of which are *proteoglycans*, fills the spaces between the fibers and limits their mobility. Proteoglycans are polysaccharide-protein complexes in which the *glycosaminoglycans* (formerly known as the acid mucopolysaccharides) represent the polysaccharide in the molecule (von Maillot *et al.*, 1981).

Cervical smooth muscle

A thin layer of smooth muscle can be identified at the periphery of the cervix. Part of it is arranged in a circular fashion. However sparse, the cervical muscle may gain functionally in importance when the connective tissue framework loses rigidity during softening. It has been claimed that the circular muscle bundles would be capable of contracting independently and of responding differently from the myometrium to certain pharmacologic agents. This, episodically, leads to the development of a spastic ring interfering with cervical dilatation. Empirically, dextropropoxyphene has been used, frequently with success, in cases of delayed progress in labor. In such instances, the lack of myometrial stimulation observed in the face of very rapid cervical dilatation, would indicate the cervix as being the site of action of the drug.

Cervical maturation

Little is known about the complicated process leading in late pregnancy to thinning, softening and dilatation of the cervix. Profound structural changes occur in the collagen matrix and in the ground substance which appear to be caused by locally produced prostacyclin and prostaglandins; rising estrogen levels and relaxin possibly play a contributory role (Calder, 1979; Ellwood *et al.*, 1981). One observes separation of the collagen bundles, less aggregation of the fibers, distension with fluid of the intervening spaces and a lesser degree of definition in the appearance of collagen.

Simultaneously, there is a sharp increase in glycosaminoglycans (von Maillot *et al.*, 1981). All of these modifications can be obtained by local administration of exogenous prostaglandins (Ellwood *et al.*, 1981; Uldbjerg *et al.*, 1981).

NEUROENDOCRINE CONTROL OF UTERINE ACTIVITY IN PREGNANCY

Mechanisms of parturition are extremely diversified among mammals. Even among primates, important differences exist. Great care must therefore be taken before extrapolating observations made in animals to man. Because of these limitations, the physiology of labor in women has not been completely elucidated. Although many substances are pharmacologically active on the uterus, only a few have a demonstrated physiologic role in human parturition.

Autonomic innervation and catecholamines

The uterus is predominantly innervated by sympathetic fibers of α (noradrenergic) and β (adrenergic) type. Parasympathetic (cholinergic) nerve fibers play a negligible role in the regulation of uterine activity. The uterus also contains norepinephrine (α-stimulant) and epinephrine (predominantly β-stimulant) derived from systemic sources. α-Adrenergic stimulation of the myometrium causes contraction, whereas β-adrenergic stimulation produces relaxation. As stated before, the relaxant effect of β-agonists is mediated by activation of adenylate cyclase and the subsequent increase in intracellular concentration of cAMP (Krall *et al.*, 1977).

There is very little α-adrenergic activity in the pregnant uterus. Norepinephrine given in pharmacologic doses stimulates the myometrium, but it plays a negligible role in parturition. The intravenous infusion of the α-blocking agent phenoxybenzamine during the early first stage of labor causes no abatement in contractile activity. Epinephrine acts on both the α- and the β-receptors. As the latter predominate, the relaxant effect of epinephrine stands out unless the β-receptors are blocked by a selective antagonist. A clearcut uterine activation is observed following administration of propanolol to pregnant women. This implies that epinephrine exerts an inhibitory effect on the uterus during pregnancy (Amy and Thiery, 1980). This effect is probably modulated by sex steroids. Experimentally, high doses of estrogens reduce within 24 hours the membrane density of β-receptors in the rat uterus, whereas progesterone restores it within the same period of time (Krall *et al.*, 1977).

Oxytocin

Role in parturition in animals

In animals, raised maternal plasma levels of oxytocin are measured during the expulsive phase of labor. This accelerated release of oxytocin is attributed to a spinal reflex, the so-called *Ferguson's reflex*, which is elicited by cervical and vaginal distension. Interruption of the reflex pathway by lumbar epidural anesthesia or by division of the spinal cord in the thoracic region causes a delay in fetal expulsion. The same effect is obtained by selective destruction of the paraventricular nuclei of the maternal hypothalamus, where oxytocin is being produced (Chard *et al.*, 1977; Flint *et al.*, 1978; Amy and Thiery, 1980).

Role in human parturition

Sensitive radioimmunoassay techniques have shown that oxytocin is released in *spurts* or *spikes* into the maternal circulation. These spurts occur throughout pregnancy and become somewhat more frequent with advancing gestational age. No surge is observed at the onset of labor, but a sharp increase in maternal plasma oxytocin does occur towards the end of labor, when the cervix and the vagina are maximally distended. Paracervical, lumbar epidural or subarachnoid anesthesia block this final oxytocin surge (Vasicka *et al.*, 1978).

The posterior pituitary gland of the human fetus releases oxytocin (and vasopressin) and its neurophysins during spontaneous labor. An arteriovenous difference of oxytocin concentration exists across the umbilical circulation which clearly indicates an origin from within the fetus. The levels increase progressively to reach a maximum at the time of delivery (Chard *et al.*, 1977). There is disagreement as to whether fetal (umbilical) arterial plasma levels of oxytocin at delivery are consistently higher than maternal levels (Dawood *et al.*, 1978; Vasicka *et al.*, 1978). Some investigators found a higher concentration of oxytocin in the fetal arterial plasma during labor and they believe that the hormone crosses the placental barrier towards the maternal compartment. After elective cesarean section performed before labor, the umbilical arterial levels of oxytocin were lower than the maternal levels. Moreover, maternal administration of oxytocin resulted in a reversal of the umbilical arteriovenous difference in oxytocin, demonstrating the possibility for this substance to cross, at least in part, the placental barrier without being inactivated (Dawood *et al.*, 1978). Another possible pathway for oxytocin of fetal origin to reach the maternal circulation has been described. Appreciable amounts of oxytocin are found in fetal urine; once in the amniotic cavity, it can conceivably cross the fetal membranes. But 90% of amniotic fluid oxytocin is biologically inactive (Amy and Karim, 1978).

A physiologic role of oxytocin of either maternal or fetal origin in human parturition is very much disputed. At the most, the hormone would have only a facilitatory function. Indeed, although maternal urinary excretion of oxytocin is augmented during intravenous infusion of as little as 1 mU/min of the oxytocic agent, no increase is seen during spontaneous labor. Moreover, neither milk ejection nor a rise in intramammary pressure is recorded and no increase of oxytocin-associated neurophysin is detected in the maternal circulation during labor. Finally, experimental injection of as much as 10 U of oxytocin into the human fetus fails to stimulate the maternal uterus (Amy and Thiery, 1980; Jacobs, 1980).

Mechanism of action

Oxytocin binds to specific cell membrane receptors in the decidua and the myometrium. The formation of these receptors probably is induced by high levels of circulating estrogens. Myometrial receptor concentration was found to increase considerably during pregnancy (Fuchs *et al.*, 1982). At an effective dose, the posterior pituitary hormone causes marked depolarization of the myometrial cell membrane and release of activator calcium from its intracellular storage sites into the cytosol. As stated before, this results in the contraction of the myofilaments contained in the cell. But, unlike prostaglandins, oxytocin does not trigger the formation of gap junctions (Huszar, 1981). Oxytocin-stimulated uterine contractions can be completely inhibited by several synthetic analogs of oxytocin, some of which are totally devoid of agonist properties (Soloff, 1976).

The response of the myometrium to oxytocin is partially suppressed by previous exposure to indomethacin. This may be the result of the decrease in the number of gap junctions induced by the prostaglandin synthesis inhibitor. On the contrary, oxytocin antagonists do not affect the myometrial action of prostaglandins (Garrioch, 1978; Whalley, 1978).

In pregnant women, the uterine sensitivity to intravenously injected test doses of oxytocin augments progressively with gestational age, the increase being more marked after 36 weeks. The response of the uterus to the hormone correlates with the ripeness of the cervix. The more the cervical dilatation and effacement, the greater the effectiveness of oxytocin. Therefore, oxytocin will induce effective labor only in late pregnancy, when the cervix is favorable (Anderson, 1980).

Prostaglandins

Biosynthesis

Prostaglandins are 20-carbon unsaturated fatty acids that are formed by enzymatic oxidation and cyclization of certain essential fatty acids. *Bis*-unsaturated prostaglandins are the most important in man. Their common obligatory precursor is arachidonic acid. The latter is found in the 2-position of cell membrane phospholipids and is liberated, in response to certain stimuli, by a lysosomal enzyme named *phospholipase* A_2. Under the influence of molecular oxygen and an array of microsomal enzymes (collectively called *prostaglandin synthetase*), in particular *cyclo-oxygenase*, arachidonic acid is converted into the highly labile endoperoxides G_2 and H_2. Further steps involve the synthesis of prostacyclin, thromboxane A_2, and prostaglandins D_2, E_2 and $F_2\alpha$ (Figure 3.3). The activity of the various terminal enzymes involved in prostaglandin synthesis varies according to the tissue considered (so that each tissue has a different profile of end products) and its particular condition at the time.

Role in parturition

Prostanoids derived from arachidonic acid play a central role in the ripening of the cervix (Calder, 1979) and in the initiation and maintenance of uterine activity during labor and abortion (Liggins *et al.*, 1977; Keirse, 1979; Amy and Thiery, 1980).

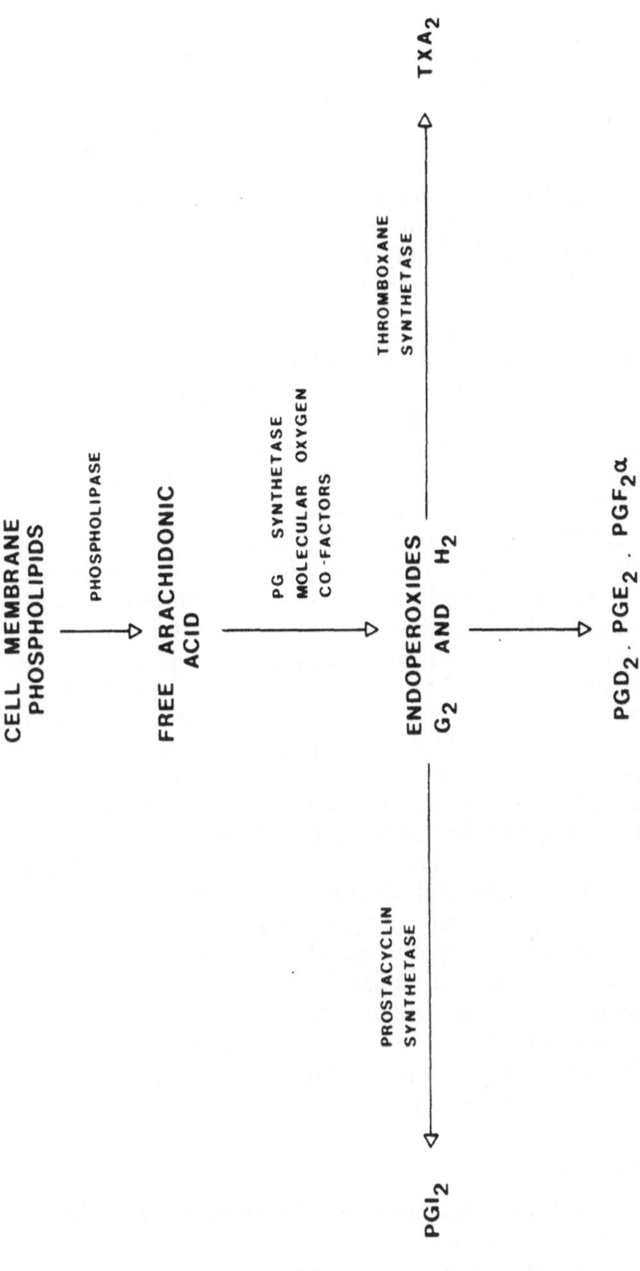

Figure 3.3 Simplified scheme of the 'arachidonic acid cascade' (biosynthesis of prostanoids). The leukotriene pathways are not represented in this diagram.

(1) Levels of prostaglandins E_2 and $F_2\alpha$ or of their metabolites in amniotic fluid, peripheral blood and urine increase during the last weeks of pregnancy, and a further rise is noted during spontaneous abortion or parturition.

(2) Prostaglandins are the only chemicals presently available that will effect softening and dilatation of the cervix, activation of the myometrium and expulsion of the conceptus, consistently and virtually at any stage of gestation.

(3) Prostaglandin synthesis inhibitors suppress uterine activity and thereby, depending on the timing of administration, postpone and/or prolong labor. These drugs also delay fetal expulsion following intra-amniotic instillation of a hypertonic solution.

Prostaglandins implicated in labor and abortion derive from esterified arachidonic acid stored in the decidua and in the fetal membranes (18 % of the total fatty acids, in contradistinction to only 0.4 % in the maternal parietal peritoneum). Some glycerophospholipids of the amnion and chorion laeve, namely *phosphatidylethanolamines*, are particularly rich in arachidonic acid. Moreover fetal membranes would possess a phospholipase A_2 specific for phosphatidylethanolamines and with greatest specifity for esterified arachidonic acid therein contained (Okazaki *et al.*, 1978). However, phospholipase A activity in the fetal membranes is probably not different during as opposed to before the onset of labor. Hence, it is unlikely that the release of free arachidonic acid is the rate-limiting factor in intrauterine prostaglandin production. The control of prostaglandin synthesis implicated in spontaneous labor and abortion is more likely to reside at the level of one or more of the enzymes responsible for conversion of arachidonic acid into prostaglandins. Combined measurements of arachidonic acid and its various metabolic products should help to elucidate this controversial matter (Keirse, 1979).

Once synthesized in chorion and decidua, prostaglandins are transported, probably by diffusion, into the myometrium, which is being activated, and into the amniotic fluid, where raised levels are being noted (Amy and Karim, 1978). During active labor, mechanical disturbance and hypoxia may augment the release of certain enzymes controlling prostaglandin synthesis thus making myometrial activity a self-perpetuating phenomenon.

It is not known what role prostaglandins of fetal origin play in parturition. The larger amounts of these chemicals detected in fetal plasma, particularly during labor, would probably to a considerable extent be inactivated by placental and maternal pulmonary 15-OH-prostaglandin dehydrogenase before reaching the myometrium.

Mechanism of action

Prostaglandins possess specific membrane-binding sites. They are not antagonized by antihistamines, atropine, serotonin antagonists, α- or β-blocking agents, or oxytocin antagonists. Prostaglandins act as the final mediators of cervical ripening and of uterine contractions. They increase the formation of gap junctions, which, on the contrary, is inhibited by indomethacin.

Prostaglandins then effect uterine stimulation by mobilization of activator calcium (Huszar, 1981).

Prostacyclin may have effects on uterine smooth muscle but sufficient data are still lacking in this regard. Thromboxane A_2 does not seem to be involved in myometrial activity.

Other utero-stimulants

Of the other endogenous substances with known oxytocic properties (acetylcholine, bradykinin, histamine, serotonin, vasopressin) none seems to be implicated in the regulation of uterine contractility.

Fetal cortisol

Role in parturition

Unlike the process in several other mammals, such as the sheep, a modification of the endocrine profile does not seem to be required for labor to start in man. Many arguments have been advanced in support of a role for the fetal hypothalamic–pituitary–adrenal axis in the timing of parturition, but several of them have limitations (Swaab *et al.*, 1977; Amy and Thiery, 1980; Anderson, 1980).

(1) Pregnancy associated with anencephaly may, in the absence of polyhydramnios, last much beyond term; furthermore it may show a degree of refractoriness to tèrmination of pregnancy or induction of labor. But this is by no means the rule. A large number of these infants are born before term, after spontaneous labor. Thus, in the absence of fetal brain, precise control over gestastional length is lost, but the mechanisms for initiating labor seem to remain intact in many pregnancies complicated by anencephaly.

(2) The weight of the fetal adrenal increases rapidly in late pregnancy. Much of this enlargement pertains to the fetal zone of the cortex, which constitutes about 80% of the gland at term and which regresses after birth.

(3) Fetal adrenal hypoplasia, without gross pituitary anomaly, is frequently but not constantly associated with post-term delivery. Furthermore, several instances of failure of cortisol production by the human fetus do not result in prolonged gestation. These include defects in steroid 21-hydroxylation, 17α-hydroxylation, 11β-hydroxylation and 3β-hydroxysteroid dehydrogenase (Pritchard and MacDonald, 1980).

(4) Fetal adrenocortical hyperplasia is frequently, but not invariably, detected in babies born prematurely for no apparent reason (as opposed to infants of similar gestational age born before term due, for instance, to abruptio placentae).

Prolonged administration of depot ACTH to anencephalic fetuses does not suffice to start labor, despite the fact that it stimulates suprarenal growth and secretory activity, as demonstrated by an increase in maternal urinary excretion of estriol. Similarly, injection of large doses of glucocorticoids to the mother or into the amniotic cavity does not consistently induce labor. In fact, this type of treatment suppresses fetal and maternal hypothalamic, pituitary and adrenal activity, and thereby reduces the amount of precursors necessary for estrogen synthesis. Thus an endocrine environment essentially different from that prevailing in physiologic circumstances is being created. In women, glucocorticoids do not induce the placental enzymes released at term in the ovine placenta, that bring about a fall in progesterone and a rise in estrogens in the maternal circulation. Biosynthesis of estrogens in late pregnancy is essentially different in the two species. In the sheep, it is predominantly a placental function, while it involves both fetal and maternal adrenal cortex as well as placenta in women (Haning *et al.*, 1978; Amy and Thiery, 1980; Anderson, 1980). Moreover, administration of pharmacologic doses of glucocorticoids is known to inhibit the release of free arachidonic acid and thus the synthesis of prostanoids. A tocolytic effect, comparable to that of ritodrine administered in therapeutic dosage, was observed following treatment of threatening preterm labor with a combination of cortisol and 17-hydroxyprogesterone caproate (Kauppila *et al.*, 1980).

Control of fetal cortisol production

Preliminary evidence (Silman *et al.*, 1977) suggests that control of suprarenal function by the pituitary is very different in the fetus from in the adult. ACTH is composed of two biologically active peptides, namely *α-melanotropin* (α-MSH) and *corticotropin-like intermediate-lobe peptide* (CLIP). Throughout most of fetal life CLIP and α-MSH are produced separately by the pituitary and they must probably be held responsible for driving the fetal zone of the adrenal cortex. Near term, however, a switch to intact ACTH occurs, which could stimulate development and activity of the definitive or adult zone. No surge in ACTH release is observed prior to parturition in the human fetus (Pritchard and MacDonald, 1980) and fetal plasma cortisol levels are no different at the onset of spontaneous labor from those recorded immediately before induction (Gennser *et al.*, 1977). However, a progressive increase in fetal plasma cortisol concentration does occur in the course of labor, part of which is of fetal origin (Campbell and Murphy, 1977) and in response to stress (Haning *et al.*, 1978).

Thus, human parturition is not triggered by a sharp rise in the secretion of cortisol by the fetal adrenal. Fetal cortisol production in primates appears to be more closely related to the functional maturation of certain organs, in preparation for extrauterine life, than to the exact timing of parturition, as in the sheep (Liggins *et al.*, 1977; Haning *et al.*, 1978; Amy and Thiery, 1980).

Sex-steroid hormones

Plasma levels of sex-steroid hormones

An increasingly potent inhibitory mechanism must be active during pregnancy to keep the uterus quiescent. By extrapolation from observations done on various animals where experimental progesterone withdrawal triggers abortion or parturition, a similar role has been claimed for this steroid hormone in human gestation (Csapo, 1977): a dynamic equilibrium would exist between progesterone and an *intrinsic myometrial stimulant*, supposedly prostaglandin $F_2\alpha$. Initiation of labor would be triggered off by progesterone withdrawal from the myometrium rather than by an increased synthesis of the prostanoid. Several investigators have also attributed a stimulatory function to estrogens. In two studies of carefully selected cases, a decrease in mean maternal plasma progesterone and a surge in mean plasma estradiol were indeed reported to occur shortly before parturition, but the changes mentioned were not observed in every patient. Moreover, plasma concentration of sex-steroid hormones serially determined in unselected cases failed to show a consistent decline in progesterone or a rise in estrone or estradiol prior to labor (Ryan, 1977; Boroditsky *et al.*, 1978; Mathur *et al.*, 1980). Thus, human parturition is not associated with abrupt changes in the maternal plasma content of the aforementioned steroids. Estriol levels do continue to rise during the last weeks of pregnancy (Boroditsky *et al.*, 1978; Mathur *et al.*, 1980) which reflects increasing fetal maturation. Estriol may possibly play a role, yet to be elicited, in the triggering mechanism of labor.

Role of progesterone

In the absence of any decrease in peripheral levels of unbound progesterone, a withdrawal of this hormone could still be achieved locally. The presence of a protein, which binds progesterone, has been described in the cytoplasm of cells from the fetal membranes. This protein increases in amount at the end of gestation, before labor. It was thought to make progesterone locally unavailable for biologic action, hence reducing its utero-relaxant effect (Schwarz *et al.*, 1976). Currently, this protein is thought to be cortisol binding globulin, which has no specific binding properties for progesterone. At any rate, even large doses of progesterone, 17-medroxyprogesterone acetate or 17α-hydroxyprogesterone caproate injected systemically or directly into the amniotic cavity or the myometrium fail to inhibit established uterine activity (Liggins *et al.*, 1977). However, these compounds may possibly delay delivery and reduce perinatal mortality when given from an early stage of pregnancy to women presenting a high risk for pre-term labor (Johnson *et al.*, 1979).

Progesterone would act either by hyperpolarization of the myometrial cell membrane or, more likely, by enhancing the binding of activator calcium to the sarcoplasmic reticulum and lowering myosin light-chain phosphorylation, as stated earlier (Carsten, 1979; Huszar, 1981).

Role of estrogens

As parturition in the human is not consistently preceded by a rise in maternal plasma concentration of estradiol, only a facilitatory role in the initiation of myometrial activity can be attributed to the estrogen (Anderson, 1980). Patients going into labor after intravaginal instillation of prostaglandin E_2 have been reported to have a significantly higher plasma estradiol content than those requiring amniotomy in addition; there would be no difference in either the plasma progesterone or the plasma prolactin levels (MacKenzie *et al.*, 1979). Maternal infusion of estradiol causes transient uterine contractility, but the activity elicited is not powerful enough to lead to delivery. Besides, labor can start spontaneously (and occasionally before term) when maternal plasma estradiol concentrations are low, such as is the case in placental sulfatase deficiency, anencephaly, death *in utero*, or after administration of large doses of glucocorticoids.

Finally, additional data are required before one may reach a conclusion as to the ripening action of estrogens on the uterine cervix. While some have claimed success following the extra-amniotic administration of estradiol or estriol, others found no significant difference between estrogen-treated women and those to whom a placebo was instilled (Thiery *et al.*, 1979; MacKenzie, 1981).

Relaxin

Relaxin is a polypeptide of 48 amino acid residues comprising two chains linked by disulfide bridges. It is produced by the corpus luteum, throughout pregnancy, and possibly by the decidua as well. Myometrial inhibitory properties have been described in some species, including man. Plasma levels in gravid women gradually decline towards term.

Relaxin induces relaxation of the ligaments of the bony pelvis in rodents; in the rat, it causes softening of the cervix. It may have a similar action in the woman, the sow and the mouse, among other species (Porter, 1981). These effects are obtained by means of an increase in the activity of collagen-degrading enzymes (von Maillot *et al.*, 1981).

CONCLUDING REMARKS

One or more mechanisms are operative by means of which myometrial contractility is inhibited for the entire duration of gestation. Progesterone from the corpus luteum is essential for the maintenance of early pregnancy. Luteectomy during the first weeks of gestation is followed by abortion in the case of persistent fall in circulating progesterone levels. Administration of exogenous progesterone to these women prevents abortion. The role of the steroid hormone at later stages of pregnancy is much more difficult to define. Endogenous epinephrine inhibits activity of the pregnant uterus; possibly relaxin plays a contributory role. Finally, prostaglandin production in the various structures enclosing the conceptus is greatly suppressed until the end of pregnancy.

An increase in uterine contractility and dramatic changes in the structure, the shape and the compliance of the cervix occur preceding parturition. No modification in the endocrine background can be held responsible for triggering these events. But both the sex steroids and the hormones of the fetal hypothalamic–pituitary–adrenal axis have a modulating effect: hormonal imbalance may greatly interfere with the timing of parturition.

Causes of abortion or pre-term delivery (e.g. chromosomal anomalies of the conceptus, fetal death, excessive uterine distension due to multiple gestation or hydramnios etc.) are extremely diversified and each has a neuroendocrine background proper. However, there is no reason to question that prostaglandins are, as in spontaneous term labor, the final common mediators of myometrial stimulation which they effect by means of formation of gap junctions and intracellular release of activator calcium. Oxytocin plays at most a facilitatory role.

Acknowledgements

This work was supported in part by a grant from the Belgian Foundation for Scientific Research (N.F.W.O.), Brussels. The authors are grateful to Ms Bea Pion and to Ms Martine Voet for expert secretarial assistance.

References

Amy, J. J. and Karim, S. M. M. (1978). Prostaglandins and other oxytocic substances in amniotic fluid. In Fairweather, D. V. I. and Eskes, T. K. A. B. (eds.) *Amniotic Fluid – Research and Clinical Application*. 2nd Edn., pp. 321–345. (Amsterdam: Excerpta Medica)

Amy, J. J. and Thiery, M. (1980). Labor – spontaneous and induced. In Aladjem, S., Brown, A. K. and Sureau, C. (eds.) *Clinical Perinatology*. 2nd Edn., pp. 362–381. (St Louis: Mosby)

Anderson, A. (1980). The genital system. In Hytten, F. and Chamberlain, G. (eds.) *Clinical Physiology in Obstetrics*, pp. 328–380. (Oxford: Blackwell Scientific)

Boroditsky, R. S., Reyes, F. I., Winter, J. S. D. and Faiman, C. (1978). Maternal serum estrogen and progesterone concentrations preceding normal labor. *Obstet, Gynecol.*, **51,** 686

Calder, A. A. (1979). Management of the unripe cervix. In Keirse, M. J. N. C., Anderson, A. B. M. and Bennebroek Gravenhorst, J. (eds.) *Human Parturition*, pp. 201–217. (Leiden: Leiden University Press)

Campbell, A. L. and Murphy, B. E. P. (1977). The maternal-fetal cortisol gradient during pregnancy and at delivery. *J. Clin. Endocrinol. Metab.*, **45,** 435

Carsten, M. E. (1976). How does calcium control uterine contraction? *Contemp. Obstet. Gynecol.*, **8,** 61

Carsten, M. E. (1979). Calcium accumulation by uterine microsomal preparations: Effects of progesterone and oxytocin. *Am. J. Obstet. Gynecol.*, **133,** 598

Chard, T., Silman, R. E. and Rees, L. H. (1977). The fetal hypothalamus and pituitary in the initiation of labour. In Knight, J. and O'Connor, M. (eds.) *Ciba Foundation Symposium 47: The Fetus and Birth*, pp. 359–370. (Amsterdam: Elsevier/North Holland/Excerpta Medica)

Csapo, A. I. (1977). The 'see-saw' theory of parturition. In Knight, J. and O'Connor, M. (eds.) *Ciba Foundation Symposium 47: The Fetus and Birth*, pp. 159–195. (Amsterdam: Elsevier/North Holland/Excerpta Medica)

Dawood, M. Y., Wang, C. F., Gupta, R. and Fuchs, F. (1978). Fetal contribution to oxytocin in human labor. *Obstet. Gynecol.*, **52,** 205

Ellwood, D. A., Anderson, A. B. M., Mitchell, M. D., Murphy, G. and Turnbull, A. C. (1981). Prostanoids, collagenase and cervical softening in the sheep. In Ellwood, D. A. and Anderson, A. B. M. (eds.) *The Cervix in Pregnancy and Labour*, pp. 57–73. (Edinburgh: Churchill Livingstone)

Flint, A. P. F., Forsling, M. L. and Mitchell, M. D. (1978). Blockade of the Ferguson reflex by lumbar epidural anaesthesia in the parturient sheep: Effects of oxytocin secretion and uterine venous prostaglandin F levels. *Horm. Metab. Res.*, **10**, 545

Forman, A., Andersson, K. E. and Ulmsten, U. (1981). Inhibition of myometrial activity by calcium antagonists. *Semin. Perinatol.*, **5**, 288

Fuchs, A. R., Fuchs, F., Husslein, P., Soloff, M. S. and Fernström, M. J. (1982). Oxytocin receptors and human parturition: A dual role for oxytocin in the initiation of labor. *Science*, **215**, 1396

Garfield, R. E. and Hayashi, R. H. (1981): Appearance of gap junctions in the myometrium of women during labor. *Am. J. Obstet. Gynecol.*, **140**, 254

Garrioch, D. B. (1978). The effect of indomethacin on spontaneous activity in the isolated human myometrium and on the response to oxytocin and prostaglandin. *Br. J. Obstet. Gynaecol.*, **85**, 47

Gennser, G., Orhlander, S. and Aneroth, P. (1977). Fetal cortisol and the initiation of labour in the human. In Knight, J. and O'Connor, M. (eds.) *Ciba Foundation Symposium 47: The Fetus and Birth*, pp. 401–420. (Amsterdam: Elsevier/North Holland/Excerpta Medica)

Haning, R. V. Jr., Barrett, D. A., Alberino, S. P., Lynskey, M. T., Donabedian, R. and Speroff, L. (1978). Interrelationships between maternal and cord prolactin, progesterone, estradiol, 13,14-dihydro-15-keto-prostaglandin $F_2\alpha$, and cortisol at delivery with respect to initiation of parturition. *Am. J. Obstet. Gynecol.*, **130**, 204

Harbon, S., Do Khac, L., Vesin, M. F. and Leiber, D. (1979). Etude des mécanismes d'action des prostaglandines dans la régulation de la contractilité du muscle utérin. In Amy, J. J. (ed.) *Les Prostaglandines et la Reproduction Humaine*, pp. 27–46. (Paris: Flammarion Médecine-Sciences)

Huszar, G. (1981). Biology and biochemistry of myometrial contractility and cervical maturation. *Semin. Perinatol.*, **5**, 216

Jacobs, H. S. (1980): Hypothalamus and pituitary gland. In Hytten, F. and Chamberlain, G. (eds.) *Clinical Physiology in Obstetrics*, pp. 383–399. (Oxford: Blackwell Scientific Publications)

Johnson, J. W., Lee, P. A., Zachary, A. S., Calhoun, S. and Migeon, C. J. (1979). High risk prematurity – progestin treatment and steroid studies. *Obstet. Gynecol.*, **54**, 412

Kauppila, A., Hartikainen-Sorri, A. L., Jänne, O. Tuimala, R. and Järvinen, P. A. (1980). Suppression of threatened premature labor by administration of cortisol and 17α-hydroxyprogesterone caproate: A comparison with ritodrine. *Am. J. Obstet. Gynecol.*, **138**, 404

Keirse, M. J. N. C. (1979): Prostaglandines et déclenchement spontané du travail. In Amy, J. J. (ed.) *Les Prostaglandines et la Reproduction Humaine*, pp. 107–140. (Paris: Flammarion Médecine-Sciences)

Krall, J. F., Mori, H. and Korenman, S. G. (1977). Molecular basis of drug action on uterine smooth muscle. In Anderson, A., Beard, R., Brudenell, J. M. and Dunn, P. M. (eds.) *Pre-Term Labour*, pp. 79–100. (London: Royal College of Obstetricians and Gynaecologists.)

Liggins, J. C., Forster, C. S., Grieves, S. A. and Schwartz, A. L. (1977). Control of parturition in man. *Biol. Reprod.*, **16**, 39

MacKenzie, I. Z. (1981). Clinical studies on cervical ripening. In Ellwood, D. A. and Anderson, A. B. M. (eds.) *The Cervix in Pregnancy and Labour*, pp. 162–186. (Edinburgh: Churchill Livingstone)

MacKenzie, I. Z., Jenkin, G. and Bradley, S. (1979). The relation between plasma oestrogen, progesterone and prolactin concentrations and the efficacy of vaginal prostaglandin E_2 gel in initiating labour. *Br. J. Obstet. Gynaecol.*, **86**, 171

von Maillot, K., Stuhlsatz, H. W. and Gentsch, H. H. (1981). Connective tissue changes in the human cervix in pregnancy and labour. In Ellwood, D. A. and Anderson, A. B. M. (eds.) *The Cervix in Pregnancy and Labour*, pp. 123–135. (Edinburgh: Churchill Livingstone)

Mathur, R. S., Landgrebe, S. and Williamson, H. O. (1980). Progesterone, 17-hydroxyprogesterone, estradiol, and estriol in late pregnancy and labor. *Am. J. Obstet. Gynecol.*, **136**, 25

Okazaki, T., Okita, J. R., MacDonald, P. C. and Johnston, J. M. (1978). Initiation of human parturition. X. Substrate specificity of phospholipase A_2 in human fetal membranes. *Am. J. Obstet. Gynecol.*, **130**, 432

Porter, D. G. (1981). Relaxin and cervical softening: a review. In Ellwood, D. A. and Anderson,

A. B. M. (eds.) *The Cervix in Pregnancy and Labour*, pp. 85–99. (Edinburgh: Churchill Livingstone)

Pritchard, J. A. and MacDonald, P. C. (1980). Williams Obstetrics. 16th Edn. (New York: Appleton-Century-Crofts)

Ryan, K. J. (1977). New concepts in hormonal control of parturition. *Biol. Reprod.*, **16,** 88

Schwarz, B. E., Milewich, L., Johnston, J. M., Porter, J. C. and MacDonald, P. C. (1976). Initiation of human parturition. V. Progesterone binding substance in fetal membranes. *Obstet. Gynecol.*, **48,** 685

Silman, R. E., Chard, T., Lowry, P. J., Mullen, P. E., Smith, I. and Young, I. M. (1977). Human fetal corticotropin and released pituitary peptides. *J. Steroid Biochem.*, **8,** 553

Soloff, M. S. (1976). Uterine receptors for oxytocin: Correlation between antagonist potency and receptor binding. *Br. J. Pharmacol.*, **57,** 381

Swaab, D. F., Boer, K. and Honnebier, W. J. (1977). The influence of the fetal hypothalamus and pituitary on the onset and course of parturition. In Knight, J. and O'Connor, M. (eds.) *Ciba Foundation Symposium 47: The Fetus and Birth*, pp. 379–393. (Amsterdam: Elsevier/North Holland/Excerpta Medica)

Thiery, M., De Gezelle, H. Van Kets, H., Voorhoof, L., Verheugen, C., Smis, B., Gerris, J., Derom, R. and Martens, G. (1979). The effect of locally administered estrogens on the human cervix. *Z. Geburtsh. Perinat.*, **183,** 448

Uldbjerg, N., Ekman, G., Malmström, A., Sporrong, B., Ulmsten, U. and Wingerup, L. (1981). Biochemical and morphological changes of human cervix after local application of prostaglandin E_2 in pregnancy. *Lancet*, **1,** 267

Vasicka, A., Kumaresan, P., Han, G. S. and Kumaresan, M. (1978). Plasma oxytocin in initiation of labor. *Am. J. Obstet. Gynecol.*, **130,** 263

Whalley, E. T. (1978). The action of bradykinin and oxytocin on the isolated whole uterus and myometrium of the rat in oestrus. *Br. J. Pharmacol.*, **64,** 21

4
Adrenergic control of uterine function

J. B. CALIXTO, Y. S. DE MEDEIROS and G. A. RAE

INTRODUCTION

A great amount of evidence, obtained from both *in vivo* and *in vitro* studies, has accumulated over the years on the importance of the endogenous catecholamines in the modulation of uterine activity. Such evidence is conflicting in several points and, most important, shows that much more information must be provided before we attain a clear picture of this modulation.

In this chapter, we have attempted to provide a comprehensive summary of what is known to occur within this modulation of uterine contractility by the catecholamines. Although most of the data presented have been furnished by studies in several animal species, we have, where possible, also included *in vivo* and *in vitro* data on human gravid and non-gravid myometrium function. Within the next few pages we will initially deal with the characterization of the various subtypes of uterine adrenoceptors, following on to how they are influenced by steroidal hormones. We will then analyse the relationship between uterine adrenoceptor activation and tissue cAMP levels. Finally, and more extensively, we will discuss the effects of β-adrenoceptor agonists upon human myometrium. Recently, this last topic has attracted much interest due to the increasing usefulness of these drugs in the management of premature labor and fetal suffering.

CHARACTERIZATION OF UTERINE ADRENOCEPTOR SUBTYPES

Uterine smooth muscle is provided with a rich adrenergic innervation which, in general, increases from the body to the cervix. This innervation originates from the sympathetic chain and inferior mesenteric ganglia formations in or near the uterine-vaginal junction. However, the density of this innervation varies among species, being greater for example in the cat than in the rabbit, guinea-pig or human uterus. In other animal species, such as the rat, uterine innervation is restricted almost entirely to the vasculature. Therefore, the concentration of norepinephrine of neuronal origin may vary considerably between species. Also, in view of the intense vascularization of the uterus, a high influence of epinephrine derived from systemic sources can be expected (Nasmyth, 1967; Zuspan *et al.*, 1981).

Both endogenous catecholamines exert their stimulant or inhibitory action upon the myometrium by interacting with either α- or β-adrenoceptors, respectively. Over the last few years it has been elegantly shown that the majority of the β-adrenoceptors are of the β_2-subtype, especially in pregnant myometrium, although a β_1-subtype population has also been detected (Larsen, 1979; Johansson *et al.*, 1980; Krall *et al.*, 1981; Hayashida *et al.*, 1982; Kenakin, 1982). Simultaneously, extensive research has been expended in characterizing the uterine α-adrenoceptor population. Since prazosin (an α_1-selective antagonist) is more effective than yohimbine (an α_2-selective antagonist) in blocking phenylephrine-induced uterine contractions, it is postulated that catecholamines contract the myometrium mainly by interaction with α_1-adrenoceptors (Hoffman *et al.*, 1981). Binding studies also show the presence of α_2-adrenoceptors, which appear to be located on nerve terminals, since their number is reduced by chemical denervation (Roberts *et al.*, 1981). To our knowledge the role of this α_2-subpopulation in uterine function has not yet been elucidated, but studies conducted in other tissues strongly suggest an important modulating function on neurotransmitter release.

It is worth mentioning that there are differences in the physiological and/or pharmacological characteristics between the longitudinal and circular layers of myometrium in several animal species including human (Kawarabayashy and Marshall, 1981; Bengtsson, 1982). In the pregnant rat, for instance, norepinephrine stimulates spontaneous contractions of the circular muscle and inhibits contractions of the longitudinal layer (Chow and Marshall, 1981). Norepinephrine increases amplitude and frequency of spontaneous contractions in both layers of the rabbit uterus but the circular muscle is much more sensitive than the longitudinal to this agonist (Chernaeva and Milenov, 1982). Therefore, there appears to be a relative dominance of α-adrenoceptors in the circular smooth muscle and of β-adrenoceptors in the longitudinal muscle. The non-pregnant human myometrium, in which the muscular layers are less well defined anatomically, also shows differences in the responsiveness of each layer to epinephrine. In this state, epinephrine stimulates the outer longitudinal myometrium but does not affect the inner segment, whereas in postpartum uterus the outer layer is relaxed and the inner contracted by this agonist (Daels, 1974).

Therefore, all subtypes of adrenoceptors are present in the uterus. Activation of α_1- and β_2-adrenoceptors by catecholamines undoubtedly promotes myometrial contraction and relaxation, respectively, in several animal species. However, the role of the α_2- and β_1-adrenoceptor subtypes on myometrium function cannot be clarified at present. Furthermore, the differences in adrenoceptor populations throughout the circular and longitudinal layers of the myometrium are likely to subserve an important physiological function.

HORMONAL INFLUENCE ON UTERINE ADRENOCEPTORS

Although there is marked interspecies variation, the responsiveness of the uterus to adrenoceptor agonists can be altered either by treatment with estrogen or progesterone, or by changes in the circulating endogenous levels of these steroids (Kuryama and Suzuki, 1976; Williams *et al.*, 1977). In the non-pregnant rabbit uterus, norepinephrine and epinephrine promote contraction whereas during pregnancy they evoke relaxation. In agreement with the rabbit, when human myometrium is predominantly under the influence of estrogen, catecholamine administration elicits an α-adrenoceptor-mediated contraction. Conversely, under progesterone predominance, these agonists induce relaxation via interaction with β-adrenoceptors (Williams *et al.*, 1977). However, both norepinephrine and epinephrine relax the rat uterus throughout all four stages of the natural estrous cycle and during pregnancy. In sharp contrast, the cat uterus, that usually relaxes upon exposure to catecholamines in the non-pregnant state, contracts during pregnancy (Nasmyth, 1967; Miller, 1967).

This striking dependence of uterine responsiveness upon hormonal state may be tentatively attributed to variations in the relative density of α- and β-adrenoceptors. Due to the great similarity between human and rabbit myometrial responses to sex steroid treatment, most of the studies on hormone-induced changes in adrenoceptor number have been conducted in the latter species. The total number of uterine α-adrenoceptors in immature rabbits treated with estrogen is three times greater than in naive animals, but the affinity of these receptors to a non-selective ligand remains unchanged. However, when estrogen treatment is followed by progesterone, α-adrenoceptor number is not significantly different from that of naive myometrium (Roberts *et al.*, 1977). A more detailed study shows that this increase in total α-adrenoceptor number is due to a selective enhancement by estrogen of the number of α_2-subtype sites without affecting the amount of α_1-adrenoceptors. Since denervation greatly reduces α_2-adrenoceptor content (Hoffman *et al.*, 1981), these receptors are assumed to be located mainly on nerve terminals. In addition, there is at present no evidence for the involvement of postjunctional α_2-adrenoceptors mediating catecholamine-induced uterine contraction. Furthermore, single or combined treatment with these steroids both fail to modify uterine β-adrenoceptor content or affinity (Hoffman *et al.*, 1981). Similar evidences are furnished by studies conducted with human myometrium strips. Throughout the menstrual cycle there is a considerable variation in α_2-adrenoceptor content whereas the α_1-adrenoceptor population remains constant (Botari *et al.*, 1982).

Although, at present, it appears unlikely that changes in adrenoceptor number and/or affinity are responsible for the hormone-induced changes in sensitivity to α- and β-adrenoceptor agonists, more studies on the effects of these steroids upon adrenoceptors of the different myometrial layers are necessary to allow a definite conclusion. As mentioned above, the responsiveness of each layer of the human myometrium to epinephrine is reversed from the non-pregnant to postpartum state. One cannot discard the possibility of a still undetected increase of adrenoceptor number and/or affinity in one layer being counterbalanced by a decrease in the other.

Another tentative explanation for this hormonal modulation of uterine responsiveness to adrenoceptor agonists could be an action upon one or more steps of the excitation–contraction coupling system beyond the receptor level. In this system, the levels of intracellular free calcium are of critical importance in regulating the magnitude of contraction and/or relaxation. Adrenergic agonists can promote contraction of the myometrium by increasing the influx or decreasing the efflux of calcium or by triggering its release from intracellular storage sites (Woodward *et al.*, 1970). There is strong evidence for a hormonal control of calcium availability for uterine contraction (Calixto *et al.*, 1979; 1982). Progesterone treatment increases superficial calcium binding in rabbit uterine strips (Rubanyi and Csapo, 1976), an effect which may account for the relative refractoriness of the tissue in this state to α-adrenoceptor agonists. However, both estrogen and progesterone inhibit contractions of the uterus by decreasing calcium mobilization in the myometrial cell (Batra and Daniel, 1971; Batra and Bengtsson, 1978; Calixto *et al.*, 1979; Aucélio *et al.*, 1981).

Several conclusions may be drawn from this topic. There is at present no convincing evidence for an action of steroidal hormones on the number or affinity of myometrial α- and β-adrenoceptors. Nevertheless, they undoubtedly modulate the responsiveness of the myometrium to catecholamines. Although some evidence exists for a regulatory role on calcium availability, further studies are needed to elucidate this mechanism. Furthermore, the increase of nerve terminal α_2-adrenoceptor content induced by estrogen treatment suggests a trophic function of this hormone upon uterine innervation.

β-ADRENOCEPTORS: RELATION TO TISSUE cAMP

In several smooth-muscle tissues, β-adrenoceptor mediated relaxation is associated with an increase of cAMP levels, either *in vivo* or *in vitro*. The uterus is not an exception to this rule (Korenman and Krall, 1977). Uterine relaxation is consistently observed after addition of membrane permeable dibutyril-cAMP or phosphodiesterase inhibitors such as papaverine or theophyline which prevent the enzymatic degradation of this nucleotide (Polácek *et al.*, 1971; Marshall and Kroeger, 1973).

The increase of intracellular cAMP associated with β-adrenoceptor activation is brought about by stimulation of a specific adenylate cyclase coupled to the adrenoceptor. The rank order of relative potencies of catecholamines in promoting uterine relaxation (isoprenaline > epinephrine > norepinephrine) and cAMP accumulation are identical. Furthermore, both effects are inhibited by addition of β-adrenoceptor blockers such as propranolol and potentiated by papaverine (for review see Marshall, 1973; Marshall and Kroeger, 1973).

In the rat, treatment with estrogen increases basal uterine cAMP levels (Rinard and Chew, 1975). Moreover, cAMP accumulation and glycogen-phosphorylase activation in response to addition of β-adrenoceptor agonists are both greater in uterine strips from estrogen treated than oophorectomized rats. As mentioned above, an additional influence of estrogen has been postulated on a step of the phosphorylase activation cascade beyond the β-adrenoceptor adenylate-cyclase complex (Rinard and Chew, 1978).

Uterine strips removed from women submitted to prolonged treatment with β-adrenoceptor agonists exhibit subsensitivity to these agents (Berg *et al.*, 1982). This refractory state seems to be related to several intracellular events. Initially there is a progressive loss of catecholamine sensitive adenylate cyclase activity, accompanied by a reduction of cAMP levels and an increase of phosphodiesterase activity. The last event to be detected is a decline in β-adrenoceptor number.

Some evidence, however, sheds doubt on the causal relationship between β-adrenoceptor mediated relaxation and cAMP accumulation (Diamond and Holmes, 1975). In depolarized uterine strips isoprenaline still promotes relaxation (Calixto and Aucélio, 1983), but fails to increase cAMP levels (Diamond and Holmes, 1975). Moreover, several compounds which contract the uterus, such as acetylcholine, prostaglandins and oxytocin, also enhance intracellular cAMP. In addition, other cyclic nucleotides, mainly cGMP, are also likely to influence uterine relaxation. Changes in cGMP to cAMP ratio may, in fact, be more important in the regulation of smooth muscle than the levels of either nucleotide alone (Kano, 1982).

INHIBITION OF MYOMETRIAL CONTRACTION BY β-ADRENOCEPTOR AGONISTS

Throughout pregnancy the pattern of uterine contractility exhibits considerable variation which is caused by the progressive change in hormonal status. This hormonal regulation of uterine mechanical activity is complex and may be partially attributed to their differential effects upon the electrical properties of each muscular layer. In this regard, the circular myometrium of the pregnant rat presents contractions of high frequency and low amplitude on day 15. These contractions, which increase in amplitude and become less frequent up to day 19, almost disappear before delivery on day 21. When delivery begins, strong regular contractions are again evident. In contrast, the contractions of longitudinal muscle on day 15 are irregular and less frequent, but of greater amplitude than those of the circular muscle. This longitudinal pattern gradually becomes more regular, culminating in uniform strong contractions on day 21. Therefore, at term, the contractile patterns of both layers are similar (Bengtsson, 1982). Altogether, such findings suggest that during pregnancy the contractions of the circular muscle impair movement of the fetuses toward the cervix, antagonizing longitudinal muscle activity. At term, the change in pattern of circular muscle contractions may result in a peristaltic type of movement causing a regular progression of fetuses toward the cervix.

In humans, when the uterus increases in size during pregnancy, the superficial longitudinal myometrium becomes more stretched than the deeper, more circular, muscle layer and is, therefore, shifted from the lower uterine segment. Close to delivery, the superficial layer is mainly restricted to the uterine fundus and corpus while the inner segments comprise most of the myometrium of the isthmic region (Bengtsson, 1982). This differential distribution of myometrial layers should certainly play an important role in the process of delivery. However, the relevance of the endogenous catecholamines in determining these variations of myometrial contractility and in the process of delivery remains, at present, an unsettled question.

There are cases though in which the pattern of contraction of the pregnant human uterus presents abnormalities. Several factors may be responsible for such cases including hormonal unbalance, local generation of prostaglandins and altered secretion or sensitivity to oxytocin (Fuchs, 1978). Since abnormal contractions during pregnancy can precipitate premature labor or induce fetal suffering, considerable effort has been expended in determining an efficient therapeutic approach to this problem. Such therapeutic schedules include administration of ethanol, magnesium sulfate, prostaglandin synthesis inhibitors, calcium antagonists and, more extensively in recent years, β-adrenoceptor agonists (Caritis *et al.*, 1979; Andersson, 1982). This later class comprises drugs such as isoxsuprine, orciprenaline, hexoprenaline and the more β_2-selective agonists salbutamol, ritodrine, terbutaline and fenoterol.

In vivo studies

Within the last decade, and despite their cardiovascular side-effects, a great amount of basic and clinical research has drawn attention to the usefulness of selective β_2-adrenoceptor agonists in the management of unwanted contractions during pregnancy. Thus, there are several reports on the successful prolongation of gestation and increase of mean birth weight by administration of isoxsuprine, ritodrine, orciprenaline, terbutaline, salbutamol and fenoterol (reviewed by Caritis *et al.*, 1979; Andersson, 1982; Ingemarsson, 1982; Persson, 1982). According to these authors this beneficial effect is critically dependent on the integrity of the membranes and is associated with long periods of intravenous infusion. Since only a few attempts have been made to evaluate directly the inhibition by these drugs of myometrial activity *in vivo* (Andersson *et al.*, 1973; Ingemarsson, 1976; Arkelund and Andersson, 1976), the evidence for the involvement of myometrial β_2-adrenoceptors in promoting this effect is scarce. To our knowledge, there are only two reports on the successful antagonism by propranolol infusion of terbutaline-induced inhibition (Arkelund and Andersson, 1976; Ingemarsson, 1979). Moreover, the increase in uterine blood flow observed in patients receiving terbutaline or ritodrine (Caritis *et al.*, 1979; Arkelund and Andersson, 1976) and of placental blood flow (Moura, 1981) should certainly contribute to the successful management of premature labor. It is difficult, however, to reach a general consensus as to the rank order of *in vivo* potency of these drugs. Major drawbacks include differences in the patients' clinical features, scheme and route of administration, and perhaps more importantly variations in the criteria used for evaluating risk of premature labor. Numerous studies lack an adequate control group. These considerations, unfortunately, raise serious problems for an appropriate statistical treatment of the accumulated data.

In vitro studies

In an attempt to overcome the paucity of reliable data concerning the influence of β-adrenoceptor agonists on uterine function *in vivo*, human uterine strips obtained through surgical section provide an interesting and simple experimental model. Regarding spontaneous contractions of pregnant uterine strips, experiments conducted in our laboratory showed that these are effectively inhibited by isoprenaline, isoxsuprine, terbutaline and orciprenaline (Figure 4.1). These experiments furnished the following rank order of relative potency: isoprenaline>>isoxsuprine>terbutaline>orciprenaline (Figure 4.2). Although this rank is consistent with an interaction with β_2-adrenoceptors, the low potency of the more selective agonists relative to isoprenaline is noteworthy and contrasts with the results obtained in other isolated tissues containing β_2-adrenoceptors (O'Donell, 1970; O'Donell and Wanstall, 1974). However, when the uterine strips are contracted by exposure to KCl-depolarizing solution, the addition of these drugs evokes variable effects. Therefore, two studies report that isoprenaline is ineffective in antagonizing this contraction (Sullivan and Marshall, 1970; Calixto and Simas, 1982), while another found that this agonist displayed full relaxant ability (Andersson *et al.*, 1973). Other β-adrenoceptor agonists promote only a moderate degree of relaxation in this condition (Calixto and Simas, 1982), although there is marked disagreement concerning terbutaline (Andersson *et al.*, 1973) (Table 4.1).

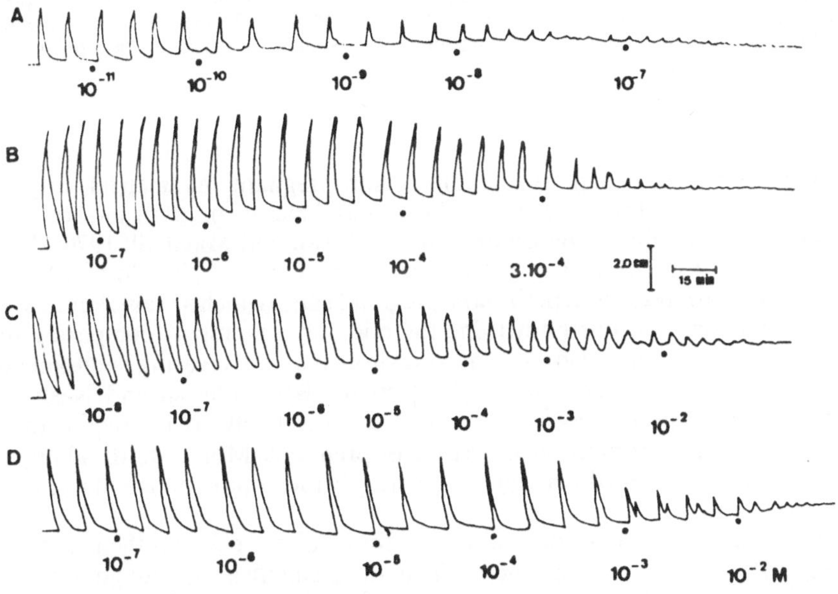

Figure 4.1 Typical isotonic record of the spontaneous contractions of strips from gravid human myometrium before and after the addition of cumulative doses of isoprenaline (A); isoxsuprine (B); terbutaline (C) and orciprenaline (D).

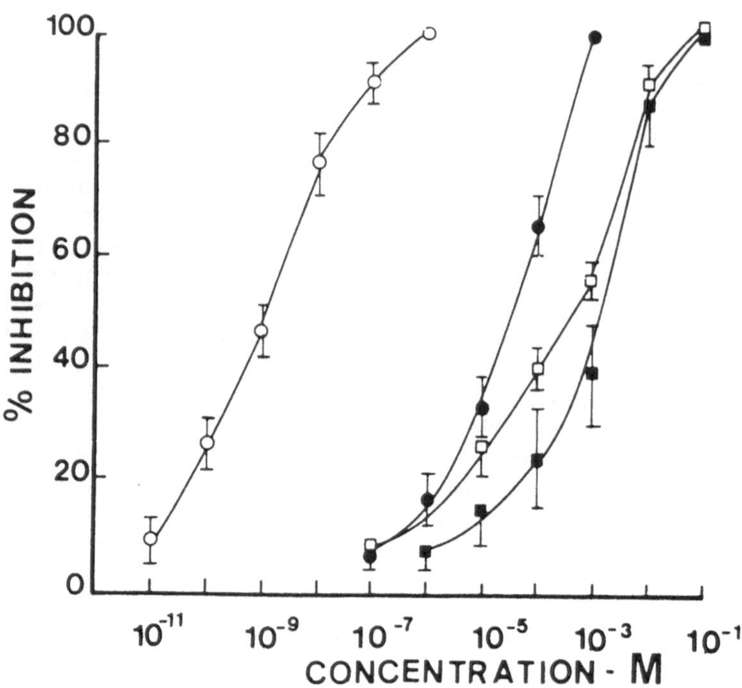

Figure 4.2 Mean inhibitory dose-response curves to isoprenaline (○——○); isoxsuprine (●——●); terbutaline (□——□) and orciprenaline (■——■) upon the spontaneous contractions of the gravid human isolated myometrium. Vertical bars represent the SEM. Each point is the mean of 7–9 experiments.

The spontaneous activity of human non-pregnant myometrial strips is greater than that of pregnant strips (Lossius and Nesheim, 1976) and is almost insensitive to inhibition by isoprenaline (Sullivan and Marshall, 1970; Berg-Johnsen, 1976). The reason for this may lie in the relative dominance of α-adrenoceptor responses in the non-pregnant state, which are also stimulated by isoprenaline. To our knowledge there is only one report comparing the ability of isoprenaline, isoxsuprine and ritodrine in decreasing spontaneous contractions of isolated non-pregnant strips (Berg-Johnsen and Nesheim, 1976). The latter two agonists, which are less likely to interact with α-adrenoceptors, were more effective than isoprenaline. Moreover, the ability of isoxsuprine to supress this activity is practically the same in pregnant and non-pregnant strips.

A critical characteristic of β-adrenoceptor mediated effects is their susceptibility to blockade by propranolol. This drug significantly antagonized the inhibitory effect of isoprenaline upon spontaneous contractions of pregnant human myometrial strips (Lossius and Nesheim, 1976; Calixto and Simas, 1982). The antagonism was dose-dependent in nature and yielded a pA_2 value compatible with that obtained in other β-adrenoceptor containing tissues

Table 4.1 Inhibitory effects of β-adrenoceptor agonists upon contraction of isolated human myometrium

Myometrium	*Agonists*	*Type of contraction*		ED_{50}(mol/l)	*% of relaxation*
Pregnant		Spontaneous	a	1.2×10^{-9}	100
			b	$\sim 3.8 \times 10^{-8}$	~ 100
	Isoprenaline	K^+-induced	a	–	no effect
			c	–	no effect
			d	–	~ 100
	Isoxsuprine	Spontaneous	a	2.6×10^{-5}	100
		K^+-induced	a	–	< 30
	Orciprenaline	Spontaneous	a	8.6×10^{-4}	100
		K^+-induced	a	–	<30
	Terbutaline	Spontaneous	a	2.5×10^{-4}	100
		K^+-induced	a	–	<30
			d		~ 100
	Isoprenaline	Spontaneous	b,e	–	<20
		K^+-induced	c	–	no effect
		Carbacol-induced	c	–	< 50
Non-pregnant	Isoxsuprine	Spontaneous	e	$\sim 10^{-5}$	80*
	Ritodrine	Spontaneous	e	–	45*

a = Calixto and Simas, 1982; b = Lossius and Nesheim, 1976; c = Sullivan and Marshall, 1970; d = Andersson *et al*, 1973; e = Berg-Johnsen and Nesheim, 1976
* Did not use doses greater than 10^{-4} mol/l

($pA_2 = 8.5$) (O'Donell and Wanstall, 1974; Larsen *et al.*, 1979; Johansson *et al.*, 1980; Patersson *et al.*, 1983). Although these results suggest a role of β-adrenoceptors in inhibiting pregnant myometrial activity, our results demonstrated that propranolol, even at extremely high concentration (10^{-4} mol/l), failed to antagonize the effects of isoxsuprine, terbutaline and orciprenaline. In non-pregnant strips, the inhibition of spontaneous contractions by isoxsuprine and ritodrine was also unaffected by propranolol (Lossius and Nesheim, 1976). However, one study using pregnant strips reports a successful blockade by propranolol of inhibition induced by terbutaline (Andersson *et al.*, 1973). Therefore, the majority of the data suggests that these β_2-selective agonists promote inhibition of human myometrial activity by a mechanism which does not involve activation of β-adrenoceptors. Further support for this view derives from the fact that these agonists are effective inhibitors of contraction in both non-pregnant and pregnant strips, while isoprenaline is only effective in the latter preparations. If one is allowed to extrapolate these observations to the *in vivo* situation, these drugs should be useful in inhibiting abnormal myometrial activity in both pregnant and non-pregnant states. The low potency exhibited by these β_2-selective agonists in *in vitro* studies may justify the requirement of long and repeated infusions of high doses of these drugs in order to successfully interrupt premature labor or avoid fetal suffering (Ingemarsson, 1979; Rydén *et al.*, 1982).

From an overview of the available *in vitro* data one may conclude that β_2-selective agonists undoubtedly suppress spontaneous myometrial contractions. However, although most of the evidence points to the non-involvement of β-adrenoceptors in promoting this effect, there are reports to the contrary. It is possible that this inconsistency derives from differences in the portion of the myometrium being studied (Pinto *et al.*, 1967) and the methodologies employed. More extensive and systematic studies are urgently needed to reach a definite conclusion as to the mode of action of these drugs.

CONCLUDING REMARKS

There is extensive evidence for the regulation of uterine function by catecholamines. In several animal species, this tissue contains both α- and β-adrenoceptors, and its responsiveness to drugs which interact with these receptors is modulated by sexual hormones.

From the data available at present, it appears that this modulation does not comprise a modification of myometrial adrenoceptor content, and is therefore possibly exerted at one or more steps situated beyond the adrenoceptor level. The great variability between species of the uterine responses to adrenoceptor agonists precludes the extrapolation of conclusions drawn in one species to another, particularly human.

Over the last two decades the development of β_2-selective agonists has provided a new therapeutic approach to the management of abnormal uterine contractions. Among situations in which these drugs have been proved useful are onset of premature labor, risk of fetal suffering and pain associated with primary dysmenorrhea. The number of reports which directly evaluate the *in vivo* effects of these agonists upon human myometrial activity is surprisingly low. Also, the few reports available on their effects *in vitro* have yielded conflicting results. Differences in the methodological approaches can possibly account for most of the contradictions observed in these later studies. Among such differences one may include: (1) portion of the myometrium used, (2) calcium level in the nutrient solution, (3) type of contraction being inhibited, (4) drug susceptibility to neuronal and extraneuronal uptake process and (5) length of the exposure period to β-adrenoceptor agonists and antagonists. Although the rank order of potencies obtained with these compounds is compatible with an action mediated through β_2-adrenoceptors, we believe that this is not the case. Our view is based on the extremely low potency of the β_2-selective compounds relative to isoprenaline and the failure of propranolol to antagonize their effects. Further support for this hypothesis derives from the contrast observed in the relaxant properties of isoprenaline and the β_2-selective agonists in pregnant and non-pregnant human myometrium. Moreover, the adequate control of abnormal myometrial contractions generally requires the continuous and/or repeated infusion of high doses of these compounds. The increase in uterine and placental blood flow associated with the administration of β_2-selective agonists may also, at least in part, account for their beneficial effect in the management of premature labor and fetal suffering. In conclusion, it is clear that many more *in vivo* and *in vitro* studies are necessary to elucidate adequately the mechanism of action of these drugs on human myometrium.

Acknowledgements

The authors are grateful to Miss Janice M. Pires and Miss Elza A. Bernardini for preparing the manuscript. Work from the authors' laboratory described in this review was supported by Conselho Nacional de Desenvolvimento Cientifico e Tecnológico (CNPq).

References

Andersson, K. E. (1982). Pharmacological inhibition of uterine activity. *Acta Obstet. Gynaecol. Scand. Suppl.*, **108,** 17

Andersson, K. E., Ingemarsson, I. and Persson, C. G. A. (1973). Relaxing effects of beta-receptor stimulators in isolated gravid human myometrium. *Life Sci.*, **13,** 335

Andersson, K. E., Bengtsson, L., Gustafson, I. and Ingemarsson, I. (1975). The relaxing effect of terbutaline on the human uterus during labor. *Am. J. Obstet. Gynecol.*, **121,** 602

Arkelund, M. and Andersson, K. E. (1976). Effects of terbutaline on human myometrial activity and endometrial blood flow. *Obstet. Gynecol.*, **83,** 673

Aucélio, J. G., Calixto, J. B. and Jurkiewicz, A. (1981). Influence of treatment with estradiol and progesterone on the contractile effects of agonists on dog uteri, after calcium removal. *Braz. J. Med. Biol. Res.*, **14,** 462P

Batra, S. and Bengtsson, B. (1978). Effects of diethyestilboestrol and ovarian steroids on the contractile responses and calcium movements in rat uterine smooth muscle. *J. Physiol.*, **276,** 329

Batra, S. C. and Daniel, E. E. (1971). Effect of multivalent cations and drugs on Ca uptake by the rat myometrial microsomes. *Comp. Biochem. Physiol.*, **38A,** 285

Bengtsson, B. (1982). Factors of importance for regulation of uterine contractile activity. *Acta Obstet. Gynaecol. Scand. Suppl.*, **180,** 13

Berg, G., Andersson, R. G. G. and Rydén, G. (1982). Effects of selective beta-adrenergic agonists on spontaneous contractions, cAMP levels and phosphodiesterase activity in myometrial strips from pregnant women treated with terbutaline. *Gynecol. Obstet. Invest.*, **14,** 56

Berg-Johnsen, P. and Nesheim, B. I. (1976). Action of isoprenaline, isoxsuprine and ritodrine in the human non-pregnant myometrium. *Acta Pharmacol. Toxicol.*, **39,** 209

Botari, S. P., Vanquelin, G., Kaivez, E., Lescrainier, J. P. and Vokaer, A. (1982). Hormonal regulation of adrenergic receptor subtypes in human myometrium. In *Proceedings of VIth International Symposium of Uterine contractility*, Brussels

Calixto, J. B., Aucélio, J. G. and Jurkiewicz, A. (1979). Relationship between modulation by estradiol, progesterone and calcium upon the pharmacological reactivity of uteri of dogs. *Res. Comm. Chem. Pathol. Pharmacol.*, **25,** 447

Calixto, J. B., Aucélio, J. G. and Valle, J. R. (1982). Effects of neonatal androgenization upon the pharmacological reactivity of dog uteri. *Arch. Int. Pharmacodyn. Ther.*, **260,** 63

Calixto, J. B. and Simas, C. M. (1982). Effect of isuprenaline, isoxsuprine, terbutaline and orciprenaline on human uteri in vitro. *Proceedings of International Symposium of Reproductive Health Care. Changing Concepts in Fertility Regulation*, Maui, Hawaii

Calixto, J. B. and Aucélio, J. G. (1983). Effect of isoprenaline adrenaline and 5-hydroxytryptamine on potassium and barium chloride-induced contraction of isolated dog uteri. *Proceedings of the VIth International Symposium of Uterine Contractility*, Brussels (In press)

Caritis, S. N., Edelstone, D. and Mueller-Henbach, E. (1979). Pharmacologic inhibition of preterm labor. *Am. J. obstet. Gynecol.*, **133,** 557

Chernaeva, L. and Milenov, K. (1982). Sensitivity of circular and longitudinal uterine muscles to noradrenaline. *Meth. Find. Exp. Clin. Pharmacol.*, **4,** 89

Chow, E. H. M. and Marshall, J. M. (1981). Effects of catecholamines on circular and longitudinal uterine muscle of the rat. *Eur. J. Pharmacol.*, **76,** 157

Daels, J. (1974). Uterine contractility patterns of the outer and inner zones of the myometrium. *Obstet. Gynecol.*, **44,** 315

Diamond, J. and Holmes, T. G. (1975). Effects of potassium chloride and smooth muscle relaxants on tension and cyclic nucleotide levels in rat myometrium. *Can. J. Physiol. Pharmacol.*, **53,** 1099

Fuchs, A. R. (1978). Hormonal control of myometrial function during pregnancy and parturition. *Acta Endocrinol. Suppl.*, **221**, 3

Hayashida, D. N., Leung, R., Goldfien, A. and Robert, J. M. (1982). Human myometrial adrenergic receptor: identification of the beta-adrenergic receptor by (^{3}H) dihydroalprenolol binding. *Am. J. Obstet. Gynecol.*, **142**, 389

Hoffman, B. B., Lavin, T. N. and Lefkowitiz, R. J. (1981). Alpha adrenergic receptor subtypes in rabbit uterus: mediation of myometrial contraction and regulation by estrogens. *J. Pharmacol. Exp. Ther.*, **219**, 290

Ingemarsson, I. (1976). Effect of terbutaline on premature labor: a double blind placebo-controlled study. *Am. J. Obstet. Gynecol.*, **125**, 520

Ingemarsson, I. (1979). Terbutaline in obstetrics. *Acta Pharmacol. Toxicol. Suppl.*, **44**, 84

Ingemarsson, I. (1982). Use of beta-receptor agonists in obstetrics. *Acta Obstet. Gynecol. Scand. Suppl.*, **180**, 29

Johansson, R. M., Andersson, R. G. G. and Wikberg, J. E. S. (1980). Comparison of beta$_1$- and beta$_2$-receptor stimulation in oestrogen or progesterone dominated rat uterus. *Acta Pharmacol. Toxicol.*, **47**, 252

Kano, T. (1982). Effects of estrogen and progesterone on adrenoceptors and cyclic nucleotides in rat uterus. *Jpn. J. Pharmacol.*, **32**, 535

Kawarabayashi, T. and Marshall, J. M. (1981). Factors influencing circular muscle activity in the pregnant rat uterus. *Biol. Reprod.*, **24**, 373

Kenakin, T. P. (1982). Theoretical and practical problems with the assessment of intrinsic efficacy of agonists: efficacy of reputed beta$_1$-selective adrenoceptor agonists of beta$_2$-adrenoceptors. *J. Pharmacol. Exp. Ther.*, **223**, 416

Krall, J. F., Barret, J. D. and Korenman, S. G. (1981). Coupling of beta-adrenoceptors in rat uterine smooth muscle. *Biol. Reprod.*, **24**, 859

Korenman, S. G. and Krall, J. F. (1977). The role of cyclic AMP in the regulation of smooth muscle cell contraction in the uterus. *Biol. Reprod.*, **16**, 1

Kuryama, H. and Suzuki, H. (1976). Changes in electrical properties of rat myometrium during gestation and following hormone treatment. *J. Physiol.*, **260**, 315

Larsen, J. J. (1979). Beta-adrenoceptors in the pregnant and non-pregnant myometrium of the goat and cow. *Acta Pharmacol. Toxicol.*, **44**, 132

Lossius, K. and Nesheim, B. I. (1976). Response of isoprenaline in the human pregnant and non-pregnant myometrium. *Acta Pharmacol. Toxicol.*, **39**, 198

Marshall, J. M. (1973). Effects of catecholamines on the smooth muscle of the female reproductive tract. *Annu. Rev. Pharmacol.*, **13**, 19

Marshall, J. M. and Kroeger, E. A. (1973). Adrenergic influences on uterine smooth muscle. *Philos. Trans. R. Soc. London.*, **265**, 135

Miller, J. W. (1967). Adrenergic receptors in myometrium. *Ann. NY Acad. Sci.*, **139**, 788

Moura, R. S. (1981). Effect of terbutaline on the human fetal placental circulation. *Br. J. Obstet. Gynaecol.*, **88**, 730

Nasmyth, P. A. (1967). The effects of adrenergic agents on smooth muscle other than those of the vascular system. In Root, W. S. and Hofman, F. G. (eds.) *Physiological Pharmacology. Vol. IV*, pp. 129–177. (New York: Academic Press)

O'Donell, S. R. (1970). A selective beta-adrenoceptor stimulant (Th 1165a) related to orciprenaline. *Eur. J. Pharmacol.*, **12**, 35

O'Donell, S. R. and Wanstall, J. C. (1974). Potency and selectivity in vitro of compounds related to isoprenaline and orciprenaline on beta-adrenoceptors in the guinea-pig. *Br. J. Pharmacol.*, **52**, 407

Patersson, J. W., Lulich, K. M. and Goldie, R. G. (1983). A comment on beta$_2$-agonists and their use in asthma. *Trends Pharmacol. Sci.*, **4**, 67

Persson, C. G. A. (1982). Some beta-adrenoceptor functions of therapeutic interest. *Acta. Obstet. Gynecol. Scand. Suppl.*, **108**, 7

Pinto, R. M., Lerner, V., Pontelli, H. and Rabow, W. (1967). Effect of estradiol-17β on oxytocin-induced contraction of three separate layers of human pregnant myometrium. *Am. J. Obst. Gynecol.*, **1**, 881

Polácek, I., Bolan, J. and Daniel, E. E. (1971). Accumulation of adenosine 3′,5′-monophosphate and relaxation in the rat uterus in vitro. *Can. J. Physiol. Pharmacol.*, **49**, 999

Rinard, G. A. and Chew, C. S. (1975). Interacting effects of estrogen progesterone and catecholamines on rat uterine cyclic AMP and glycogen phosphorilase. *Life Sci.*, **16,** 1507

Rinard, G. A. and Chew, C. (1978). Uterine cyclic AMP formation: biphasic effect of estrogen on catecholamine sensitivity. *Life Sci.*, **22,** 2043

Roberts, J. M., Insel, P. A. and Goldifien, R. D. (1977). Alpha-adrenoceptors but not beta-adrenoceptors increase in rabbit uterus with oestrogen. *Nature (Lond.)*, **270,** 624

Roberts, J. M., Insel, P. A. and Goldifien, A. (1982). Regulation of myometrial adrenoceptors and adrenergic response by sex steroids. *Mol. Pharmacol.*, **20,** 52

Rubányi, G. and Csapo, A. I. (1976). The 'activator-Ca' of the pregnant and post-partum rabbit uterus. *Life Sci.*, **19,** 1239

Rydén, G., Andersson, R. G. G. and Berg, G. (1982). Is the relaxing effect of beta-adrenergic agonists on the human myometrium only transitory? *Acta Obstet. Gynaecol. Scand. Suppl.*, **108,** 47

Sullivan, S. F. and Marshall, J. M. (1970). Quantitative evaluation of effects of exogenous amines on contractility of human myometrium in vitro. *Am. J. Obstet. Gynecol.*, **107,** 139

Williams, L. T. and Lefkowitz, R. J. (1977). Regulation of rabbit myometrial alpha adrenergic receptors by estrogen and progesterone. *J. Clin. Invest.*, **60,** 815

Woodward, D. L., Bose, D. and Innes, I. R. (1970). The effects of calcium on the contraction of the splenic capsular smooth muscle. *Fed. Proc.*, **29,** 669

Zuspan, F. P., O'Shaughnessy, R. W., Insel, J. J. and Zuspan, M. (1981). Adrenergic innervation of uterine vasculature in human term pregnancy. *Am. J. Obstet. Gynecol.*, **13,** 678

Part II

Etiology

5
Occupational factors and reproductive outcome

I. FIGÁ-TALAMANCA and L. SETTIMI

Numerous environmental risks damage the reproductive system, causing various negative outcomes. Research in this area has emphasized the study of congenital malformations. Other negative outcomes, however, such as embryonic loss, pre- or post-implantation, might be considered significant, because of their severity from the biological point of view and their more frequent occurrence. It is estimated, for example, that 60–70% of all conceptions terminate in spotaneous abortion (Roberts and Lowe, 1975).

Occupational risks may be responsible for a variety of reproductive disturbances, including disturbances of the menstrual cycle, of the endocrine function and of the libido of both males and females. Some occupational exposures may determine the reduction of fertility of both sexes, while others may cause genetic damage to the germ cells. After conception, negative outcomes include spontaneous abortion, stillbirth, prematurity, malformations, developmental anomalies and childhood cancer. Parental occupational exposures may also indirectly harm the newborn child through contaminated clothing or through breast milk.

Occupational factors may affect the reproductive system by a variety of mechanisms; the same agent may produce different negative outcomes, depending on the stage of development of the embryo. Mutagenes may result in either the death of the germ cell or the development of a defective embryo. Germ cells may be carriers of point mutations as well as alterations in the number of chromosomes. Two percent of humans are carriers of point mutations, while 6.8% of newborns are affected by numerical errors of the chromosomes such as trisomies. Such events are much more frequent among abortuses, about half of whom are carriers of chromosome aberrations (DHSS, 1981). Among surviving fetuses, the frequency of chromosome aberrations decreases with gestational age because of selective fetal mortality (Hook, 1981).

After the zygotic phase, environmental agents may damage the somatic fetal cells directly (as in the case of ionizing radiation) or through the placenta. Our present knowledge of transplacental toxicity is derived primarily from animal studies. The outcome of such an event may be either lethal (spontaneous abortion of stillbirth) or teratogenic.

Laboratory animal assays, routinely used to test the teratogenicity of new drugs, are now also used for the evaluation of occupational risks. Such tests involve the treatment of male and female animals prior to and during pregnancy. Other tests recently developed include the study of the alteration of the germ cells, of the sex hormones, as well as studies of behavioral toxicology to evaluate the risk of occupational hazards.

Studies involving humans examine the damage among exposed individuals (e.g. sperm, menstrual cycle or hormonal alterations) or the frequency of negative reproductive outcomes, such as infertility, spontaneous abortion, prematurity, congenital malformations. Case control studies have been used to study rare events such as childhood tumors or certain congenital malformations (e.g., of the CNS). Such studies, usually based on clinical records or registries, cannot always define adequately the parental occupational risks *post factum*. Longitudinal studies, which usually provide valid data on occupational exposures, require careful monitoring not only of the reproductive events of the population under study, but also of the developing infants up to school age (Christianson *et al.*, 1981). These requirements cause such studies to be particularly costly.

Epidemiologic studies have successfully identified reproductive risks when exposure to such risks is massive (e.g. exposures to polychlorinated biphenyls (PCB_s), methylmercury, ionizing radiation), or when such exposure is very specific (e.g. viruses, diethylstilbestrol (DES); thalidomide or other drugs). Work environmental risks, however, are often moderate and multiple and generally affect a small number of people. In addition, negative reproductive events, with the exception of spontaneous abortion, are relatively infrequent. As a consequence, it is often difficult to establish a cause–effect relationship between a reproductive pathology and occupational exposures.

Despite these difficulties, scientific research on the subject has grown rapidly in recent years. In the following pages an attempt is made to summarise the most significant studies published to date. The findings are also presented in tabular form, Table 5.1 showing the effects of occupational risks on the reproductive system, and Tables 5.2 and 5.3 on the conceptus. For each occupational risk examined, we have tried to summarize results from both animal and human studies, and to illustrate the many questions still left unanswered.

CHEMICAL AGENTS

Chemical agents are probably the most diffused and least understood hazards of the work environment. It is estimated that 1000 new compounds enter the environment each year. A large proportion of these compounds are used exclusively in the work environment. Only a few of these compounds have been studied for carcinogenic and reproductive effects.

Cadmium

Cadmium has an affinity for male gonads and for the placenta (Pařízek, 1964). It is probable that the fetotoxic effects, observed in animals treated with cadmium, are primarily due to the placental damage rather than to a direct effect of cadmium (Levin and Miller, 1981). A study conducted in the USSR revealed that infants of women professionally exposed to cadmium have, on the average, a lower birth weight than infants of women not exposed (Tsvetkova, 1970). Animal studies illustrate the teratogenic effect of cadmium administered during the latter phases of the organogenesis. Characteristically, it causes malformations of the anterior extremities (Messerle and Webster, 1982). Such an effect, however, has been observed at exposure levels which exceed those considered safe for the work environment.

Organic mercury

Accidental mass exposures of humans to methyl mercury have shown the fetotoxic and teratogenic effects of this substance which tends to accumulate in the CNS, especially the brain. Infants exposed *in utero* present mental retardation, ataxia, tremors, convulsions and chorea (Koos and Longo, 1976). Methyl mercury is also excreted in the maternal milk (Mansour *et al.*, 1973). Exposure levels which are non-toxic to animals may nevertheless increase the frequency of resorption and low birth weight (Masatoshi *et al.*, 1978). Similar observations apply to ethyl and phenyl mercury (Koos and Longo, 1976).

Nickel

Nickel, a known carcinogenic agent, has not been studied for human reproductive damage. Nickel salts cause testicular damage to animals (Waltscheva *et al.*, 1972), while nickel carbonyl causes malformations when administered to pregnant rats (Sunderman *et al.*, 1979). Embryotoxic effects have also been observed after administration of nickel chloride (Gilani and Marano, 1980). Nickel tends to accumulate in the pituitary gland (Parker and Sunderman, 1974) interfering with the production of prolactin (La Bella *et al.*, 1973). The embryotoxic and fetotoxic activity of the substance may be attributed to interference with the maternal hormonal equilibrium (Sunderman *et al.*, 1978).

Lead

Lead is probably the most studied metal from the occupational health point of view. The reproductive effects demonstrated in both animals and humans include disturbances of gonadal function, infertility, embryotoxic and teratogenic effects on the fetus (Rom, 1980). Professionally exposed males with lead blood levels between 23 mg/100 ml and 75 mg/100 ml present asthenospermia, hypospermia and teratospermia (Lancranjan *et al.*, 1975a).

Exposed females show anovulatory cycles and disturbances in the development of the corpus luteum (Panova, 1972). Experimental exposures of rats and monkeys produce similar effects (Rom, 1980). The ability of lead to pass the placental barrier has been demonstrated in both humans and animals and it is proportionate to the concentration of lead in the maternal blood (Lauwerys *et al.*, 1978). Fetal exposure may result in growth retardation and in embryotoxic and teratogenic effects, particularly of the CNS (Gerber *et al.*, 1980). Historically, lead is considered an abortifacient. Such effect, however, has not been demonstrated in humans exposed in recent times. Nevertheless, among exposed pregnant women, lead placental levels were higher in those whose pregnancy terminated with a stillbirth than in those who had a livebirth (Khera *et al.*, 1980).

Chloroprene

This compound, which is similar to vinyl chloride from the chemical point of view, is used in the production of synthetic materials (neoprene). Human studies suggest that chloroprene may affect spermatogenesis and reproductive outcomes. Animal studies have shown that exposure to 0.5 parts/10^6 of chloroprene causes testicular atrophy and reduction of the number and the motility of the spermatozoa. Exposure of pregnant females causes excess embryonic mortality, especially prior to the implantation (Infante, 1980).

Vinyl chloride

This compound is a potent carcinogen and mutagen for both man and animals. The epidemiologic data concerning the embryotoxic and teratogenic properties of vinyl chloride are inconclusive. Two successive studies examining the reproductive outcome of the wives of exposed workers found an increase in spontaneous abortion and in birth defects, especially of the CNS (Wagoner and Infante, 1980). The teratogenic effects of vinyl chloride have, however, not been confirmed by other studies (Edmonds *et al.*, 1978). An animal study had demonstrated the induction of angiosarcoma in pups of pregnant rats exposed to vinyl chloride (Maltoni and Lefemine, 1974).

Polychlorinated biphenyls (PCB_s)

The first observations on human toxicity of these compounds were conducted in Japan in 1968 after a massive intoxication through the consumption of contaminated oil. Infants born to intoxicated pregnant women presented low birth weight, anomalous skin pigmentation and skeletal abnormalities (Karatsune *et al.*, 1972). Animal studies have shown disturbances of the estrus, reduction of fertility and increases in resorbtion and malformations (NIOSH, 1977; Mauks *et al.*, 1981). Similarly to other chlorinated hydrocarbons, PCB_s are excreted through the mammary gland. Breast fed infants present blood concentrations of PCB_s as high as or even higher than that of their mothers (Yakushiji *et al.*, 1979).

DDT

The ability of dichloro-diphenyl-trichloro-ethane (DDT) to interfere with the metabolism of steroid hormones has been documented by several studies (Kupfer and Bulger, 1976). Several animal studies have shown that DDT interferes with sexual maturation of both males and females (NIOSH, 1978). An epidemiologic study among female workers exposed to 1–2 mg of DDT per day showed an increased risk for spontaneous abortion and for low birth weight of infants (Nikitina, 1974). It has also been demonstrated that in contaminated areas, DDT and its metabolites are excreted by the mammary glands in the breast milk (Krauthacker *et al.*, 1980). Other common organochlorinated pesticides such as chlordane are also considered suspected transplacental carcinogens for human beings (Infante *et al.*, 1978).

Dibromochloropropane (DBCP)

Although not as dangerous as other pesticides, this compound has been found mutagenic and carcinogenic for laboratory animals. One study among males working in a DBCP production plant found that exposure to 300 parts/10^6 had caused sterility, in some cases irreversible, to about one third of these men (Whorton, 1980). The mechanism of action of this substance is not known.

Carbon disulfide

Carbon disulfide is used commonly in the production of viscose rayon. Negative health effects of exposed workers include disturbances of the nervous and cardiovascular system. Reproductive health effects have been observed among both male and female textile workers. Primary gonadal insufficiency has been observed among men even at relatively low exposure levels (Lancranjan, 1972; Wägar *et al.*, 1981). These findings have been confirmed by animal studies (Youdzik, 1971). As for female exposure, according to studies conducted in the USSR women exposed to less than 20 mg/m^3 of carbon disulfide develop disturbances of the ovarian function and experience irregularities of the menstrual cycle more frequently than control groups (Vasilyeva, 1973) as well as increased abortivity and prematurity (Petrov, 1969). Exposure of pregnant animals has resulted in increased fetal deaths, prematurity and abnormalities of the CNS (Tabacova *et al.*, 1978). According to recent animal studies, low dose, non-toxic maternal exposures may produce malfunction of the hepatic drug-metabolizing system, deviations in lipid metabolism and neurobehavioral disturbances (Tabacova *et al.*, 1981).

Anesthetic gases

Since the original observation in 1967 that anesthetic gases may have negative reproductive effects on operating room personnel, over ten major epidemiologic studies have been conducted on the topic (Edling, 1980). Most studies confirm the existence of an increased risk for spontaneous abortion among the females exposed professionally. Some studies have also found increased risk for malformations (Corbett *et al.*, 1974; Corbett, 1976; Pharoah *et al.*, 1977; Rosenberg and Vanttienen, 1978) while others have not confirmed such findings (Cohen *et al.*, 1980). A number of studies have also shown an increased risk for low-birth weight of infants of mothers working in the operating room (Knill-Jones *et al.*, 1972; Rosenberg and Kirves, 1973, Pharoah *et al.*, 1977).

Studies on males exposed professionally to anesthetic gases have not yielded conclusive evidence on reproductive damage while animal studies confirm the fetotoxicity of these gases. Halothane, for example, administered prior or during pregnancy at concentrations above 0.30 % reduces fertility and increases the frequency of fetal deaths, of prematurity and of malformations, while exposure of male animals results in reduction of fertility. Anesthetic gases such as chloroform, trichloroethylene and enflurane have been shown to cause alterations of the sperm morphology (Smith *et al.*, 1978; Land *et al.*, 1979). Generally, experimental studies have shown that among the anesthetic gases, halothane and nitrous oxide may be dangerous for reproduction, while xenon methoxyflurane and enflurane did not show any fetotoxic effects (Lane *et al.*, 1979; Wharton *et al.*, 1978, 1981).

The mechanism of action of anesthetic gases on the reproductive system is not sufficiently understood. The most commonly observed pathology may be due to a direct action of these gases and their metabolites on the fetus. Studies on the mutagenic properties of nitrous oxide have been negative, reinforcing the direct action hypothesis (Baden and Monk, 1981). However, the direct action hypothesis does not explain the reduction in fertility observed in exposed animals. An alternative hypothesis is that some of the observed effects may be associated with preconception exposure and others with exposure during the pregnancy (Reiber-Strobino *et al.*, 1978). In addition, it may be interesting to consider possible synergistic effects with other professional risks such as ionizing radiation. This hypothesis was tested in a study of reproductive outcomes of hospital female employees exposed at various single or combined environmental risks. The women at the greatest risk for all types of reproductive disturbances are those exposed to both anesthetic gases and ionizing radiation (Figá-Talamanca, 1981).

Smoking

Smoking, although not an occupational hazard, is included in this review because it is a common habit among working men and women. Cigarette smoke, in addition to being associated with a long list of neoplastic and cardiovascular diseases, is also known to enhance the pathogenicity of a number of occupational hazards such as uranium, vinyl chloride, asbestos, arsenic, (Hoffman and Wynder, 1976). In terms of reproductive effects, the best documented risk of pregnant smokers is that of low birth weight of the infant. Other effects more recently studied include perinatal mortality, spontaneous abortion and congenital malformations (Kline *et al.*, 1977,

Himmelberger *et al.* 1978). The risk of spontaneous abortion is further increased for women smokers who also consume alcohol (Harlap and Shiono, 1980).

Other chemical agents

Other substances have been found associated with negative reproductive outcomes mostly in experimental animals (Hemminki, 1980). These include the following. *Acrylonitrile*, a substance used in the production of plastics and fibers, has been found to be teratogenic to rats at dose levels similar to those considered acceptable for human exposure. The teratogenic effect is attributed to the production of cyanide and its metabolites (Calvin *et al.*, 1981). *Methacrylate esters*, another group of substances widely used in industry and in dentistry, have teratogenic effects on rats. *Phthalate esters* are normally used as additives of plastic products. Laboratory studies showed that these substances are teratogenic for the chicken and for the rat embryo (Hemminki, 1980). Benzene vapors inhaled by pregnant rats at levels over 50 parts/10^6 cause a decrease of maternal and infant weight (Kuna and Karpt, 1981).

Other substances tested for reproductive effects include the *chlorinated aliphatic* solvents (Hemminki, 1980) and *borate*. Infertility associated with oligospermia and decreased libido has been reported among workers and in populations exposed to boron (Krasovskii *et al.*, 1976). Testicular dysfunction has been reported in rats following exposure to sodium borate (Lee *et al.*, 1978).

Recent research on *n*-hexane, a known neurotoxic agent, has shown that 2,5 hexanediol, a metabolite of *n*-hexane, causes testicular damage (Cavanagh and Bennetts, 1981).

PHYSICAL AGENTS

Ionizing radiation

Among the physical risks of the occupational environment, ionizing radiation is probably the best known. The first international protective norms were in fact established half a century ago. Present day norms limit the annual dose of the professionally exposed to 5 rem. Preventive measures have greatly reduced the incidence of disease caused by chronic exposure to ionizing radiation. However, the problem remains pertinent because of potential accidental exposures which might endanger both the occupationally exposed and the general population.

The reproductive effects of elevated doses of radiations have been extensively studied among the survivors of Hiroshima and Nagasaki. These studies showed increase of spontaneous abortion, of neonatal deaths and malformations, especially microcephaly and mental retardation (Hunt, 1978). However, the reproductive effects of small frequent exposures to radiation, as in the professionally exposed population, are not well known. Epidemiologic studies on the pregnancy outcome of radiologists (Dreyer and Friedlander, 1982) are not conclusive. Animal studies have furnished more definitive information. Experimental exposure of animals to low doses of radiation prior to conception showed a greater mutational sensitivity of sperm as compared to egg cells (Hunt, 1978). Dose levels producing dominant or recessive mutation as well as reciprocal translocations to sperm cells (resulting in early fetal death or malformations) have no such effect on the exposed female germ cells. This might in part explain why epidemiologic studies (which often cannot detect recessive mutations or early fetal deaths) have not been able to identify reproductive damage to radiologists.

Direct fetal exposure studied among women exposed for medical reasons is associated with CNS malformations, especially microcephaly. These effects were observed when the exposure occurred during the 4–11th weeks of gestation and at doses over 2.5/Gy. In later stages of gestation (12–19 weeks), such doses were associated with an increased risk of mental retardation (UN Scientific Committee on the Effects of Atomic Radiation, 1977). In addition, exposure of the fetus to diagnostic radiation has also been associated with an increased risk of developing leukemia in latter life (Hunt, 1978).

The accumulated experimental and epidemiological evidence now permits a cost–benefit analysis of the medical use of ionizing radiation. However, this cannot be applied to low dose radiation exposure in the work setting. In addition, other problems such as latency periods and synergistic effects with other environmental risks like chemical agents, smoking etc. are not known.

Other physical risks

Although *noise* and *vibration* are common objects of study for the occupational health specialist, they have rarely been studied in relation to reproduction. Animal studies have been shown that exposure to noise is associated with irregularities of the estrus cycle (Singh, 1972) with early fetal mortality (Staples, 1975) and with permanent damage of the auditory apparatus of the fetus (Cook, 1979). In man the studies conducted so far suggest that noise and vibration probably harm the fetus indirectly by interfering with the blood circulation of the maternal pelvic area. Epidemiologic studies of women operators of agricultural machines (Frolova, 1975) and of other types of vehicles (Bohm, 1964; Samoilova and Marinova, 1978), as well as of women exposed to noise in industry (Carosi and Calabro, 1968) or at home (Ando and Hattori, 1977; Jones, 1978) have shown an increased risk for negative reproductive effects such as subfertility, menstrual irregularities, spontaneous abortions, prematurity, malformations and reduction of the placental lactogen serum level. However, the presence of multiple risk factors in such settings (e.g. physical stress, environmental pollution) do not allow to draw conclusions on the role of noise *per se*.

The effects of vibrations independently of noise have rarely been studied. One Eastern European study has shown that women already affected occupationally by vibration disease presented serious reproductive pathology including toxemia, delivery complications and high perinatal mortality (Gratsianskaya *et al.*, 1974).

Continuous exposure to *high temperature* may also be a risk factor for the reproductive function. High temperature inhibits spermatogenesis. Surprisingly there are no epidemiologic data on the subject (Dukes-Dobos, 1981). Reliable data on the effects of high temperature on women workers are also completely lacking. Laboratory studies have shown that non-acclimatized animals exposed daily to 38.5 °C for 55 min experience reduction of copulation and of fertility. Female exposure to such conditions results in irregularity of the estrus cycle and fetal mortality (Knecht *et al.*, 1978).

Microwaves were first observed to cause alterations of spermatogenesis in 1974 (Lancranjan *et al.*, 1975b). Animal studies conducted recently show that high exposure levels to microwaves, by increasing the tissue temperature, may cause developmental anomalies of the nervous system (Berman *et al.*, 1982). Microwave exposure within the daily limits established by NIOSH (10 mW/cm^2 for less than 6 min), have not been shown to be associated at present with cardiovascular disease or with negative reproductive effects (Stellman and Stellman, 1980).

Two other occupational risks might be considered in relation to reproduction: physical stress and shift work.

The degree to which *stressful physical work* may be hazardous to the reproductive function has been studied primarily among women athletes. These studies have shown that physical work in the first part of pregnancy does not effect negatively the reproductive outcome (Hunt, 1979). Similar results were also obtained from animal studies. Intense physical work in the later part of pregnancy in non-exercised animals was shown to be associated with weight reduction of both the mother and the infant. Perinatal mortality too was higher among these animals (Terada, 1974). Epidemiologic studies of pregnant women workers have shown that, with the exception of an increased sense of fatigue in the last weeks of pregnancy, from the physiologic point of view a pregnant woman adapts completely to her usual work activity (Granati and Lenzi, 1976). Some counter-indications have been noted, however, for a fixed work position (always standing or always seated), which has been associated with an increased risk for threatened abortion and for immaturity (Berlinguer *et al.*, 1981). Most studies on physical activity in pregnancy have been conducted among well-nourished healthy women and therefore cannot be generalized to women working under hazardous and stressful conditions in industry and in agriculture, as is largely the case in many developing countries.

Shiftwork has been shown to influence the endocrine rhythm inducing the state of desinchronosis. Human studies have been conducted on volunteers rather than on workers. There is, however, sufficient evidence to suggest that women undergoing forced alteration of their circadian rhythm (e.g. airline hostesses, nurses) often complain of generic malaise and menstrual irregularities (Preston *et al.*, 1973). The degree and long term consequences of such pathology is, however, still not well defined (Angeli, 1980).

CONCLUDING REMARKS AND FUTURE RESEARCH

The main findings from both experimental and epidemiologic studies for the various major occupational risks previously discussed, are summarized in

Table 5.1 Occupational factors affecting the reproductive system

Chemical agents/ physical agents	*Ovarian function*		*Testicular function*		*Sterility subfecundity*	
	Animal	*Human*	*Animal*	*Human*	*Animal*	*Human*
CHEMICAL AGENTS						
Metals						
Cadmium	+ Pařízek (1964)					
Organic mercury			+ Lee and Dixon (1975)		+ Lee and Dixon (1975)	
Nickel			+ Waltscheva *et al.* (1972)		+ Waltscheva *et al.* (1972)	
Lead	+ Jacquet and Gerber (1977)	+ Panova (1972)		+ Lancranjan *et al.* (1975a)	+ Varma *et al.* (1974)	
Organic compounds						
Chloroprene			+ Infante (1980)	+ Infante (1980)	+ Infante (1980)	
DDT	+ NIOSH (1978)		+ NIOSH (1978)			
Dibromochloro-propane			+ Whorton (1980)	+ Whorton (1980)		+ Whorton (1980)
Polychlorinated biphenyls	+ NIOSH (1977)				+ NIOSH (1977)	
Borate			+ Lee *et al.* (1978)	+ Krasovskii *et al.* (1976)		
Carbon disulfide		+ Vasilyeva (1973)	+ Youdzik (1971)	+ Lancranjan *et al.* (1972) + Wägar *et al.* (1981)		
n-hexane			+ Cavanagh and Bennetts (1981)			

Anesthetic gases			+Land *et al.* (1979)		+Land *et al.* (1979) +Lane *et al.* (1979) +Wharton *et al.* (1978)	
PHYSICAL AGENTS						
Ionizing radiation			+UN (1977)	+Manson and Simons (1979)	+UN (1977)	+/−Hunt (1978)
Noise	+Singh (1972)	+/−Singh (1972) +/−Frolova (1973)			+Singh (1972)	+/−Carosi and Calabro (1968)
Vibration		+Singh (1972) +Frolova (1973)				
Microwaves	+Leach (1980)		+Leach (1980) +Goud *et al.* (1982)	+Lancranjan *et al.* (1975b)	+Goud *et al.* (1982)	
High temperatures	+/−Knecht *et al.* (1978)		+Knecht *et al.* (1978)	+/−Dukes-Dobos (1981)	+Knecht *et al.* (1978)	
Stressful physical work	+Zucher and Charmichael (1981)	+Preston *et al.* (1973)	+Zucher and Charmichael (1981)			

\+ positive findings
+/− inconclusive findings

Tables 5.1–5.3. The number of occupational risks so far examined for possible reproductive effects is limited. The available evidence for the risks examined is still scarce. Evident gaps in our knowledge may be observed even for some of the most common work exposures such as the monomers or the low dose radiation. These gaps are particularly disturbing considering that some of these substances (e.g. vinyl chloride or chloroprene) have chemical similarities with known mutagenic and teratogenic agents. The studies conducted so far have tended to concentrate on particular aspects of reproduction, often giving priority to the teratogenic effect. This emphasis has limitations from the point of view of research methodology as well as from the point of view of prevention. It is known for example that malformations are a relatively infrequent event. A significant number of malformations may fail to be detected unless one includes in the study an examination of abortuses (which are often malformed) and a follow-up of infants into school age.

From the point of view of prevention, a congenital defect is the last manifestation of a pathologic process which ideally should be arrested at an earlier stage. When experimental or epidemiologic evidence has identified a potential reproductive risk, research endeavors should be concentrated on the study of the whole spectrum of possible manifestations such as endocrinologic and menstrual effects, spermatogenesis etc. Such effects must be studied in both the experimental and the epidemiologic setting. Epidemiologic data alone have often not been sufficient to evaluate the possible risk of exposed individuals. This is particularly true of studies based on data banks (e.g. tumor registries or registries of birth defects) which often do not provide sufficient information on the exact environmental exposures of the individuals involved. A Finnish study of spontaneous abortions among various professional categories linking health and work registries provides an example of these difficulties (Hemminki *et al.*, 1980). Abortion frequencies resulted most highly among two professional categories which have little in common: agricultural workers and students. This probably reflects the fact that the professional classification provided by the social security registry does not reflect distinct or determinant environmental risks.

Similar difficulties arise in the interpretation of the relationship between infantile tumors and paternal or maternal occupation. The first study on this topic concluded that the paternal professions at risk included mechanics, machinists, miners and painters – professions which presumably had, in common, exposure to aromatic hydrocarbons (Fabia and Thuy, 1974). In a similar study in Finland, the paternal professions identified at risk included farmer, driver, mechanic and painter. The maternal professions were pharmacist, clerk, baker and industrial worker (Hemminki *et al.*, 1981).

The priority for future research is to plan studies which can provide useful data from the point of view of social planning and prevention. To achieve this, laboratory studies must simulate the work environment as much as possible. This means that experimental conditions should take in consideration: (1) the frequent combination of risks present in the work environment, (2) the doses at which workers are exposed and (3) the multiplicity of pathologic outcomes, reproductive and non-reproductive.

Epidemiologic studies, on the other hand, should give priority to risks

Table 5.2 Occupational factors related to embryonic and fetal wastage

Chemical agents/ physical agents	*Resorption or spontaneous abortion*		*Perinatal death*	
	Animal	*Human*	*Animal*	*Human*
CHEMICAL AGENTS				
Metals				
Cadmium			+ Levin and Miller (1981)	
Organic mercury	+ Spyker and Smithberg (1971)			
Lead	+ Wide and Nebon (1977)	+ Khera *et al.* (1980)	+ Gerber *et al.* (1980)	+ Khera *et al.* (1980)
Organic compounds				
Chloroprene	+ Infante (1980)	+ Infante (1980)		
Vinyl chloride		+ Infante *et al.* (1976)		
Polychlorinated biphenyls	+ NIOSH (1977)		+ NIOSH (1977)	
Carbon disulfide	+ Tabacova *et al.* (1978)	+ Petrov (1969)		
Anesthetic gases	+ Wharton *et al.* (1978) + Lane *et al.* (1979)	+ Cohen *et al.* (1980) + Corbett *et al.* (1974) + Knill-Jones *et al.* (1975) + Rosenberg and Kirves (1975) + Rosenberg and Vanttienen (1978)	+ Wharton *et al.* (1978) + Lane *et al.* (1979)	
Smoking		+ Kline *et al.* (1977) + Himmelberger *et al.* (1978)	+ Hoffman and Cambell (1977)	+ Underwood *et al.* (1965)
PHYSICAL AGENTS				
Ionizing radiation	+ UN (1977)	+ Hunt (1978)	+ UN (1977)	+ Hunt (1978)
Noise	+ Staples (1975)	+ Hunt (1979)		
Vibration		+ Hunt (1979)		
Microwaves	+ Goud *et al.* (1982)	+ Goud *et al.* (1982) + Berman *et al.* (1978)		
High temperatures	+ Knecht *et al.* (1978)		+ Knecht *et al.* (1978)	
Stressful physical work			+ Terada (1974)	

Table 5.3 Occupational factors related to developmental anomalies

Chemical agents/ physical agents	*Low birth weight*		*Birth defects*		*Infantile tumors*	
	Animal	*Human*	*Animal*	*Human*	*Animal*	*Human*
CHEMICAL AGENTS						
Metals						
Cadmium	+ Levin *et al.* (1981)		+ Messerle and Webster (1982)			
Organic mercury	+ Spyker and Smithberg (1971)	+ Spyker and Smithberg (1971)	+ Koos and Longo (1976)			
Nickel			+ Sunderman *et al.* (1978)			
Lead	+ Gerber *et al.* (1980)	+ Khera et al. (1980)	+ Gerber *et al.* (1980)			+/− Kantor *et al.* (1979)
Organic compounds						
Acrylonitrile	+ Calvin *et al.* (1981)	+ Calvin *et al.* (1981)				
Methacrylate esters			+ Hemminki (1980)			
Polychlorinated biphenyls	+ NIOSH (1977)	+ NIOSH (1977)	+ Mauks *et al.* (1981)	+ NIOSH (1977)		
Carbon disulfide	+ Tabacova *et al.* (1978)	+ Petrov (1969)		+ Tabacova *et al.* (1981)		
Anesthetic gases	+ Wharton *et al.* (1978) + Lane *et al.* (1979)	+ Knill-Jones *et al.* (1972) + Pharoah *et al.* (1977) + Rosenberg and Kirves (1973)	+ Wharton *et al.* (1978) + Lane *et al.* (1979) + Smith *et al.* (1978)	+ Knill-Jones *et al.* (1972) + Ad Hoc Com. (1974)	+ Corbett *et al.* (1976)	

Smoking	+ Hoffman and Wynder (1976)	US DHEW (1976)		+ Himmelberger *et al.* (1978)	
PHYSICAL AGENTS					
Ionizing radiation		+ UN (1977)	+ Hunt (1978)		+ Hunt (1978)
Noise		+ Hunt (1979)	+ Cook (1979)	+/− Jones (1978)	
Vibration		+ Hunt (1979)			
Microwaves	+ Leach (1980) + Goud *et al.* (1982)		+ Leach (1980) + Berman *et al.* (1978) + Inouye *et al.* (1982)		
High temperatures	+ Knecht *et al.* (1978)	+/− McDonald (1958)		+/− McDonald (1958)	
Stressful physical work	+ Terada (1974)				

already identified by laboratory studies and be designed in such a way as to eliminate confounding of the environmental variables. This requires identifying more precisely both the hazardous agent and the exposed population. Such studies would allow not only the evaluation of occupational health hazards, but also the establishment of a much needed criteria for the prevention of reproductive pathology.

Acknowledgement

This work was partially supported by the Italian National Research Council (CNR) Progetto Finalizzato Biologia della Riproduzione.

References

Ad Hoc Committee on the Effects of Trace Anesthetics (1974). Occupational disease among operating room personnel: a national study. *Anesthesiology*, **41**, 321–340

Ando, Y. and Hattori, H. (1977). Effects of noise on human placental lactogen (HPL) levels in maternal plasma. *Br. J. Obstet. Gynaecol.*, **84**, 115

Angeli, A. (1980). Ritmi endocrini in rapporto all'alternanza sonnoveglia. *Atti del Simposio Nazionale Lavoro a Turni Cronobiologia e Protezione della Salute*, Verona, 14 marzo 1980

Baden, J. and Monk, S. (1981). Mutagenicity and toxicity studies with high pressure nitrous oxide. *Toxicol. Lett.*, **7**, 259

Berlinguer, G., Figá-Talamanca, I. and Schirripa, P. (1981). Indagine sulla salute riproduttiva delle lavoratrici dell'artigianato. *Epideminol. Prevenz.*, **14**, 53

Berman, E., Kinn, J. B. and Carter, H. B. (1978). Observations of mouse fetuses after irradiation with 2.45 GHz microwave radiation. *Health Phys.*, **35**, 791

Bohm, F. (1964). The effect of vehicle vibration on the genitalia of female driving personnel. *Z. Gesamte Hyg.*, **10**, 720

Calvin, C. W., Ferm, V. H. and Smith, R. P. (1981). Teratogenic effects of aliphatic nitriles. *Teratology*, **23**, 317

Carosi, L. and Calabro, F. (1968). Fertilitá di coppie esposte a rumore industriale. *Folia Med.*, **51**, 264

Cavanagh, J. B. and Bennetts, R. J. (1981). On the patterns of changes in the rat nervous system produced by 2,5 hexanediol. *Brain*, **104**, 297

Christianson, R., Van den Berg, J. Milkovich, L. and Oechsli F. W. (1981). Anomalies among white and black live births with long term follow up. *Am. J. Public Health*, **71**, 1333

Cohen, E. N., Gift, H. C., Brown, B. W., Greenfield, W., Wu, M. L., Jones, T. W., Whitcher, C. E., Driscoll, E. J. and Brodsley, J. B. (1980). Occupational disease in dentistry and chronic exposure to trace anesthetic gases. *J. Am. Dent. Assoc.*, **101**, 21

Cook, R. O. (1979). Effects of prenatal noise exposure in the learning level of guinea pigs. *Environ. Health Perspect.*, **33**, 341

Corbett, T. H. (1976). Cancer and congenital anomalies associated with anesthetics. *Ann. NY Acad. Sci.*, **271**, 58

Corbett, T. H., Cornell, R. G., Endres, J. L. and Lieding, K. (1974). Birth defects among children of nurse anesthetists. *Anesthesiology*, **41**, 341

DHSS (Department of Health and Social Security) (1981). Guidelines for the testing of chemicals for mutagenicity. Report on Health and Social Subjects, 24. (London: HMSO)

Dreyer, N. A. and Friedlander, E. (1982). Identifying the health risks from very low dose sparsely ionizing radiation. *Am. J. Public Health*, **72**, 585

Dukes-Dobos, F. N. (1981). Hazards of heat exposure. A review. *Scand. J. Work Environ. Health*, **7**, 73

Edling, C. (1980). Anesthetic gases as an occupational hazard. A review. *Scand. J. Work Environ. Health*, **6**, 85

Edmonds, L. D., Anderson, C., Flynt, J. W. and James, L. M. (1978). Congenital central nervous system malformations and vinyl chloride monomer exposure: a community study. *Teratology* **17,** 137

Fabia, J. and Thuy, T. B. (1974). Occupation of father at time of birth of children dying of malignant diseases. *Br. J. Prev. Soc. Med.,* **28,** 98

Figá-Talamanca, I. (1981). Indagine epidemiologica sugli esiti riproduttivi del personale femminile esposto ai rischi nell'ambiente ospedaliero. *Quaderni Stat. San.,* **IV,** 1

Frolova, T. P. (1975). Features specific for the effect of vibration on the pelvis at different periods in the menstrual cycle. *Gig. Truda Prof. Zabol.,* **19,** 14

Gerber, G. B., Léonard, A. and Jacquet, P. (1980). Toxicity; mutagenicity and teratogenicity of lead. *Mutat. Res.,* **76,** 115

Gilani, S. H. and Marano, M. (1980). Congenital abnormalities in nickel poisoning in chick embryos. *Arch. Environ. Contam. Toxicol.,* **9,** 17

Goud, S. N., Rani, V., Réddy, P. P., Saddi, O. S., Rao, M. S. and Saxeno, V. K. (1982). Genetic effects of microwave radiation in mice. *Mutat. Res.,* **103,** 39

Granati, A. and Lenzi, R. (1976). Lavoro e funzione di maternitá. *39° Congresso Nazionale della Societá Italiana di Medicina del Lavoro e di Igiene Industriale,* Fiuggi, 16–18 sett., Ist. Med. Sociale, Roma

Gratsianskaya, L. N., Eroshenko, E. A. and Libertovich, A. P. (1974). Influence of high-frequency vibration on the genital region in females. *Gig. Truda Prof. Zabol.,* **18,** 70

Harlap, S. and Shiono, P. H. (1980). Alcohol smoking and incidence of spontaneous abortion in the first and second trimester. *Lancet,* **2,** 173

Hemminki, K. (1980). Occupational chemicals tested for teratogenicity. *Int. Arch. Occup. Environ. Health,* **47,** 191

Hemminki, K., Niemi, M. L., Saloniemi, I., Vainio, H. and Hemminki, E. (1980). Spontaneous abortion by occupation and social class in Finland. *Int. J. Epidemiol.,* **9,** 149

Hemminki, K., Saloniemi, I., Salonem, T., Portanen, T. and Vainio, H. (1981). Childhood cancer and parental occupation in Finland. *J. Epidemiol. Community Health,* **35,** 11

Himmelberger, D., Byron, W., Brown, E. and Cohen, E. (1978). Cigarette smoking during pregnancy and the occurrence of spontaneous abortion and congenital abnormality. *Am. J. Epidemiol.,* **108,** 470

Hoffman, D. C. and Wynder, E. L. (1976). Smoking and occupational cancers. *Prev. Med.,* **5,** 245

Hoffmann, D. J. and Cambell, K. I. (1977). Postnatal toxicity of carbon monoxide after pre and post natal exposure *Toxicol. Lett.,* **1,** 147

Hook, E. (1981). Prevalence of chromosome abnormalities during human gestation and implications for studies of environmental mutagens. *Lancet,* **2,** 169

Hunt, R. V. (1979). *Work and the Health of Women,* pp. 105–107. Boca Raton, Fl: CRC Press

Hunt, V. (1978). Occupational radiation exposure of women workers. *Prev. Med.,* **7,** 294

Infante, P. F. (1980). Chloroprene: adverse effects on reproduction. In *Proceedings of a Workshop on Methodology for Assessing Reproductive Hazards in the Workplace,* pp. 87–101. US DHHS (NIOSH) Publication no. 81–100

Infante, P. F., Wagonen, J. K. and Waxweiler, R. J. (1976). Carcinogenic, mutagenic and teratogenic risks associated with vinyl chloride. *Mutat. Res.,* **41,** 131

Infante, P. F., Epstein, S. S. and Newton W. A. (1978). Blood dyscrasias and childhood tumors and exposure to chlordane and heptachlor. *Scand. J. Work Environ. Health,* **4,** 137

Inouye, M., Galvin, M. and McRee, D. (1982). Effects of 2.45 GHz microwave radiation on the development of Japanese quail cerebellum. *Teratology,* **25,** 115

Jacquet, P. and Gerber, G. B. (1977). Plasma hormone levels in normal and lead treated mice. *Experientia,* **33,** 1375

John, J. A., Smith, F. A., Leong, B. K. J and Schwetz, B. A. (1977). The effects of maternally inhaled vinyl chloride on embryonal and fetal development in mice, rats and rabbits. *Toxicol. Appl. Pharmacol.,* **39,** 497

Jones, F. N. (1978). Residence under an airport landing pattern as a factor in teratism. *Arch. Environ. Health,* **33,** 10

Kantor, A. F., McCrea Curner, M. G., Meigs, J. W. and Flannery, J. T. (1979). Occupations of fathers of patients with Wilm's tumor. *J. Epidemiol. Commun. Health,* **33,** 253

Karatsune, M., Yoshimura, T., Matzuzaka, J. and Yamaguchi, A. (1972). Epidemiologic study on Yusho, a poisoning caused by ingestion of rice oil contaminated with a commercial brand of polychlorinated biphenyls. *Environ. Health Perspect.,* **1,** 119

Khera, A. K., Wibberly, D. G. and Dathan, J. G. (1980). Placental and stillbirth tissue lead concentrations in occupationally exposed women. *Br. J. Ind. Med.*, **37**, 394

Kline, A. J., Stein, S., Susser, M. and Warburton, D. (1977). Smoking: a risk factor for spontaneous abortion. *N. Engl. J. Med.*, **297**, 793

Knecht, E. A., Wright, G. L. and Toraason, M. A. (1978). Periodic short-term heat exposure in male and female rats. *Can. J. Physiol. Pharmacol.*, **56**, 747

Knill-Jones, R. P., Moir, D. B., Rodriques, L. V. and Spence A. A. (1972). Anaesthetic practice and pregnancy: a controlled study of women anaesthesists in the U.K. *Lancet*, **1**, 1326

Knill-Jones, R. P., Newman, B. J. and Spence, A. A. (1975). Anaesthetic practice in pregnancy: a controlled survey of male anaesthesists in the U.K. *Lancet*, **2**, 807

Koos, B. J. and Longo, L. D. (1976). Mercury toxicity in pregnant women, fetus and new born infant. *Am. J. Obstet. Gynecol.*, **1**, 390

Krasovskii, G. N., Varshavskaya, S. P. and Borisova, A. F. (1976). Toxicologic and gonadotropic effects of cadmium and boron relative to standard of these substances in drinking water. *Environ. Health Perspect.*, **13**, 69

Krauthacker, B., Alebic-Kolbah, T., Buntíc, A., Tkalčevć, B. and Reiner, E. (1980). DDT residues in samples of human milk and mother's and cord blood serum, in a continental town in Croatia (Yugoslavia). *Int. Arch. Occup. Environ. Health*, **46**, 267

Kuna, R. A. and Karpt, R. W. (1981). The embryotoxic teratogenic potential of benzene vapor in rats. *Toxicol. Appl. Pharmacol.*, **57**, 1

Kupfer, D. and Bulger, W. H. (1976). Interactions of chlorinated hydrocarbons with steroid hormones. *Fed. Proc.*, **35**, 2603

La Bella, F. S., Dular, R., Vivian, S. and Queen, G. (1973). Prolactin secretion is specifically inhibited by nickel. *Nature (Lond.)*, **245**, 330

Lancranjan, I. (1972). Alterations of spermatic liquid in patients chronically poisoned by carbon disulfide. *Med. Lav.*, **63**, 29

Lancranjan, I., Papescu, H. I., Gavanesu, O., Klepsch, I. and Sabanescu, M. (1975*a*). Reproductive ability of workmen occupationally exposed to lead *Arch. Environ. Health*, **30**, 396

Lancranjan, I., Maicanescu, M., Rafaila, E., Klepsch, I. and Popescu, H. I. (1975*b*). Gonadic function in workmen with long-term exposure to micro-waves. *Health Phys.*, **29**, 381

Land, P. C., Owen, E. L. and Linde, H. W. (1979). Mouse sperm morphology following exposure to anesthetics during early spermatogenesis. *Anesthesiology*, **51**, Suppl. S259

Lane, G. A., Nahrwold, M. L., Tait, A. R., Taylor, B. S., Beaudoin, A. R. and Chonen, P. J. (1979). 'Nitrous oxide is teratogenic: xenon is not!' *Anesthesiology*, **51**, Suppl. S260

Lauwerys, R., Roels, H. and Hubermont, G. (1978). Placental transfer of lead mercury, cadmium and monoxide in women. I. comparison of the frequency distribution of the biological indices in maternal and umbilical cord blood. *Environ. Res.*, **15**, 278

Leach, W. M. (1980). Genetic growth and reproductive effects of micro-wave radiation. *Bull, NY Acad. Med.*, **56**, 249

Lee, I. P. and Dixon, R. L. (1975). Effects of mercury on spermatogenesis studied by velocity sedimentation cell separation and serial mating. *J. Pharmacol. Exp. Ther.*, **194**, 171

Lee, I. P., Shering, R. J. and Dixon, R. L. (1978). Evidence for induction of germinal aplasia in male rats by environmental exposure to boron. *Toxicol. Appl. Pharmacol.*, **23**, 557

Levin, A. A. and Miller, R. K. (1981). Fetal toxicity of cadmium in rats: decreased utero-placental blood flow, *Toxicol. Appl. Pharmacol.*, **58**, 297

McDonald, H. D. (1958). Women at work. Maternal health and congenital defects. A prospective investigation. *N. Engl. J. Med.*, **258**, 767

Maltoni, C. and Lefemine, G. (1974). Le potenzialitá dei saggi sperimentali nella predizione dei rischi oncogeni ambientali. Un esempio: il cloruro di vinile. *Rend. Sci. Fis. Mat. Nat. (Lincei)*, **66**, 1

Manson, J. and Simons, R. (1979). Influence of environmental agents on male reproductive failure. In Hunt, V. (ed.) *Work and the Health of Women*, pp. 155–175. (Boca Raton. Fl: CRC Press)

Mansour, M., Dyer, N., Hoffman, L., Schulert, A. and Brill, A. (1973). Maternal fetal transfer of organic and inorganic mercury via placenta and milk. *Environ. Res.*, **6**, 479

Masatoshi, F., Toyoaki, F. and Shuichi, H. (1978). Embriotoxic effects of methylmercuric chloride administered to mice and rats during organogenesis. *Teratology*, **18**, 353

Mauks, T. A., Kimmel, G. L. and Staplest, R. E. (1981). Influence of symmetrical polychlorinated biphenyl isomers on embryo and fetal development in mice. *Toxicol. Appl. Pharmacol.*, **61,** 269

Messerle, K. and Webster, W. S. (1982). The classification and development of cadmium induced limb defects in mice. *Teratology*, **25,** 61

Nikitina, Y. I. (1974). Course of labor and puerperium in the vineyard workers and milkmaids in Crimea. *Gig. Truda Prof. Zabol.*, **18,** 17

NIOSH (1977). *Criteria for a Recommended Standard . . . Occupational Exposure to PCBs.* DHEW (NIOSH) Publication no 77-225

NIOSH (1978). *Special Occupational Hazard Review DDT.* DHEW (NIOSH) Publication no. 78–200, 78–85

Panova, Z. (1972). Early changes in the ovarian function of women in occupational contact with inorganic lead. Works of the United Research Institute of Hygiene and Industrial Safety, Sofia, Bulgaria, 161–166

Pařízek, J. (1964). Vascular changes at sites of oestrogen biosynthesis produced by parenteral injection of cadmium salts: the destruction of placenta by cadmium salts. *J. Reprod. Fertil.*, **7,** 263

Parker, K. and Sunderman, W. (1974). Distribution of ^{63}Ni in rabbit tissues following intravenous injection of ^{63}Ni Cl_2. *Res. Commun. Chem. Pathol. Pharmacol.*, **7,** 755

Petrov, M. V. (1969). Some data on the course and termination of pregnancy in female workers of the viscose industry. *Pediatr. Akush. Gynekol.*, **3,** 50

Pharoah, P. O. D., Alberman, E., Doyle, P. and Chamberlain, G. (1977). Outcome of pregnancy among women in anesthetic practice. *Lancet*, **1,** 34

Preston, F. S., Bateman, S. L., Short, R. V. and Wilkinson, R. T. (1973). Effects of time changes on the menstrual cycle length and on performance in airline stewardesses. *Aerospace Med.*, **44,** 438

Reiber-Strobino, B., Kline, J. and Stein, Z. (1978). Chemical and physical exposure of parents: effects on human reproduction and offspring. *J. Early Hum. Dev.*, **1,** 371

Roberts, C. J. and Lowe, C. R. (1975). Where have all the conceptions gone? *Lancet*, **1,** 498

Rom, W. (1980). Effect of lead on reproduction. In *Proceedings of a Workshop on Methodology for Assessing Reproductive Hazards in the Workplace*, pp. 33–40. US DHHS (NIOSH) Publication no. 81–100

Rosenberg, P. and Kirves, A. (1973). Miscarriages among operating theatre staff. *Acta Anaesthesiol. Scand. Suppl.*, **53,** 37

Rosenberg, P. H. and Vanttienen, H. (1978). Occupational hazards to reproduction and health in anesthetists and pediatricians. *Acta Anaesthesiol. Scand.*, **22,** 202

Samoilova, G. S. and Marinova, G. (1978). Effect of industrial vibration on specific functions of a woman's body. *Gig. Sant.*, **6,** 27

Singh, K. B. (1972). Effect of sound on the female reproductive system. *Am. J. Obstet. Gynecol.*, **112,** 981

Smith, R., Bowman, R. E. and Katz, J. (1978). Behavioural effects of exposure to halothane during early development in the rat. *Anesthesiology*, **49,** 319

Spyker, J. M. and Smithberg, M. (1971). Effects of methylmercury on prenatal development in mice. *Teratology*, **5,** 181

Staples, R. E. (1975). Teratogenic potential of noise in mice and rats. *Toxicol. Appl. Pharmacol.*, **33,** 123

Stellman, J. and Stellman, S. (1980). Health effects of radiofrequency radiation in a cohort of physical therapists. *Am. J. Epidemiol.*, **112,** 442

Sunderman, F. W., Shen, S. K., Mitchell, J. M., Allpass, P. R. and Damjanov, I. (1978). Embryotoxicity and fetal toxicity of nickel in rats. *Toxicol. Appl. Pharmacol.*, **43,** 381

Sunderman, F. W. Jr., Allfais, P. R., Mitchell, J. M., Baselt, R. C. and Albert, D. M. (1979). Eye malformations in rats. Induction by prenatal exposure to nickel carbonyl. *Science*, **203,** 550

Tabacova, S., Hinkova, L. and Balaboeva, L. (1978). Carbon disulphide teratogenicity and postnatal effects in rats. *Toxicol. Lett.*, **2,** 129

Tabacova, S., Hinkova, L., Nikiforov, B. and Balaboeva, L. (1981). Hazards for the progeny after maternal exposure to low carbon disulphide concentrations. *G. Ital. Med. Lav.*, **3,** 121

Terada, M. (1974). Effects of physical activity before pregnancy on fetuses of mice exercised forcibly during pregnancy. *Teratology*, **10,** 141

Tsvetkova, R. P. (1970). Influence of cadmium compounds on the generative function. *Gig. Truda Prof. Zabol..*, **14,** 31

Underwood, P. B., Hester, L. L., Lafittee, J. Jr. and Gregg, K. V. (1965). The relationship of smoking to the outcome of pregnancy. *Am. J. Obstet. Gynecol.*, **91,** 270

UN Scientific Committee on the Effects of Atomic Radiation (1977). Report. *Sources and Effects of Ionizing Radiation.* (New York: UN)

US DHEW (Department of Health, Education and Welfare) (1976). *Health Consequences of Smoking.* (Washington: US Govt. Printing Office)

Varma, M. M., Joschi, S. R. and Adeyemi, A. O. (1974). Mutagenicity and infertility following administration of lead subacetate to Swiss male mice. *Experientia,* **30,** 486

Vasilyeva, I. A. (1973). Effects of small concentration of carbon disulfide and hydrogen sulfide on the menstrual function of women and the estrus cycle of experimental animals. *Gig. Sant.*, **7,** 24

Wägar, G., Tolonen, M. and Helpio, E. (1981). Endocrinological studies of Finnish viscose rayon workers exposed to carbon disulfide. *G. Ital. Med. Lav.*, **3,** 103

Wagoner, K. J. and Infante, P. F. (1980). A review of the methodologic approach in the assessment of the association between vinyl chloride exposure and reproductive hazards. In *Proceedings of a Workshop on Methodology for Assessing Reproductive Hazards in the Workplace,* pp. 43–49. US DHHS (NIOSH) Publication no. 81–100

Waltscheva, V., Slateva, M. and Michailov, I. V. (1972). Testicular changes due to long-term administration of nickel sulfate. *Pathol. Exp.*, **6,** 116

Wharton, R., Mazze, R., Baden, J. M., Hitt, B. A. and Dooley, J. R. (1978). Fertility, reproduction and postnatal survival in mice chronically exposed to halothane. *Anesthesiology,* **48,** 167

Wharton, R., Mazze, R. and Wilson, A. (1981). Reproductive and fetal development in mice chronically exposed to enflurane. *Anesthesiology,* **54,** 505

Whorton, D. (1980). Dibromochloropropane (DBCP). In *Proceedings of a Workshop on Methodology for Assessing Reproductive Hazards in the Workplace,* pp. 103–109. US DHHS (NIOSH) Publication no. 81–100

Wide, M. and Nebon, O. (1977). Differential susceptibility of the embryo to inorganic lead during preimplantation in the mouse. *Teratology,* **16,** 273

Yakushiji, T., Watanabe, K., Kuwabara, S., Yoshida, K. Koyama and Kunita, N. (1979). Levels of polychlorinated biphenyls (PCB_s) and organochlorine pesticides in human milk and blood collected in Osaka Prefecture from 1972 to 1977. *Int. Arch. Occup. Environ. Health,* **43,** 1

Youdzik, M. (1971). Histology and histochemistry of rat testicles as affected by carbon disulphide. *Pol. Med. J.*, **10,** 133

Zucher, I. and Charmichael, M. (1981). Circadian rhythms, brain peptides and reproduction. In Martin, J. B., Reichlin, S. and Bick, K. L. (eds.) *Neurosecretion and Brain Peptides,* pp. 459–473. (New York: Raven Press)

6
Spontaneous abortion following ovulation induction

N. J. SPIRTOS, M. F. HAYES, D. M. MAGYAR and N. J. COSSLER

Infertility is generally defined as the absence of known conception following 12 months of unprotected sexual intercourse. The etiology of this disorder may reside equally within the male or the female. Of the female factors, anovulation or oligo-ovulation play a significant role as the causative mechanism in the inability to achieve pregnancy.

The basic abnormality in ovulatory dysfunction may reside discretely within the hypothalamus, the anterior pituitary or the ovary, or it may be consequent to inappropriate feedback signals to the central nervous system and the hypothalamic–pituitary–ovarian axis. Regardless of the underlying mechanism, ovulation induction using pharmacologic agents constitutes the mainstay of treatment for infertility secondary to abnormal ovulatory function. As with any therapeutic regime, the drugs utilized in ovulation induction have limitations and potentially hazardous complications.

The major complications of ovulation induction include the increased risk of multiple pregnancies and spontaneous abortions. These two areas will be discussed for each of the three most commonly used ovulation inducing agents, i.e. bromocriptine, clomiphene citrate and human menopausal gonadotropins. Prior to this discussion a review of the risk of spontaneous abortion and multiple gestation occurring in the general population will be covered as a basis for comparison.

SPONTANEOUS ABORTION IN THE GENERAL POPULATION

Reproduction in the human female involves an intricate and delicate interplay between the central nervous system, hypothalamus, pituitary, ovaries, fallopian tubes, uterus and cervix. If these mechanisms are not operating in synchrony, the reproductive process will be inhibited. The degree of inhibition will ultimately determine whether sterility, infertility or reproductive wastage will occur. The following discussion will focus on the various factors involved in spontaneous abortions occurring in the general population.

In 1966, the World Health Organization defined 'spontaneous abortion' as the non-induced separation from the mother of the product of conception before it is sufficiently mature to lead an independent life (often considered to be at approximately the 28th week of fetal life) (Lauritsen, 1977). As improved obstetrical and neonatal care has developed over recent years, this arbitrary point in time has been lowered. Since the gestational age at which the fetus, upon delivery, ceases to be an abortus and becomes an infant is difficult to define, many states require a birth certificate for any pregnancy at 20 weeks gestational age or more, or for any fetus that weighs 500 g or more (Pritchard and McDonald, 1980). Spontaneous abortions have been divided into early abortions, occurring during the first 16 weeks of pregnancy, and late abortions, occurring between the 17th and 20th weeks of pregnancy (Lauritsen, 1977). This line of demarcation was chosen to reflect the observation that a high proportion of early abortuses are chromosomally abnormal, whereas abortions at 17–20 weeks are for the most part chromosomally normal abortuses, some of which may be prevented by treatment of the mother (Lauritsen, 1977). As used here, the term spontaneous abortion will refer to fetal loss prior to 20 weeks of gestation.

It is estimated that approximately 15% of all recognized pregnancies terminate in a spontaneous abortion (Lauritsen, 1977; US Department of Health and Human Services, 1982; Reid *et al.*, 1972). The normal incidence of clinically apparent abortion among first pregnancies in women under age 30 years is in the range of 8.3–11.0% (Jansen, 1982). The pregnancy loss rate seems to increase with increasing age of the mother (US Department of Health and Human Services, 1982). The loss rate for women whose most recent previous pregnancy had ended with a spontaneous abortion is about double the rate of those women whose most recent pregnancy ended in a livebirth (US Department of Health and Human Services, 1982). Other statistics from the US Department of Health and Human Services show that 15% of married women have had one pregnancy loss, about 4% have had two and about 3% have had three or more. The percent of wives who have had one or more pregnancy loss increases from 12% of wives 15–24 years of age to 31% of wives 35–44 years of age, and from 11% of wives with no children ever born to 31% of wives with three or more children (US Department of Health and Human Services, 1982).

Thus, spontaneous abortion is a very common occurrence in the general population and seems to vary with maternal age and parity, as well as with prior reproductive history.

The early detection of pregnancy and early fetal wastage

Although the frequency of clinically recognized spontaneous abortion in the general population is often assumed to be known, the actual rate is difficult to determine since some patients do not seek medical services and abort completely at home (Rock and Zacur, 1983). Other women may experience an unusually long menstrual cycle followed by an episode of heavy vaginal bleeding which may represent an occult spontaneous abortion or, alternatively, an anovulatory cycle with subsequent shedding of a lush, proliferative endometrium. The differentiation, based on clinical assessment alone, may be impossible unless a very sensitive pregnancy test is performed prior to the bleeding episode.

One means of detection of early fetal wastage may be provided by measuring the production of the pregnancy-specific protein, early pregnancy factor (EPF). EPF can be detected in serum within 48 hours of fertilization (Rolfe, 1982). Of 28 cycles in which intercourse took place at the time of ovulation, EPF was detected in 18. However, EPF production continued to be detectable for more than 14 days in only four cases. Successful pregnancy was maintained in two of these, while in the other two disappearance of EPF preceded miscarriage. In the remaining 14 cases, EPF disappeared from the serum before the onset of menstruation (Rolfe, 1982), which suggests that a high incidence of early embryonic loss exists normally in nature.

A radioimmunoassay for the beta-subunit of human chorionic gonadotropin (B-hCG) can be used to detect a conception 6–10 days after fertilization. Using this assay, it was observed that only 87 of 152 conceptions (57 %) advanced beyond 20 weeks gestation, a postconceptual pregnancy loss rate of 43 % (Miller *et al.*, 1980). Of the lost conceptions, 50 (33 %) were diagnosed only by raised B-hCG levels, whereas the remaining 15 (11 %) produced both clinical and biochemical evidence of pregnancy. The apparent spontaneous abortion rate based on clinical evidence of pregnancy was 13.7 %, a figure consistent with the accepted norm.

Using a statistical model, married women aged 20–29 in England and Wales were found to abort 78 % of their conceptions (Roberts and Lowe, 1975). If this hypothesis is correct, most conceptual losses must occur before pregnancy is diagnosed and often before the first missed menstrual period (Miller *et al.*, 1980).

In vitro fertilization and embryo transfer

With the advent of *in vitro* fertilization and embryo transfer (IVF-ET) new insight into the rates of pregnancy success and failure has been gained. Using a sensitive and specific radioimmunoassay to measure hCG in overnight urine samples in women undergoing IVF-ET, it was observed that 60–65 % of uterine blastocysts either failed to implant or failed to produce measureable hCG (Lopata *et al.*, 1982). Secondary to this high pregnancy wastage, only 5–20 % of embryos arising from IVF progress to term pregnancy following embryo transfer (Lopata *et al.*, 1982; Wallach, 1982).

Following exposure to spermatozoa *in vivo*, the probability of a livebirth is stated to be 0.31 (Biggers, 1981). Logically, it would seem reasonable to expect that, if 100 % efficiency in ovum retrieval and embryo transfer could be achieved, the pregnancy outcome in IVF-ET could not be more efficient than that which would occur normally (Wallach, 1982). Since embryonic loss in women is high in the early stages of pregnancy during the normal reproductive process (roughly 65 % of human embryos are lost by 14 weeks after ovulation), a finite level of successful birth after IVF-ET may fall in the range of 30–35 % (Wallach, 1982). This estimation correlates well with the 60–65 % failure rate of uterine blastocysts noted previously.

Psychological aspects of spontaneous abortion

Women who have had three or more consecutive spontaneous abortions are classified as habitual aborters (Pritchard and McDonald, 1980). The etiologic factors of habitual abortion are beyond the scope of this chapter and are discussed in detail elsewhere (Pritchard and McDonald, 1980; Stenchever, 1983; Rock and Zacur, 1983; Moghissi, 1982; King *et al.*, 1982). The risk of a future spontaneous abortion does not appear increased by prior history; it is approximately 24 % after one, 26 % after two, 32 % after three and 26 % after four spontaneous abortions (Warburton and Fraser, 1961). The need to explain this concept to couples who have just suffered a pregnancy loss is obvious. Further, it is vitally important to remember that these couples need supportive therapy. Women who have undergone a fetal loss often describe themselves as unhappy, depressed, hostile or anxious (Seibel and Graves, 1980). Approximately 25 % admit to having a psychiatric problem and another 25 % feel they were personally responsible for the miscarriage. Recognition and attention to these facts enables the obstetrician-gynecologist to offer better patient care in the form of reassurance and information at several points of interaction with the patient experiencing a spontaneous abortion (Seibel and Graves, 1980).

Threatened abortion

Although there is no effective intervention to prevent a spontaneous first trimester abortion from occurring, certain pertinent points need to be emphasized. Threatened abortion is a frequent cause of first trimester bleeding, occurring in 16 % of all pregnancies (Hertig and Livingstone, 1944). The prognosis for a pregnancy complicated by early bleeding is somewhat controversial, but of 266 patients admitted with threatened abortion, 135 (50.8 %) aborted, while 131 (49.2 %) gave birth to 106 full term children and 25 premature children (Johannsen, 1970). A history of bleeding during pregnancy has been found, by some investigators, to be more frequent in children with congenital anomalies of the central nervous system and/or psychomotor retardation (33 %) and in children with congenital anomalies of other systems (29 %) than in control children (12 %) (Ornoy *et al.*, 1976). However, another author has not observed uterine bleeding early in pregnancy to be associated with an increased risk of producing a chromosomally abnormal child (Lauritsen, 1977).

Once a pregnancy threatens to abort, couples frequently experience increased anxiety concerning both possible fetal wastage and fetal outcome should the pregnancy continue – this anxiety is only compounded if there was a previous infertility history. Reassurance and emotional support is the mainstay of treatment: however, hormonal studies and ultrasonography may be performed to determine the viability of the fetus. Although multiple abnormal serum estradiol levels strongly suggest the absence of fetal development and a blighted ovum, no single hormonal level will clearly distinguish between a blighted ovum and a potentially salvagable threatened abortion (Schweditsch *et al.*, 1979). Serial serum levels of hCG may be useful to determine fetal viability. It is known that the doubling time of hCG with an early embryo is approximately 48 hours. If two quantitative serum hCG levels are evaluated exactly 48 hours apart, a rise of at least 66% between the two samples is a good prognostic sign of fetal well-being (Kadar *et al.*, 1981).

Ultrasonography may also be used to detect early fetal viability (Jouppila *et al.*, 1980). At 9 weeks gestation, a negative ultrasonic detection of fetal life signs has been associated with an unsuccessful pregnancy outcome in 100% of the cases. On the other hand, the ultrasonic demonstration of fetal life can predict delivery in 90% of cases despite symptoms of threatened abortion (Jouppila *et al.*, 1980).

The performance of these diagnostic tests may greatly reassure an anxious couple experiencing a threatened abortion. If fetal viability is not found, however, active intervention may eliminate the pronounced uterine hemorrhage that can accompany an incomplete or complete abortion.

In summary, then, clinical and subclinical spontaneous abortions occur frequently in nature. The human reproductive process is, on the one hand, highly inefficient with respect to production rates but, on the other hand, highly efficient in filtering the gene pool to ultimately produce chromosomally normal individuals in the majority of cases.

MULTIPLE PREGNANCIES IN THE GENERAL POPULATION

A major factor that ultimately contributes to the spontaneous abortion rate in the general population is the spontaneous occurrence of multiple pregnancies. The rate of spontaneous twinning in the pregnant population is 1.05–1.35% and that of triplets is 0.010–0.017% (Guttmacher, 1953). The expected incidence of high multiple births can be calculated by using Hellin's hypothesis: if the twinning rate in a population is known, the frequency of twins = 'n', that of triplets = 'n^2', and that of quadruplets = 'n^3' (Schenker *et al.*, 1982).

The frequency of monozygotic twins is fairly constant throughout the world, being in the range of one in 286 (0.3–0.4%), while dizygotic twinning varies between races and generally increases with maternal age (Benirschke and Kim, 1973; Bulmer, 1970; Myrianthopoulos, 1970). Besides the well-known association between dizygotic twinning and maternal age, other associated factors include maternal parity, maternal weight and height, and familial occurrence of dizygotic twins in the mother's family (Hémon *et al.*, 1979). The ratio of monozygotic to dizygotic twins in the United States is generally thought to be approximately 1:2 (Myrianthopoulos, 1970).

The rate of twinning in pregnancies which spontaneously abort has been found to be one in 35 (Livingston and Poland, 1980). This figure was calculated from the 53 pairs of twins obtained during examination of 1939 spontaneously aborted complete embryos and fetuses. The ratio of monozygotic to dizygotic twin abortuses was 17.5/1. These observations suggest that twinning, particularly the monozygotic form, occurs much more frequently than has been previously assumed from newborn data, and that embryonic and fetal mortality is much higher in twins than singletons. Approximately 88% of the twin embryos and 21% of the twin fetuses were found to be abnormal. Other investigators have also found that twins, especially monozygotic twins, have a higher congenital anomaly rate than singletons (Hendricks, 1966; Hay and Wehrung, 1970; Onyskowova *et al.*, 1971; Myrianthopoulos, 1975).

As most epidemiologic studies of twins exclude pairs with no liveborn members, the twinning rate and mortality rate of twins may both be underestimated (Livingston and Poland, 1980). With the use of ultrasound to detect early embryonic twins, a closer approximation to the true overall rates of twinning and spontaneous pregnancy losses may be estimated. Abnormal multiple pregnancies can also be diagnosed successfully by ultrasound (Kurjak and Latin, 1979). The most frequently observed abnormality is a normal pregnancy and a synchronous blighted ovum. Others include twin blighted ova, blighted ovum and missed abortion, missed abortion in both gestational sacs, two embryonic echoes with the development of only one baby, normal fetus and an anencephalic twin, normal fetus and fetus papyraceous and triplets with two fetuses papyraceous. One or more gestational sacs may, thus, be resorbed during pregnancy without any adverse effect on the coexisting normal fetus (Kurjak and Latin, 1979). Unless these ultrasonic findings are incorporated into the observed rates of multiple pregnancies and embryonic losses, the subsequent calculated rates will be lower than the actual incidence that occurs in future.

The dizygotic twinning rate

From an epidemiologic perspective, therefore, the factors which induce the resorption of the zygote and/or cause fetal death will modify the observed dizygotic twinning rate at delivery (Lazar *et al.*, 1978). The dizygotic twinning rate (DZTR) can be calculated as follows: for a given population, let 'f' equal the number of fertilized women, 'k' the frequency of double ovulations, 's' the probability of non-abortion (or 'success') of a zygote, 'n' the number of single deliveries, and 'dz' the number of dizygotic twin deliveries, assuming independent 'successes' of the two ova of a double ovulation. This may be written as:

$$n = f \times s \tag{1}$$

and

$$dz = k \times f \times s^2 \tag{2}$$

The DZTR is then given by:

$$t = (dz/n) = k \times s \tag{3}$$

The DZTR is, therefore, proportional to the frequency of double ovulation and to the probability of non-abortion (Lazar *et al.*, 1978). In contrast with others, the DZTR has been found by some authors actually to decrease at higher maternal ages as a result of increasing spontaneous abortion after the age of 35 years, which is the precise age when the frequency of lethal chromosomal anomalies begins to increase sharply (Lazar, 1976; Lazar *et al.*, 1978, 1971).

MULTIPLE PREGNANCIES FOLLOWING OVULATION INDUCTION

The spontaneous reproductive wastage of multiple concepti, therefore, is of major concern as this increased inherent risk is not amenable to current therapy. As ovulation-inducing drugs are used to promote follicular maturation and extrusion of a mature ovum, the risks of multiple pregnancies and subsequent spontaneous abortions are increased against a background of already high reproductive loss.

The dramatic increase in multiple pregnancies after the use of some ovulation-inducing agents is undoubtedly due to fraternal (dizygotic) twinning consistent with superovulation (Kistner, 1975). The magnitude of increase in the incidence of multiple pregnancies among patients in whom ovulation is induced varies among different etiologic anovulatory groups, the various types of ovulation-inducing preparations and the different schedules of treatment (Schenker *et al.*, 1982).

Even with appropriate monitoring techniques, multiple ovulation and multiple pregnancies cannot be predicted or entirely prevented (Wu, 1975). Multiple gestations ranging from twins to nonuplets have occurred in response to ovulation induction (Benirschke and Kim, 1973; Carey, 1976). The occurrence of a multiple pregnancy represents an extremely high risk situation for both the mother and the unborn fetuses. The potential maternal complications include iron deficiency anemia, pregnancy-induced hypertension, hydramnios, premature rupture of the membranes, premature labor, placenta previa and placental abruption (Cetrulo *et al.*, 1980). The fetal complications result mainly from high pregnancy wastage and prematurity. The discussion to follow will concentrate on the incidence and etiology of spontaneous abortions occurring following ovulation induction using bromocriptine, clomiphene citrate and human menopausal gonadotropin.

Bromocriptine

The first ovulation-promoting drug to be discussed is the semisynthetic brominate ergot alkaloid, bromocriptine (Parlodel, Sandoz Pharmaceuticals, East Hanover, NJ). Bromocriptine (2-bromo-α-ergocriptine mesylate) has a molecular weight of 750.72 and is rapidly and almost completely absorbed from the gastrointestinal tract in man (Del Pozo and Fluckiger, 1979; Parkes, 1977). Peak plasma level is reached in 2–3 hours but small traces persist for up to 24 hours (Kinch, 1982). The major route of elimination of bromocriptine is via the biliary tree (Mehta and Tolis, 1979).

Bromocriptine's action is thought to relate to its centrally active dopamine agonist properties (Del Pozo and Fluckiger, 1979). At the level of the pituitary, there is good evidence that lactotrophs contain dopamine receptors and that bromocriptine acts via these receptors in an agonist fashion (Kinch, 1982). Dopamine, itself, is thought to be the neurotransmitter, prolactin-inhibiting factor (Speroff *et al.*, 1978*a*), and bromocriptine, as a dopamine agonist, has been demonstrated to lower prolactin levels through this inhibitory control mechanism. Most bioaminergic neurons modify anterior pituitary function only by influencing hypophysiotropic neurosecretion (Kinch, 1982). The apparent exception is dopamine, which can exert direct effects on the pituitary that are inhibitory to prolactin and to release of thyroid-stimulating hormone (Kinch, 1982).

Women with inappropriate, non-puerperal hyperprolactinemia may present with amenorrhea and/or galactorrhea, oligomenorrhea, dysfunctional uterine bleeding, hirsutism, luteal phase defect and infertility (Jones, 1979). A prospective study to determine the incidence of hyperprolactinemia in 113 infertile women revealed that 22 (19.5 %) had elevated levels of serum prolactin and that five (4.4 %) with hyperprolactinemia had neither abnormal menstrual function nor galactorrhea (Kredentser *et al.*, 1981).

The pathophysiology of menstrual irregularity in hyperprolactinemic women is difficult to establish because it is not known whether the excessive prolactin or the associated dopamine deficiency, or both, are responsible for the abnormality (Jones, 1979). Prolactin is intimately associated with steroidogenesis in both the adrenal gland and ovary. As prolactin receptors have been identified in the adrenal gland and ovary, as well as in the breast and endometrium, hyperprolactinemia may stimulate or depress vital enzyme systems and steroidogenic pathways that may disrupt the orderly and physiologic events of the menstrual cycle (Jones, 1979). The anovulation or luteal phase inadequacy that occurs may contribute to the problem of infertility or early spontaneous abortion. A relative hypothalamic dopamine deficiency might cause both an elevated prolactin level and failure of the luteinizing hormone surge, resulting in either polycystic ovary syndrome or a luteal phase defect. A more severe dopamine deficiency might be associated with low follicle-stimulating hormone and luteinizing hormone levels (Jones, 1979). Thus, the effects of hyperprolactinemia may operate at both the central level by interfering with gonadotropin secretion and at the local level by disrupting the enzymatic or steroidogenic pathways.

Bromocriptine is approved for the use in the amenorrhea/galactorrhea syndrome and female infertility associated with hyperprolactinemia in the absence of a demonstrable pituitary tumor (Sandoz Pharmaceuticals, 1982). Bromocriptine has also been used successfully in many studies treating women with documented prolactinomas (Ho Yuen *et al.*, 1982; Sobrinho *et al.*, 1981; Baskin and Wilson, 1981; Archer *et al.*, 1982). It has been stated that the induction of ovulation using bromocriptine in hyperprolactinemic women is not associated with an increased risk of spontaneous abortions, multiple pregnancies or congenital malformations (Sandoz Pharmaceuticals, 1977; Griffith *et al.*, 1978). Examination of the outcome of 448 pregnancies in mothers who had been given bromocriptine at some stage in the early weeks of pregnancy revealed a 9% spontaneous abortion rate, a 1.6% twin-birth rate, and a 2.9% malformation rate (Griffith *et al.*, 1978). In reviewing 1233 pregnancies in which anovulatory hyperprolactinemic women were treated with bromocriptine, the spontaneous abortion rate was 11.8%, a rate comparable to that found among pregnant women under 30 years of age (Jansen, 1982).

Thus, the spontaneous abortion rate of bromocriptine-treated hyperprolactinemic women appears nearly the same as the rate in normal control populations. The apparent explanation lies in the fact that as elevated prolactin levels are normalized, ovulation and proper steroidogenesis follows, thus allowing optimal growth and development of the conceptus. The euprolactinemic pregnancy should now be subject to all events that would occur normally in nature, irrespective of the previous hyperprolactinemia.

Clomiphene citrate

The second ovulation-inducing drug to be discussed is clomiphene citrate (Clomid, Merrell-National Laboratories). Structurally, clomiphene (1-{p-(β-diethylaminoethoxy) phenyl}-1,2-diphenyl-2-chloroethylene) is closely related to both diethylstilbestrol and chlorotrianisene (Tace) (Huppert, 1982). Clomiphene is a non-steroidal agent possessing estrogenic and antiestrogenic properties (Natrajan and Greenblatt, 1979). The commercially available compound, clomiphene citrate, is an equal mixture of the *cis* and *trans* isomers of clomiphene and is readily absorbed orally and excreted principally in the feces (Natrajan and Greenblatt, 1979).

The mechanism of action by which clomiphene brings about release of gonadotropins is not clearly understood(Natrajan and Greenblatt, 1979), but it is thought that clomiphene acts at the level of the hypothalamus by competing with endogenous estradiol for estrogen-receptor binding sites (Huppert, 1982). Clomiphene does not competitively inhibit the action of estrogen at the receptor level, but rather modifies hypothalamic activity by affecting the concentration of the intracellular estrogen receptors, thus reducing the concentration of cytoplasmic estrogen receptors through the inhibition of the process of receptor replenishment (Speroff *et al.*, 1978*b*). Therefore, the hypothalamus cannot perceive or act upon the true endogenous estrogen level in the circulation (Speroff *et al.*, 1978*b*). Thinking that the estrogen level in the circulation is low, the homeostatic negative feedback relationship between estrogen and gonadotropins is activated, leading to the secretion of gonadotropin-releasing hormone (GnRH) into the portal system (Speroff *et al.*, 1978*b*). GnRH then stimulates the anterior pituitary to augment its secretion of follicle-stimulating hormone (FSH) and luteinizing hormone (LH). The rise in gonadotropins stimulates a set of follicles to begin growth and maturation which ultimately leads to subsequent ovulation through a process similar to that which occurs naturally (Speroff *et al.*, 1978*b*).

The augmented gonadotropin stimulation of multiple ovarian follicles may ultimately lead to superovulation and fraternal twinning after clomiphene therapy. The stated incidence of multiple pregnancies varies greatly from one

Table 6.1 Incidence of multiple pregnancies and spontaneous abortions following clomiphene citrate therapy

	Multiple pregnancy rate (%)	*Spontaneous abortion rate* (%)
Drake *et al.* (1978)	0	12
Gorlitsky *et al.* (1978)	2	9
Correy *et al.* (1982)	4	10
Rust *et al.* (1974)	4	21
Kistner (1975)	6	17
Hack *et al.* (1972)	8	—
Hull *et al.* (1979)	13	13
Adashi *et al.* (1979)	13	27
Garcia *et al.* (1977)	—	25
Gysler *et al.* (1982)	—	14
Ruiz-Velasco *et al.* (1979)	—	15
Greenblatt and Dalla Pria (1971)	8	—
Merrell-National Labs (1972)	9	—

author to another. The rates of multiple pregnancies (Table 6.1) range between zero to as high as 13% (Drake *et al.*, 1978; Gorlitsky *et al.*, 1978; Correy *et al.*, 1982; Rust *et al.*, 1974; Kistner, 1975; Adashi *et al.*, 1979; Hull *et al.*, 1979; Hack *et al.*, 1972). The most consistent figures seem to be approximately 6–8% (Kistner, 1975; Merrell-National Laboratories, 1972; Greenblatt and Dalla Pria, 1971). The majority of the multiple pregnancies are twins but the incidences of triplets, quadruplets and quintuplets are 0.5%, 0.3% and 0.13% respectively (Merrell-National Laboratories, 1972).

The use of clomiphene citrate has been associated with a similar variation in stated incidence of spontaneous abortions ranging between 9% and 27% (Hull *et al.*, 1979; Rust *et al.*, 1974; Gorlitsky *et al.*, 1978; Correy *et al.*, 1982; Gysler *et al.*, 1982; Drake *et al.*, 1978; Garcia *et al.*, 1977; Adashi *et al.*, 1979; Ruiz-Velasco *et al.*, 1979) (Table 6.1). Although these figures may seem exaggerated as compared to the spontaneous abortion rate in the general population, it must be remembered that fetal wastage is approximately 22.3% in a previously infertile population of women (Buxton and Southam, 1958).

Etiology of abortion following clomiphene citrate

The possible association between clomiphene citrate and increased fetal wastage may be partly explained by the fact that multiple gestations have higher embryonic mortality than singletons (Livingston and Poland, 1980). Another plausible explanation to account for the apparent increased abortion rate in clomiphene-induced pregnancies may be abnormal corpus luteum function (Jones *et al.*, 1970). Thirty-two of the 70 women treated with clomiphene citrate developed abnormal luteal function. Three of these 32 patients became pregnant and all three aborted. The numbers of women showing defective luteal function seems, therefore, higher in clomiphene treated women than might be expected in an unselected series of infertility patients. This defect is found to occur spontaneously in 3.5–10.7% of patients with primary infertility (Jones and Pourmond, 1962; Gillam, 1955). In women with secondary infertility and repeated abortions, the incidence is between 25% and 35% (Jones and Pourmond, 1962; Jones and Delfs, 1951). The defective luteal phase may be related to suboptimal FSH stimulation early in the cycle or an inadequate cyclic LH stimulation as a preovulatory LH surge (Kistner, 1966). This defective pituitary stimulation of the developing follicle may not allow proper ovulation and luteinization to occur. The abnormal corpus luteum, therefore, may be unable to support the growth and development of an implanted blastocyst or embryo, resulting in a spontaneous first trimester abortion. Atrophy of the endometrium, overripeness of a defective ovum or chromosomal abnormality of the ovum have also been suggested to explain the high frequency of spontaneous abortions in first clomiphene citrate cycles as compared to subsequent cycles (Toshinobu *et al.*, 1979). Again, there is no satisfactory explanation to account for this phenomenon.

Human menopausal gonadotropin

The third, and final, ovulation-inducing drug to be discussed is human menopausal gonadotropin (HMG). Human menopausal gonadotropin (Pergonal, Serono Laboratories) is a highly purified, standardized and essentially non-antigenic drug that acts directly at the ovarian level to induce follicular maturation (Spadoni *et al.*, 1974). HMG is an extremely potent pharmacologic agent that can be associated with such potentially serious complications as ovarian hyperstimulation, multiple pregnancies and increased fetal wastage (Thompson and Hansen, 1970).

The multiple pregnancy rate ranges between 17% and 40.0% (Jewelewicz, 1975; Thompson and Hansen, 1970; Spadoni *et al.*, 1974; Oelsner *et al.*, 1978; Gemzell, 1978; Schwartz *et al.*, 1980; Hack *et al.*, 1970) (Table 6.2). Women with negligible endogenous estrogen activity and low gonadotropin levels (group I)

Table 6.2 Incidence of multiple pregnancies and spontaneous abortions following HMG therapy

	Multiple pregnancy rate (%)	*Spontaneous abortion rate* (%)
Jewelewicz (1975)	17	24
Schwartz *et al.* (1980)	31	28
Oelsner *et al.* (1978)	33	28
Spadoni *et al.* (1974)	31	12
Thompson and Hansen (1970)	19	28
Ben-Rafael *et al.* (1983)	—	29*
		12†
Gemzell (1978)	30	22
Hack *et al.* (1970)	40	29

* Following first HMG conception; † following second HMG conception

have higher multiple pregnancy rates than women with normal gonadotropin levels and distinct endogenous estrogen activity in whom all other treatments have failed (group II). The difference in the multiple pregnancy rate between group I (38%) and group II (15.7%) women has been demonstrated to be statistically significant (Oelsner *et al.*, 1978). As expected, the vast majority of multiple pregnancies involve twin births (Oelsner *et al.*, 1978; Thompson and Hansen, 1970), and thus the same maternal and fetal complications exist as discussed previously.

The incidence of spontaneous abortions following HMG therapy ranges between 12% and 29% (Spadoni *et al.*, 1974; Schwartz *et al.*, 1980; Gemzell, 1978; Thompson and Hansen, 1970; Ben-Rafael *et al.*, 1983; Oelsner *et al.*, 1978; Hack *et al.*, 1970) (Table 6.2). It is of interest to note that the abortion rate has been found to be higher in group II women than in group I women, the rates being 41.7% and 22.8% respectively (Oelsner *et al.*, 1978). One might expect that in women who are amenorrheic and lack endogenous estrogen activity (group I), pregnancy induced by treatment might be more endangered than in patients who have not endured prolonged estrogen deficiency and its consequences, as in group II (Oelsner *et al.*, 1978). These observed differences cannot, at this time, be adequately explained.

Despite the high incidence of fetal loss following gonadotropin therapy, the etiologic factors that contribute to this loss remain unknown (Ben-Rafael *et al.*, 1983). In 203 women who conceived following gonadotropin therapy, the abortion rate was 28.5%. However, in 84 women who conceived a second time, also with gonadotropin treatment, the abortion rate was only 11.9% (Ben-Rafael *et al.*, 1983). This difference is of particular note because it is generally thought that the rate of abortion tends to increase with each successive abortion (Polland *et al.*, 1977).

Etiology of abortion following HMG

There are several theoretical causes to explain the high abortion rate in gonadotropin-induced pregnancies. It is possible that exogenous stimulation of the ovaries may sometimes result in a faulty ovum ill-prepared for fertilization (Oelsner *et al.*, 1978). Postovulatory aging of the oocyte, leading to an abnormal blastula, has also been suggested (Butcher, 1975; Polland *et al.*, 1977). Another reason for the high incidence of abortions may be the relative hyperestrogenism in induced ovulations. The high estrogen levels could cause abnormally high tubal motility resulting in accelerated passage of the fertilized ovum and its premature arrival in a uterine cavity not yet ready for implantation (Oelsner *et al.*, 1978). Some ovulations induced by gonadotropins may be followed by insufficient corpus luteum formation incapable of supporting an early pregnancy (Oelsner *et al.*, 1978). Since most of the abortions of multiple pregnancies following ovulation induction with gonadotropin therapy occur late, an anatomical factor as opposed to a physiological factor may be responsible (Gemzell and Roos, 1966). Cervical incompetence resulting in high intrauterine pressure may, thus, play a role in midtrimester abortions of multiple pregnancies (McGowan, 1970). Using gonadotropin therapy, one abortion was noted to occur in 20 singleton conceptions, three abortions in 14 sets of twins, and seven abortions in nine sets of triplets (Gemzell and Roos, 1966). Using human menopausal gonadotropin and human chorionic gonadotropin therapy, three of five second-trimester abortions were multiple pregnancies (Caspi *et al.*, 1976). The incidence of abortions has been found to be 17.5% in pregnancies without hyperstimulation and 33.3–35% with hyperstimulation (Gemzell, 1977). Others have noted two late abortions of quintuplets, one of quadruplets and two of triplets, indicating that the risk of fetal loss is directly proportional to the number of fetuses (Schenker *et al.*, 1982). As human fetal loss is significantly higher in multiple gestations than in singletons, this single factor is an important cause of the increased pregnancy wastage following gonadotropin-induced pregnancy. As the abortion rate increases accordingly with the increased rate of multiple pregnancy, the abortion rate among pregnancies induced by clomiphene citrate is lower when compared to those induced by gonadotropin preparations (Schenker *et al.*, 1982). Without modern treatment, the fetal loss attributed to the increased abortion rate and prematurity is 31% in triplets and 51% in quadruplets (Friedman and Little, 1958).

PREVENTATIVE MEASURES

In order to decrease the rate of spontaneous abortion following ovulation induction, the rate of multiple pregnancies must also decline. The use of ultrasound can assist, not only in the detection of hyperstimulation, but also in the more accurate timing of the ovulatory dose of human chorionic gonadotropin (hCG). By withholding the hCG when three or more ovulations are possible, the conception of more than twins may, thus, be avoided (O'Herlihy *et al.*, 1982). Ultrasound appears to be useful for monitoring induction of ovulation with human menopausal gonadotropin as it provides more accurate information on follicular number and size than can be obtained by estrogen determinations alone (Haning *et al.*, 1982).

Other preventative measures to reduce the multiple pregnancy rate and minimize both the maternal and fetal risks have included changing the FSH:LH ratio of the gonadotropin preparations, diminishing the dose of hCG and substituting pituitary LH for hCG (Schenker *et al.*, 1982). None of these manoeuvers has, thus far, proved very successful. Luteinizing hormone-releasing hormone (LHRH) administration, however, may increase the chances that only a single preovulatory follicle will develop (Seibel *et al.*, 1983), thus lowering the subsequent incidence of multiple pregnancy. LHRH may well be the ovulation-inducing drug of the future if the delivery system can be refined to make it highly reliable and widely available (Ory, 1983; Yen, 1983).

Unless real-time, linear array or sector scanning ultrasound equipment is available to measure follicular number and diameter, the only means available today to monitor gonadotropin induction of ovulation is urinary or plasma estrogen determinations. Multiple pregnancies occur more frequently when estrogen levels are markedly elevated (Buxton and Hermann, 1961). Some authors have observed a reduction in multiple pregnancy rate (from 33% fo 15%) with no real change in the pregnancy rate (45% to 41%) if daily estrogen monitoring is utilized (Gemzell *et al.*, 1968; Gemzell and Roos, 1966; Gemzell, 1975, 1977). These relationships are tenuous, as much controversy exists over the value of estrogen monitoring in regards to the prevention of hyperstimulation and multiple pregnancy. Multiple pregnancies can occur in spite of hormone levels that are nearly as low as those found during spontaneous ovulation (Schenker *et al.*, 1980). Thus, although multiple pregnancy cannot be entirely eliminated, the following recommendations should be followed: hCG should be administered only when the level of plasma estradiol is approximately 300–600 pg/ml, which normally occurs in the preovulatory phase of the normal menstrual cycle. When urinary estrogens are measured the level should be between 100 and 150 μg per 24 h prior to the administration of hCG (Schenker *et al.*, 1982).

CONCLUDING REMARKS

The induction of ovulation using clomiphene citrate and human menopausal gonadotropin can be a hazardous proposition culminating in a high incidence of reproductive failures, multiple pregnancies and ovarian hyperstimulation. Prior to initiating any ovulation induction protocol, the infertile couple should be warned of these potential complications so the excitement of a much-awaited pregnancy is not suddenly transformed into disappointment and despair if fetal wastage should occur.

References

Adashi, E. Y., Rock, J. A., Sapp, K. C., Martin, E. J., Wentz, A. C. and Jones, G. S. (1979). Gestational outcome of clomiphene-related conceptions. *Fertil. Steril.*, **31,** 620

Archer, D. T., Lattanzi, D. R., Moore, E. E., Harger, J. H. and Herbert, D. L. (1982). Bromocriptine treatment of women with suspected pituitary prolactin-secreting micoadenomas. *Am. J. Obstet. Gynecol.*, **143,** 620

Baskin, D. S. and Wilson, C. B. (1981). Bromocriptine treatment of pituitary adenomas. *Neurosurgery*, **8,** 741

Benirschke, K. and Kim, C. K. (1973). Multiple pregnancy. *N. Engl. J. Med.*, **288,** 1276, 1329

Ben-Rafael, Z., Dor, J., Mashiach, S., Blankstein, J., Lunenfeld, B. and Serr, D. M. (1983). Abortion rate in pregnancies following ovulation induced by human menopausal gonadotropin/human chorionic gonadotropin. *Fertil. Steril.*, **39,** 157

Biggers, J. D. (1981). In vitro fertilization and embryo transfer in human beings, *N. Engl. J. Med.*, **304,** 336

Bulmer, M. G. (1970). *The biology of Twinning in Man.* Chap. 4, pp. 68–94. (Oxford: Clarendon Press)

Butcher, R. L. (1975). The role of intrauterine environment and intrafollicular aging of the oocyte on implantation rates and development. In Blandau, R. J. (ed.) *Aging Gametes – Their Biology and Pathology*, p. 201. (Basel: Karger)

Buxton, C. L. and Herman, W. (1961). Induction or ovulation in the human with human gonadotropins. *Am. J. Obstet, Gynecol.*, **81,** 584

Buxton, C. L. and Southam, A. L. (1958). In *Human Infertility*. 1st Edn., p. 18. (New York: Hoeber)

Carey, H. M. (1976). Induction of ovulation resulting in nonuplet pregnancy. *Aust. N.Z. J. Obstet. Gynaecol.*, **16,** 200

Caspi, E., Ronen, J., Schreyer, P. and Goldbery, M. D. (1976). The outcome of pregnancy after gonadotropin therapy. *Br. J. Obstet. Gynaecol.*, **83,** 967

Cetrulo, C. L., Ingardia, C. J. and Sbarra, A. J. (1980). Management of multiple gestation. *Clin. Obstet. Gynecol.*, **23,** 533

Correy, J. F., Marsden, D. E. and Schokman, F. C. M. (1982). The outcome of pregnancy resulting from clomiphene-induced ovulation. *Aust. N.Z. J. Obstet. Gynaecol.*, **22,** 18

Del Pozo, E. and Fluckiger, E. (1979). Pharmacological aspects of the prolactin inhibitor bromocryptine. In Tolis, G., Labrie, F., Martin, J. B. and Naftolin, F. (eds.) *Clinical Neuroendocrinology: A Pathophysiological approach*, p. 429. (New York: Raven Press)

Drake, T. S., Tredway, D. R. and Buchanan, G. C. (1978). Continued clinical experience with an increasing dosage regimen of clomiphene citrate administration. *Fertil. Steril.*, **30,** 274

Friedman, G. A. and Little, W. A. (1958). The twin delivery: factors influencing second twin mortality. *Obstet. Gynecol.*, **13,** 611 (Survey)

Garcia, J., Jones, G. S. and Wentz, A. C. (1977). The use of clomiphene citrate. *Fertil. Steril.*, **28,** 707

Gemzell, C. A. (1975). Induction of ovulation. *Acta. Obstet. Gynaecol. Scand.* (Suppl.), **47,** 1

Gemzell, C. A. (1977). Induction of ovulation with human gonadotropins. *J. Reprod. Med.*, **18,** 155

Gemzell, C. A. (1978). Experience with the induction of ovulation. *J. Reprod. Med.*, **21,** 205

Gemzell, C. A. and Roos, P. (1966). Pregnancies following treatment with human gonadotropins with special reference to the problem of multiple births. *Am. J. Obstet. Gynecol.*, **94,** 490

Gemzell, C. A., Roos, P. and Loeffler, F. E. (1968). Follicle stimulating hormone extracted from human pituitary. In Behrman, S. J. and Kistner, R. W. (eds.) *Progress in Infertility*, p. 375. (Boston: Little, Brown)

Gillam, J. S. (1955). Study of the inadequate secretion phase endometrium. *Fertil. Steril.*, **6,** 18

Gorlitsky, G. A., Kase, N. G. and Speroff, L. (1978). Ovulation and pregnancy rates with clomiphene citrate. *Obstet. Gynecol.*, **51,** 265

Greenblatt, R. B. and Dalla Pria, S. (1971). Clomiphene in women. In Jöel, C. A. (ed.) *Fertility Disturbances in Men and Women*, pp. 541–556 (Basel, Munich, Paris, New York: Karger)

Griffith, R. W., Turkalj, I. and Braun, P. (1978). Outcome of pregnancy in women given bromocriptine. *Br. J. Clin. Pharmacol.*, **5,** 227

Guttmacher, A. F. (1953). The incidence of multiple births in man and some other unipareae. *Obstet. Gynecol.*, **2,** 22

Gysler, M., March, C. M., Mishell, D. R. and Bailey, E. J. (1982). A decade's experience with an individualized clomiphene treatment regimen including its effect on the postcoital test. *Fertil. Steril.*, **37,** 161

Hack, M., Brish, M., Serr, D. M., Insler, V. and Lunenfeld, B. (1970). Outcome of pregnancy after induced ovulation. Follow-up of pregnancies and children born after gonadotropin therapy. *J. Am. Med. Assoc.*, **211,** 791

Hack, M., Brish, M., Serr, D. M., Insler, V., Salomy, M. and Lunenfeld, B. (1972). Outcome of pregnancy after induced ovulation. Follow-up of pregnancies and children born after clomiphene therapy. *J. Am. Med. Assoc.*, **220,** 1329

Haning, R. V., Austin, C. W., Kuzman, D. L., Shapiro, S. S. and Zweibel, W. J. (1982). Ultrasound evaluation of estrogen monitoring for induction of ovulation with menotropins. *Fertil. Steril.*, **37,** 627

Hay, S. and Wehrung, D. A. (1970). Congenital malformations in twins. *Am. J. Hum. Genet.*, **22,** 662

Hémon, D., Berger, C. and Lazar, P. (1979). The etiology of human dizygotic twinning with special reference to spontaneous abortion. *Acta Genet. Med. Gamellol.*, **28,** 253

Hendricks, C. H. (1966). Twinning in relation to birth weight, mortality and congenital anomalies. *Obstet. Gynecol*, **27,** 47

Hertig, A. T. and Livingstone, R. G. (1944). Medical prognosis; spontaneous, threatened and habitual abortion; their pathogenosis and treatment, *N. Engl. J. Med.*, **230,** 797

Ho Yuen, B. Cannon, W., Sy, L., Booth, J. and Burch, P. (1982). Regression of pituitary microadenoma during and following bromocriptine therapy: persistent defect in prolactin regulation before and throughout pregnancy. *Am. J. Obstet. Gynecol.*, **142,** 634

Hull, M. G. R., Savage, P. E. and Jacobs, H. S. (1979). Investigation and treatment of amenorrhea resulting in normal fertility. *Br. Med. J.*, **1,** 1257

Huppert, L. C. (1982). Induction of ovulation with clomiphene citrate. In Wallach, E. E. and Kempers, R. D. (eds.) *Modern Trends in Infertility and Conception Control.* Vol. 2, pp. 153–160. (Philadelphia; Harper & Row)

Jansen, R. P. (1982). Spontaneous abortion incidence in the treatment of infertility. *Am. J. Obstet. Gynecol.*, **143**, 451

Jewelewicz, R. (1975). Management of infertility resulting from anovulation. *Am. J. Obstet. Gynecol.*, **122**, 909

Jones, G. S. (1979). Hyperprolactinemia: an extension of the galactorrhea-amenorrhea syndrome. *Ob/Gyn Digest*, **21**, 21

Jones, G. S. and Delfs, E. (1951). Endocrine patterns in term pregnancies following abortion. *J. Am. Med. Assoc.*, **146**, 1212

Jones, G. S., Maffezzoli, R. D., Strott, C. A., Ross, G. T. and Kaplan, G. (1970). Pathophysiology of reproductive failure after clomiphene-induced ovulation. *Am. J. Obstet. Gynecol.*, **108**, 847

Jones, G. S. and Pourmond, K. (1962). An evaluation of etiologic factors and therapy in 555 private patients with primary infertility. *Fertil. Steril.*, **13**, 398

Johannsen, A. (1970). The prognosis of threatened abortion, *Acta Obstet. Gynaecol. Scand.*, **49**, 89

Jouppila, P., Huhtaniemi, I. and Tapanainen, J. (1980). Early pregnancy failure: study by ultrasonic and hormonal methods. *Obstet. Gynecol.*, **55**, 42

Kadar, N., Caldwell, B. V. and Romero, R. (1981). A method of screening for ectopic pregnancy and its indications. *Obstet. Gynecol.*, **58**, 162

Kinch, R. A. (1982). The use of bromocriptine in obstetrics and gynecology. In Wallach, E. E. and Kempers, R. D. (eds.). *Modern Trends in Fertility and Conception Control*. pp. 161–168. (Philadelphia: Harper and Row).

King, C. R., Pernoll, M. L. and Prescott, G. (1982). Reproductive wastage. In Wynn, R. M. (ed.) *Obstetrics and Gynecology Annual*. Vol. 11, pp. 59–109. (Norwalk, Conn: Appleton-Century-Crofts)

Kistner, R. W. (1966). Use of clomiphene citrate, human chorionic gonadotropin and human menopausal gonadotropin for induction of ovulation in the human female. *Fertil. Steril.*, **17**, 569

Kistner, R. W. (1975). Induction of ovulation with clomiphene citrate. In Behrman, S. J. and Kistner, R. W. (eds.) *Progress in Infertility*. 2nd Edn., pp. 509–536. (Boston: Little, Brown)

Kredentser, J. V., Hoskins, C. F. and Scott, J. Z. (1981). Hyperprolactinemia – a significant factor in female infertility. *Am. J. Obstet. Gynecol.*, **139**, 264

Kurjak, A. and Latin, V. (1979). Ultrasound diagnosis of fetal abnormalities in multiple pregnancy. *Acta Obstet. Gynecol. Scand.*, **58**, 153

Lauritsen, J. G. (1977). Genetic aspects of spontaneous abortion. *Dan. Med. Bull.*, **24**, 169

Lazar, P. (1976). Effet des avortements spontanés sur la fréquence des naissances gémellaires, *C. R. Acad. Sci. (D) Paris*, **282**, 243

Lazar, P., Gueguens, S., Boue, J. and Boue, A. (1971). Sur la distribution des âges de 715 mères ayant eu un avortement spontané précoce. *C.R. Acad. Sci. (D) Paris*, **272**, 2852

Lazar, P., Hemon, D. and Berger, C. (1978). Twinning rate and reproduction failures. *Prog. Clin. Biol. Res.*, **24**, 125

Livingston, J. E. and Poland, B. J. (1980). A study of spontaneously aborted twins. *Teratology*, **21**, 139

Lopata, A., Martin, M., Oliva, K. and Johnston, I. (1982). Embryonic development and blastocyst implantation following in vitro fertilization and embryo transfer. *Fertil. Steril.*, **38**, 682

McGowan, G. W. (1970). Cervical incompetence in multiple pregnancy. *Obstet. Gynecol.*, **35**, 589

Mehta, A. E. and Tolis, G. (1979). Pharmacology of bromocriptine in health and disease. *Drugs*, **17**, 313

Merrell-National Laboratories Product Information Bulletin (1972)

Miller, J. F., Williamson, E., Glue, J., Gordon, Y. B., Grudzinskas, J. G. and Sykes, A. (1980). Fetal loss after implantation: a prospective study. *Lancet*, **2**, 554

Moghissi, K. S. (1982). What causes habitual abortion? *Contempor. Ob/Gyn*, **20**, 45

Myrianthopoulos, N. C. (1970). An epidemiologic survey of twins in a large, prospectively studied population. *Am. J. Hum. Genet.*, **22**, 611

Myrianthopoulos, N. C. (1975). Congenital malformations in twins: epidemiologic survey. *Birth Defects: Original Article Ser.* **XI**, 8

Natrajan, P. K. and Greenblatt, R. B. (1979). Clomiphene citrate. In Greenblatt, R. B. (ed.) *Induction of Ovulation*, pp. 35–76 (Philadelphia: Lea & Febiger)

Oelsner, G., Serr, D. M., Mashiach, S., Blankenstein, J., Snyder, M., Lunenfeld, B. (1978), The study of induction of ovulation with menotropins: analysis of results of 1897 treatment cycles, *Fertil. Steril.*, **30,** 538–544

O'Herlihy, C., Evans, J. H., Brown, J. B., Chi de Crespigny, L. J. and Robinson, H. P. (1982). Use of ultrasound in monitoring ovulation induction with human pituitary gonadotropins. *Obstet. Gynecol.*, **60,** 577

Onyskowova, Z., Dolezal, A. and Jedlicka, V. (1971). The frequency and the character of malformations in multiple birth (a preliminary report). *Teratology*, **4,** 496

Ornoy, A., Benady, S., Kohen-Raz, R. and Russell, A. (1976). Association between maternal bleeding during gestation and congenital anomalies in the offspring. *Am. J. Obstet. Gynecol.*, **124,** 474

Ory, S. J. (1983). Clinical uses of luteinizing hormone-releasing hormone. *Fertil. Steril.*, **39,** 577

Parkes, D. (1977). Bromocriptine. *Adv. Drug Res.*, **12,** 247

Polland, B. J., Miller, J. R., Jones, D. C. and Trimble, B. K. (1977). Reproductive counseling in patients who have had a spontaneous abortion. *Am. J. Obstet. Gynecol.*, **127,** 685

Pritchard, J. A. and McDonald, P. C. (1980). Abortion. In Pritchard, J. A. and McDonald, P. C. (eds.) *Williams Obstetrics*, pp. 587–601. (New York: Appleton-Century-Crofts)

Reid, D. E., Ryan, K. J. and Benirschke, K. (1972). *Principles and Management of Human Reproduction*, p. 255. (Philadelphia, London, Toronto: Saunders)

Roberts, C. J. and Lowe, C. R. (1975). Where have all the conceptions gone? *Lancet*, **1,** 498

Rock, J. A. and Zacur, H. A. (1983). The clinical management of repeated early pregnancy wastage. *Fertil. Steril.*, **39,** 123

Rolfe, B. E. (1982). Detection of fetal wastage. *Fertil. Steril.*, **37,** 655

Ruiz-Velasco, V., Rosas-Arceo, J. and Matute, M. M. (1979). Chemical inducers of ovulation: comparative results. *Int. J. Fertil*, **24,** 61

Rust, L. A., Israel, R. and Mishell, D. R. (1974). An individualized graduated therapeutic regime for clomiphene citrate. *Am J. Obstet. Gynecol.*, **120,** 785

Sandoz Pharmaceuticals (1977). Outcome of pregnancy in mothers taking Parlodel: status report. December 1976, January 10, 1977

Sandoz Pharmaceuticals (1982). Parlodel. *Physicians Desk Reference*. Vol. 36, pp. 1684–1686. (Oradell, NJ: Medical Economics Company)

Schenker, J. G., Laufer, N., Weinstein, D. and Yarkoni, S. (1980). Quintuplet pregnancy. *Eur. J. Obstet. Gynecol. Reprod. Biol.*, **10,** 257

Schenker, J. G., Yarkoni, S. and Granat, M. (1982). Multiple pregnancies following induction of ovulation. In Wallach, E. E. and Kempers, R. D. (eds.) *Modern Trends in Infertility and Conception Control*. Vol. 2, pp. 134–152. (Philadelphia: Harper & Row)

Schwartz, M., Jewelewicz, R., Dyrenfurth, I., Tropper, P. and Van de Wiele, R. L. (1980). The use of human menopausal and chorionic gonadotropins for induction of ovulation. *Am. J. Obstet. Gynecol.*, **138,** 801

Schweditsch, M. O., Dubin, N. H., Jones, G. S. and Wentz, A. C. (1979). Hormonal considerations in early normal pregnancy and blighted ovum syndrome. *Fertil. Steril.*, **31,** 252

Seibel, M. and Graves, W. L. (1980). The psychological implications of spontaneous abortions. *J. Reprod. Med.*, **25,** 161

Seibel, M. M., Kamrava, M., McArdle, C. and Taymor, M. L. (1983). Ovulation induction and conception using subcutaneous pulsatile luteinizing hormone-releasing hormone. *Fertil. Steril.*, **61,** 292

Sobrinho, L. G., Nunes, M. C., Calhaz-Jorge, S., Mauricio, J. C. and Santos, M. A. (1981). Effect of treatment with bromocriptine on the size and activity of prolactin producing pituitary tumours. *Acta Encdocrinol.*, **96,** 24

Spadoni, L. R., Cox, D. W. and Smith, D. C. (1974). Use of human menopausal gonadotropin for the induction of ovulation. *Am. J. Obstet. Gynecol.*, **120,** 988

Speroff, L., Glass, R. H. and Kase, N. G. (1978*a*). Neuroendocrinology. In Speroff, L., Glass, R. H. and Kase, N. G. (eds.) *Clinical Gynecologic Endocrinology and Infertility*, pp. 27–48. (Baltimore: Williams & Wilkins)

Speroff, L., Glass, R. H. and Kase, N. G. (1978*b*), Induction of ovulation. In Speroff, L., Glass, R. H. and Kase, N. G. (eds.) *Clinical Gynecologic Endocrinology and Infertility*, pp. 375–391. (Baltimore: Williams & Wilkins).

Stenchever, M. A. (1983). Habitual abortion. *Contemp.* Ob/Gyn, **21,** 162

Thompson, C. R. and Hansen. L. M. (1970). Pergonal (menotropins): a summary of clinical experience in the induction of ovulation and pregnancy. *Fertil. Steril.*, **21**, 844

Toshinobou, T., Seiichiro, F., Noriaki, S. and Kihyoe, I. (1979). Correlation between dosage or duration of clomid therapy and abortion rate. *Int. J. Fertil.*, **24**, 193

US Department of Health and Human Services (1982). Reproductive impairments among married couples. *United States, Vital and Health Statistics, Series 23*, No. 11, December 1982, pp. 5–31. (Hyattsville, MD: National Center for Health Statistics)

Wallach, E. A. (1982). In vitro fertilization and embryo transfer in 1982 – random thoughts. *Fertil. Steril.*, **38**, 656

Warburton, D. and Fraser, F. C. (1961). On the probability that a woman who has had a spontaneous abortion will abort in subsequent pregnancies. *J. Obstet. Gynaecol. Br. Commonw.* **68**, 784

Wu, C. (1975). Plasma estrogen monitoring of ovulation induction. *Obstet. Gynecol.*, **46**, 294

Yen, S. S. C. (1983). Clinical applications of gonadotropin-releasing hormone and gonadotropin-releasing hormone analogs. *Fertil. Steril.*, **39**, 257

7
Early embryonic loss: physiology

E. S. E. HAFEZ

PATTERNS OF EMBRYONIC MORTALITY

Gestation refers to the period from implantation of the blastocyst in the endometrium until the termination of pregnancy. The term 'conception' is not an appropriate physiological term due to difficulty in the clinical evaluation of any spontaneous embryonic loss which may occur before implantation of the blastocyst (Figure 7.1). Such conceptus has no apparent effect on the length of the subsequent menstrual cycle. Three embryonic developmental stages are recognized: (1) two-cell, four-cell, eight-cell, 32-cell and early morula, (2) late morula and preimplantation blastocyst and (3) postimplantation development of blastocyst (Figure 7.1). This is followed by the 'fetus' from completed organogenesis until the completion of pregnancy. The onset of embryonic mortality depends on the time at which the corpus luteum is exhausted. In cases of spontaneous abortion, evidence of luteal insufficiency follows evidence of abnormal trophoblast function (Exalto *et al.*, 1982).

Two distinct patterns in spontaneous abortions have been identified (Edmonds *et al.*, 1982): one in which trophoblastic activity is normal and a second in which hCG production is always poor. The former conceptions seem to be associated with abnormal development of the fetus and suffer subsequent maternal rejection, whereas the latter are caused by poor implantation and subsequent conceptus failure. A large number of implanted blastocysts are lost almost exclusively during the early stages of gestation.

Degeneration at the morula and blastocyst stages are associated with various morphological characteristics (Table 7.1). Asymmetrical blastomere in size and shape, multinucleation, and nuclear fragmentation are the most common morphological characteristics.

The presence of a retarded or deformed embryo during the first month of gestation may be associated with a normal or abnormal corpus luteum and endometrium (Boyd and Hamilton, 1970). The incidence of placental involvement in defective embryos is considerably greater in the human than in non-human primates (Hendrickx and Binkerd, 1980). The physiological and clinical significance of this phenomenon is unknown.

Recurrent abortion is characterized by various parameters: repeated abortion, abortion of chromosomally normal conceptions late in gestation,

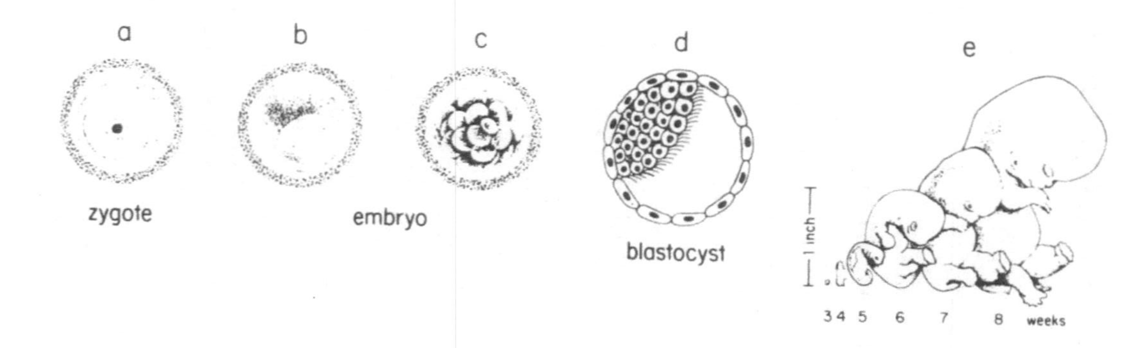

Figure 7.1 Terminology of early embryonic and fetal development. (**a**) Zygote: note male and female pronuclei in fertilized egg, Embryo: two-cell egg; (**b**) morula; (**c**) preimplantation blastocyst; (**d**) fetus with completed organogenesis. Very early embryonic loss, not associated with a change in menstrual regulation, the morula and blastocyst are extracted. Termination of pregnancy (spontaneous or voluntary) occurs in various stages of fetal development. (Drawing not to scale.).

Table 7.1 Morphological characteristics of human defective embryos during the first month of gestation

Stage of embryo	*Major morphological characteristics*
Morula and blastocyst; preimplantation (1 week of gestation)	(1) Blastomeres of variable, non-uniform size (2) Cellular debris in the morula (3) Collapse of the degenerated blastocyst within an oblong-shaped zona pellucida (4) Indistinct foamy blastomeres (5) Disintegrating mitotic figure (6) Fragmentation of cytoplasmic and nuclear material (7) Abnormal shape of morula or blastocyst
Postimplantation (2–4 weeks of gestation)	(1) Presence of vacuoles in the syncytium, as a result of phagocytosis or degenerative changes (2) Retardation or asymmetry of embryonic disc (3) Alterations in the thickness of the embryonic disc (4) Abnormalities of the amnion, trophoblast and chorion (5) Presence of syncytiotrophoblast only (6) Poor trophoblast and no embryo (7) Relatively good trophoblast but no chorionic cavity (8) Trophoblastic hypoplasia (9) Shallow implantation, with maloriented embryonic disc (10) Irregular or deformed amniotic cavity (11) Embryo retarded and asymmetrical; yolk sac defective. (12) Yolk sac defective with a thick plate and no lumen; small amniotic cavity (13) Small embryonic disc; trophoblast and amniotic cells retarded (14) Embryo retarded and atypical in form, collapsed and blood-filled; atypical implantation and chorion

Data from Boyd and Hamilton (1970); Corner and Bartelmez (1954); Benirschke and Driscoll (1967); Hendrickx and Binkerd (1980); unpublished data from IVF/Andrology International

abortion at the same stage of gestation in each pregnancy, a tendency to deliver premature livebirths, and difficulty in achieving conception. Products of abnormal early gestation show several trophoblastic structures: (1) amniotic sacs covered by chorion frondosum of chorion laeve; empty, with stunted embryonic growth or with normal development, (2) hydropic and (3) molar degeneration. Trophoblastic topography of a rare partial mole, with a coexistent viable fetus, is shown in Figure 7.2.

ESTIMATES OF EARLY EMBRYONIC MORTALITY

The rate of early embryonic mortality ranges from 25 to 78%. A large percentage of early embryonic death is unavoidable and should be regarded as a normal way of eliminating unfit genotypes in each generation. In several cytogenetic and epidemiological studies, no less than 50% of clinically recognizable spontaneous abortuses are chromosomally abnormal. Most of the abnormalities which are identified are never seen among liveborn individuals.

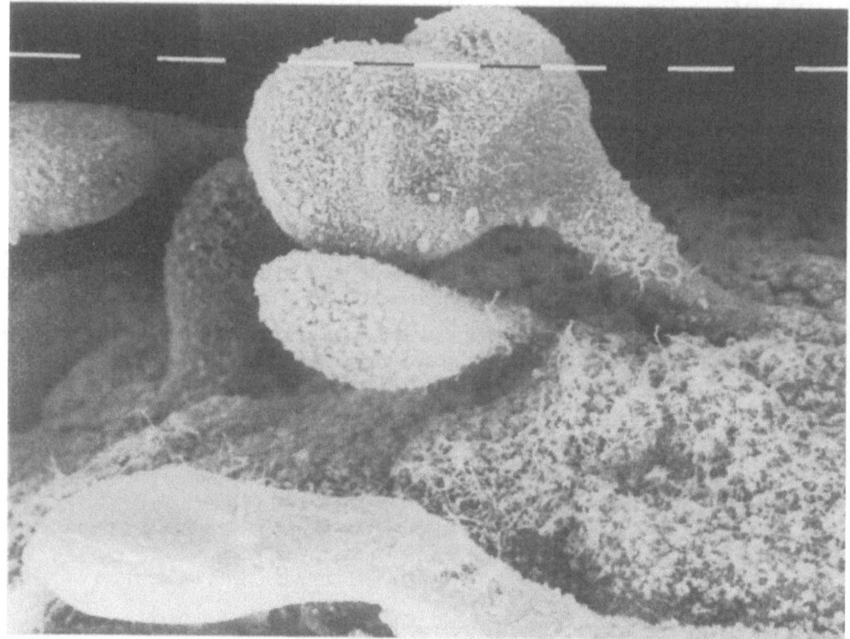

Figure 7.2 Scanning electron micrograph of partial hydatidiform mole from a patient who delivered, in the 28th week of pregnancy, an immature fetus which soon died. The fetus was followed by a placenta which was both macroscopically and microscopically normal. However, directly after the birth of the placenta, a multitude of grape-like vesicles was delivered. The placenta was within the normal range for immaturity: many trophoblastic sprouts on long chorionic villi showing abundant microvillous surface pattern. The molar syncytiotrophoblast showed many sprouts, which were rather flat in comparison to cylindrical in the normal prophoblast. The syncytial surface was covered by closely packed and frequently branching pleomorphic microvilli. (P. Kenemans, H. P. van Geyn and E.S.E. Hafez.)

The risk of pregnancy in exposed ovulatory cycles is estimated to be 60% (Edmonds *et al.*, 1982). This is similar to the estimated maximum fertility rate of 58% (Hertig *et al.*, 1952); however, 62% of all detected pregnancies terminated prior to 12 weeks. Some 92% of these losses occur subclinically without the knowledge of the mother. Embryonic and early fetal loss occurs in approximately one out of two pregnancies (Shepard and Fantel, 1979). Approximately 15% of pregnancies terminate in recognizable spontaneous abortion (Warburton and Fraser, 1964; Roth, 1963). If the woman is pregnant and has missed one menstrual cycle she has a 30% chance of aborting. Some women with occult pregnancy do not realize that a delayed heavy menstruation is an early subclinical abortion (Roth, 1963; Braunstein *et al.*, 1977).

Spontaneous menstrual abortions represent 21% of a total of 90 observed pregnancies and 321 cycles (Chartier *et al.*, 1979). The chances of a woman producing one viable offspring per menstrual cycle is approximately 25% (Henry, 1965; Sheps, 1965; Vessey *et al.*, 1964). Some 15% of clinically recognized pregnancies terminate in spontaneous abortion (Roth, 1963; Warburton *et al.*, 1964). Seventy-eight percent of fertilizations fail to result in live birth (Roberts and Lowe, 1975). Embryonic mortality occurs in 40% by the time of the expected menstrual cycle (Hertig *et al.*, 1952). When this is combined with the percentage of patients who fail to have a successful pregnancy after a missed period (French and Bierman, 1962), postimplantation embryo loss appears to be almost four times the figure accepted for spontaneous abortion (Edmonds *et al.*, 1982).

Study and analysis of the abortus have allowed identification of a number of new embryonic and fetal syndromes. Careful description and classification combined with continued monitoring of abortuses are an important adjunct to reproductive counseling and an important defense against teratogenic exposure. It is through this study that the etiology and ultimately the control of preventable pregnancy wastage will be understood and implemented (Shepard and Fantal, 1979).

Figure 7.3 demonstrates the controversies in the calculation of gestational age according to WHO, USA and Japanese criteria, in relation to perinatal terminology.

1st lunar month					5th lunar month				6th lunar month			
1	2	3	4	U.S.A. criteria	17	18	19	20	21	22	23	24
0	1	2	3	W.H.O. and Japanese criteria	16	17	18	19	20	21	22	23

abortion (in Japan) up to day 167

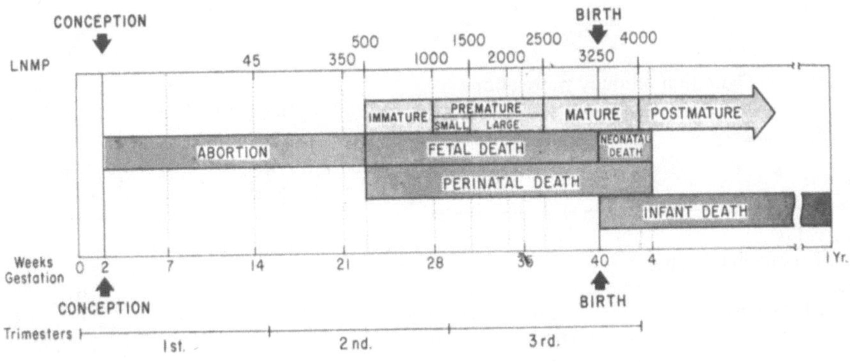

Figure 7.3 *Top*: Controversies in the calculation of gestational age according to WHO, USA, and Japanese criteria. *Bottom*: Graphic display of perinatal nomenclature (from Pernoll, 1980).

ETIOLOGY OF EARLY EMBRYONIC LOSS

Early embryonic loss is common in all mammalian species, particularly in litter species and man. In women, this embryonic loss is influenced by genetic and environmental (radiation, excessive smoking) factors, developmental mechanisms, anatomical anomalies of the female reproductive system, endocrine imbalance, infectious disease, previous induced abortion and/or immunological factors.

Early embryonic loss may also be due to errors of gametogenesis, defects in fertilization, developmental abnormalities after fertilization such as mosaicism or differentiation failure. It is also possible that early embryonic loss is due to asynchronous implantation in relation to the progestational development of the endometrium. The cause of repetitive spontaneous abortion is often unknown, but may be due to several genetic, anatomical, endocrine, microbiological and immunological factors affecting the female reproductive system.

Embryonic mortality may be due to a teratogenic insult early in embryonic development when the undifferentiated embryonic cells are refractory to teratogenesis. Interference with development during the periods of histogenesis and functional maturation causes growth retardation associated with disturbed physiological integrity. Several maternal factors may affect embryonic loss, such as diet, drugs, hormones, chemicals, radiation, hyperthermia, general health, infections, psychological stress, and specific uterine conditions, related to placenta.

Epidemiological studies

Several case reports and studies on very small samples and studies not subject to statistical analysis have implicated numerous causes of recurrent abortion: thyroid disorders, abnormalities of the uterus, fibroids or developmental defects, and inheritance of unbalanced chromosome rearrangements. Extensive subsequent investigations with large samples utilizing various epidemiological parameters (Table 7.2) did not substantiate these early reports.

Table 7.2 Definition of study populations

Study pregnancy		*Groups*	
	Repeaters abortion	*Multiparae livebirth*	*Sporadics abortion*
Gravidity	⩾ 3	⩾ 3	⩾ 3
Prior spontaneous abortions	⩾ 2	0	0
Prior livebirths	⩽ number of prior spontaneous abortions	⩾ 2	⩾ 1

Strobino *et al.*, 1980

Strobino *et al.* (1980) summarized the independent variables used in the discriminate analysis of repeat abortion:

Gravidity
maternal age
ethnicity – white, black, hispanic, other
maternal weight
age at menarche
length of menstrual cycle
length of menstrual flow
interval to conception – length of time during which intercourse took place without birth control prior to conception
male infertility

Chronic disorder – hormonal (diabetes or thyroid disorder)
other chronic disorders (anemia, hypertension, arthritis)
gynecological disorders – infectious origin (venereal diseases, pelvic inflammatory disease, tube obstruction)
gynecological disorders – structural defects (incompetent cervix or uterine anomalies)
other gynecological disorders (polyps, fibroids, cysts, etc.)
usual alcohol use
cigarette smoking
gestation at abortion
abortion rate in patient's mother

Genetic factors

Early prenatal loss is associated with defective embryogenesis, and spontaneous or teratogen induced cytogenic defects (Benirschke and Driscoll, 1967).

The principal genetic causes of embryonic death are lethal factors carried by the spermatozoa and/or the egg. Lethal factors are genes, or combinations of genes, which cause death in the next generation before the reproductive phase is reached. Lethal factors often exert their effect at a particular phase of embryonic development that is characteristic for each factor.

Several genetic mechanisms of different degrees of manifestation and penetrance cause early embryonic death, e.g. mutations, deletions, replication, translocation and inversion. Sex limited lethal factors are associated with the autosomes but cause death in one sex only. Conditional lethal factors exert their effects only in certain circumstances whereas sex-linked lethal factors are associated with differential segments of the sex chromosomes. Recessive lethal genes involve incompatibility between the spermatozoon and the egg.

Chromosomal anomalies

There are remarkable differences in the rate of chromosome anomalies reported in different studies. This variability may be due to: (1) differences in the frequency of the anomaly at fertilization, (2) variability in the incidence rate of abnormal conceptions surviving to term, (3) differences in the rates of loss in early or biochemical pregnancies and/or (4) differences in the rates at which specimens are obtained or successfully karyotyped (Warburton *et al.*, 1980).

The frequency of chromosomal anomalies in spontaneous abortion during the first 7 weeks of gestation is much lower than during later gestations. This is somewhat surprising since it is widely believed that the proportion of chromosomally abnormal abortions increases as gestational age decreases (Warburton *et al.*, 1980). This low rate may be due to the retention of chromosomally abnormal specimens *in utero* for several weeks after implantation. Such embryos may sustain very early placèntal growth even though they will degenerate within 8–10 weeks of gestation.

Structural anomalies of the chromosomes include translocation, deletions, rings and inversions of chromosomes during either mitosis or meiosis. Such anomalies affect individual autosomes or sex chromosomes. A balanced translocation occurs in some 3% of individuals and 6.2% of couples with repetitive early embryonic loss. There seems to be an excess of translocation carriers among couples experiencing recurrent abortion (Sinet *et al.*, 1973; Papp *et al.*, 1974; Byrd *et al.*, 1977; Kajii and Ferrier, 1978; Mennuti *et al.*, 1978).

Different types of chromosomal anomalies causing embryonic loss (Table 7.3) are due to different mechanisms: (1) an error during oogenesis resulting in a chromosomally abnormal ovum, (2) an error during spermatogenesis resulting in a chromosomally abnormal sperm, (3) an error of fertilization or (4) an error during early stages of cleavage of the zygote (Jacobs and Hassold, 1980).

Most of the chromosome abnormalities in spontaneous abortion are rarely, if ever, found among liveborn babies. They included various autosomal trisomies, triploidy, tetraploidy and double aneuploidy. Most of the abortuses with these lethal chromosome abnormalities are represented in either an empty sac or a totally disorganized embryo. It seems that the incidence of chromosome abnormalities and trisomy in spontaneous abortions increases with maternal age. There is also increased frequency of chromosome abnormalities in couples who have had multiple miscarriages. Trisomies are noted with chromosomes 13, 16, 18, 21, and 22, trisomy 16 being most frequent.

Table 7.3 Some chromosomal anomalies associated with spontaneous embryonic mortality

Anomaly	*Definition*	*Chromosome numbers*
Monosomy	absence of one chromosome	45
Trisomy: Single	one additional chromosome	47
Double	two additional chromosomes	48
Polyploidy	One or two additional haploid sets	69 or 92
Structural anomaly of chromosomes	unbalanced chromosome constitution	46, or 45, or 47

Jacobs and Hassold, 1980

In habitual spontaneous abortion, chromosomal factors (balanced translocation) of the couple may be involved. Indeed, in those couples ascertained for two or more miscarriages plus an abnormal (multiple congenital malformation) child, the frequency of reciprocal translocations ranges from 3 to 31 %.

Effects of inbreeding

The effects of inbreeding on embryonic loss occur during early stages of cleavage; thus, embryos are reabsorbed causing biochemical pregnancy. Inbreeding associated with increased homozygosity is caused by greater genetic similarity between relatives than between randomly chosen individuals. Thus an inbred embryo may have two alleles at a locus which are identical by descent, having been derived from the same gene in a common ancestor of the parents (MacCluer, 1980). The probability that the two alleles at a locus are identical by descent is known as 'coefficient of inbreeding' (Tables 7.4, 7.5).

The magnitude of the inbreeding effect on homozygosity at any locus is a function of both the degree of inbreeding and the allele frequencies at the locus (Table 7.5). Whatever the gene frequency, the offspring of first cousins are more likely to be homozygous than are the offspring of unrelated parents (Crow and Kimura, 1970).

Table 7.4 Probability of being homozygous recessive for the offspring of unrelated parents and of first cousins

Gene frequency	*Probability of homozygosity when parents are* Unrelated	*First Cousins*	*Ratio*
0.1	0.01	0.016	1.6
0.01	0.0001	0.00072	7.2
0.005	0.000025	0.000335	13.4
0.001	0.000001	0.000063	63

Crow and Kimura, 1970

Table 7.5 Coefficients of (autosomal) inbreeding for offspring of various mating types

Mating	*Coefficient*
Parent–offspring	1/4
Brother–sister	1/4
Half-sib	1/8
Uncle–niece or aunt–nephew	1/8
First cousin	1/16
First cousin once removed	1/32
Second cousin	1/64

MacCluer, 1980

Neural tube defects

In the USA, neural tube defects occur in one or two in every 1000 live births (Table 7.6). The polygenic/multifactorial inheritence of these disorders allows prepregnancy genetic counseling and the determination of certain risk estimates. A positive family history in either parent is associated with a 1% risk of occurrence of a neural tube defect in the offspring.

Neural tube defects (NTD) result from failure of the neural tube to diffuse during early embryogenesis. These malformation are associated with anencephaly, various types of spina bifida and lumbar meningomyelocele.

In cases of neural tube defects, the levels of α-fetoprotein are elevated in maternal serum and amniotic fluid. Closed defects, including those associated with hydrocephalus, are not associated with abnormal levels of α-fetoprotein. High levels of α-fetoprotein occur in cases of multiple pregnancy and certain fetal abnormalities such as omphalocele, congenital nephrosis, Turner's syndrome with cystic hygroma, trisomy-13, fetal bowel obstruction and teratoma (ACOG, 1982).

Table 7.6 Neural tube defects in the United States (approximately 6000/year)

Type (degree)		*Prognosis*	
	Incidence/ 1000 births	*Neonatal death (%)*	*Long term disability (%)*
1. Anencephaly	0.6–0.8	100	0
2. Spina bifida (open)	0.5–0.8	33	65*
3. Spina bifida (closed)	0.1–0.14	7	10*
Total	1.2–1.7	60	60*

* Disability has been reported including lower limb paralysis, sensory loss, chronic bladder or bowel problems, club foot, scoliosis, meningitis, hydrocephalus, and mental retardation (ACOG, 1982).

Genotype of the male

A considerable part of embryonic death is attributable to the male or to the mating system. Genetic factors that are transmitted by the male to the embryo may be further classified into three classes according to the time in the life cycle at which they are acquired: (1) factors which are inherited by the male from his parents, (2) factors which arise in the spermatogenic tissue and (3) factors which rise in spermatozoa after their release from the testis (Bishop, 1964).

The inherited genotype of the male may include a variety of genetic factors which lead to incompatibility and early embryonic loss. The resulting incompatibility may be between spermatozoa and mother, between spermatozoa and egg; or between zygote and mother. The lethal factors inherited by a male from his parents may include dominant lethal factors of less than full penetrance, and factors (such as translocation) that become dominant lethals as a result of chromosome rearrangements at meiosis, and dominant factors of various kinds that are lethal in the homozygous state.

Uterine anomalies

Anatomical anomalies include incompetent cervix and structural defects of the uterus, such as bicornuate uterus or fibroids. Uterine malformations are associated with habitual abortion during the late first or second trimester. Laparoscopy and hysteroscopy are used to detect specific malformation. Echotomography with frontal sections is used to assess anomalies of the uterus and urinary tract. Various techniques of metroplasty have been used to correct uterine malformation. Surgical correction using hysteroscopy may be adequate for certain minor abnormalities.

Immunological parameters

Spontaneous recurrent abortion is frequent in women with autoimmune disease. Circulating autoantibodies and immuno complexes are usually associated with organ-specific and non-organ-specific autoimmune diseases. In both spontaneous and induced abortion, Rh-negative women have a great risk of immunization to the Rh_0 (D) antigen except when the fetal Rh type also is Rh-negative. Post-abortum immunization is due to failure to administer anti-Rh prophylaxis. Maternal sensitization is influenced by several mechanisms: (1) frequency of fetal–maternal transfusion, (2) individual variation in ability of Rh-negative individuals to respond to Rh antigens, (3) strength of Rh-antigen on fetal erythrocytes and (4) concomitant ABO protection. RhIG prophylaxis prevents primary sensitization of mothers and costs far less than treatment of infants with hemolytic disease of the newborn.

Infections

Asymptomatic bacteriospermia is very common in men and pathogenic strains are frequent. Single and recurrent abortions are caused by various infections in pregnant women and by asymptomatic infection in the male reproductive organs. Long term treatment of male partners with antibiotics is recommended.

ENDOCRINE PROFILES

The functions of the corpus luteum, trophoblast, and placenta and embryo are influenced by chorionic gonadotropin (hCG) prolactin (hPL), progesterone (P) and estrogens. HCG, hPL and progesterone levels reflect the placental and/or corpus luteum function whereas estrogen levels are influenced partly by the fetal conditions.

Chorionic gonadotropin (hCG)

HCG is normally secreted by the cytotrophoblast, and syncytiotrophoblast of the placenta, by tumours developing from these cell types (gestation trophoblastic neoplasms) (Odell *et al.*, 1967), by teratomas of the ovary, testis or pineal, by hepatoblastomas, and by some carcinomas of the lung, stomach, pancreas and colon. HCG can be detected in maternal blood approximately 9 days following the preovulatory LH surge coinciding with the time of implantation. Following a successful implantation, there is a rapid rise in hCG levels. This characteristic rise is not noted in women whose pregnancy is clinically diagnosed, who subsequently had spontaneous abortions. Several investigators measured levels of hCG to evaluate the course of pregnancy and maintenance of the corpus luteum (Mishell *et al.*, 1974; Corker *et al.*, 1976). However, the structural similarity between hCG and hLH has presented analytic difficulties. The slope of the regression line derived from hCG levels during the first 3 weeks of pregnancy is significantly lower in pregnancies which aborted before the 60th day than in normal pregnancies (Chartier *et al.*, 1979).

HCG measurements provided information that is qualitative (diagnosis of unknown pregnancies) and quantitative (prediction of ovum vitality) (Chartier *et al.*, 1979). Several measurements of hCG have been used to assess early embryonic loss in women. Urine samples obtained from a control group of sterilized women with normal ovulatory menstrual cycles enabled a concentration limit of 56 iu/l to be determined so that any non-trophoblastic hCG or other cross-reacting compounds could be accounted for (Edmonds *et al.*, 1982). Diagnosis of early pregnancy was applied to various populations of infertile women desirous of having children. In some of the cycles examined, a high LH-hCG activity appears during the days preceding menstruation (Chartier *et al.*, 1979; Bloch, 1976).

Normal levels of relaxin are associated with low hCG levels. The corpus luteum continues to function for some time after spontaneous abortion. Subnormal levels of relaxin seem to reflect inadequate luteal stimulation due to low hCG production by placental malfunction. Thus, luteal failure is a consequence, rather than a cause, of the abortion process.

Doubling time of hCG level

The doubling time of hCG concentration in healthy pregnancies is shorter than in clinically confirmed pregnancies that abort during the first 60 days following the thermal nadir. The increase in plasma hCG level is correlated to the doubling time of trophoblastic calls (Braunstein *et al.*, 1977). This doubling time increases in cases of primary failure of ovum development due to an intrinsic defect. The slope of the plasma hCG curve during the first 3 weeks of gestation has diagnostic value. Repeated measurement of hCG activity during the luteal phase was made using semilogarithmic coordinates (Roger *et al.*, 1982).

It is possible to calculate the growth curve and the doubling time of the hCG level which is an index of trophoblastic growth. Normal pregnancies have an average doubling time not significantly different whether ovulation had been spontaneous or induced (1.4 and 1.5 days, respectively). The same is true of the twin pregnancies (1.6 days), the pregnancies with hypotrophic fetuses (1.2 days) and those which aborted after more than 2 months (1.4 days). On the other hand, pregnancies which abort before 60 days have an average doubling time significantly higher than that of normal pregnancies.

Other hormones

Prolactin (hPL) is used as a marker of placental function, and estriol as that of fetal condition. The levels of these hormones can be plotted on two-dimensional monitoring tables. Semiquantitative sensitive kits for hPL have been commercialized. The minimum detectable assay range of these kits is 0.02 μg/ml. The lower limit of physiologically normal hPL level is 0.02 μg/ml in 6th and 7th week of gestation, and 0.04 μg/ml in 8th and 9th week.

In cases of spontaneous abortion, low values for the diameter of gestational sac and levels of hPL, HCG and 17β-estradiol are usually the first abnormalities detected either in cases with an empty sac or, when an embryo is present, even before embryonic death. Certain types of morphological abnormalities (e.g. triploidy) seem to have characteristic 'growth patterns'. Before the 8th week of pregnancy the determination of β-hCG, in combination with P and estradiol (E_2), is most valuable in women with a history of abortion, and in women with uterine bleeding (Gerhard and Runnebaum, 1982). During the 9th–12th weeks of pregnancy, ultrasound examinations are usually sensitive enough to detect pregnancy disorders. However, in women with irregular menstrual bleeding the estimations of β-hCG and P (or E_2) are reliable criteria for the viability of early pregnancies.

Early pregnancy factor (EPF)

Early pregnancy factor (EPF) is a pregnancy-dependent protein, detectable in blood serum within 24 h of fertilization, and for approximately the first two thirds of pregnancy. In experimental animals the production of EPF depends on the presence of a viable embryo, whereas the removal of the embryo causes the disappearance of EPF from the serum within 6–24 h. The appearance of EPF is not induced by either intercourse or ovulation alone, thus suggesting that the presence of EPF is indicative of fertilization. The kinetics of EPF production, namely rapid appearance after fertilization and rapid disappearance after removal or death of the embryo, indicate its potential use as a means of detecting fertilization and monitoring embryonic development during early stages of pregnancy (Rolfe *et al.*, 1982). This test can be used to the discrimination between failure of fertilization and failure of implantation.

SENSITIVITY OF PREGNANCY TESTS

The various techniques used for the detection of early pregnancy vary in their simplicity, reliability and sensitivity. Serial estimation of hCG is recommended, since monoclonal antibodies can provide a constant and high discrimination towards LH. Radioimmunoassay (RIA) techniques are simpler than radioreceptor assays (van Weeman *et al.*, 1982). Changes have been made from classical rabbit antisera to mouse monoclonal antibodies for production of pregnancy tests (Pregnosticon all-in, Plantotest). New monoclonal tests include: (1) a reverse passive hemagglutination test for hCG with a sensitivity of 50 iu/l (Neo-Pregnosticon); (2) homogeneous sol particle immunoassay (SPIA) for hCG resulting in a color change which can be detected quantitatively (photometer; range 50–1000 iu/l with undiluted sample) or qualitatively (eye; sensitivity threshold 500 iu/l) (Table 7.7). These two tests show 5 % cross-reaction with LH, require minimal handling, and can be read in 2 hours or less. The SPIA can easily be run on automated equipment.

Pregnancy detection tests were evaluated on urine of pregnant and non-pregnant women. One hundred percent correct results were obtained with Neo-Pregnosticon, 99.9 % correct results with SPIA (colorimetry) and 99.6 % correct results with SPIA (eye reading) (Table 7.7). 'Trophoblastic' HCG is first detected at the level of 55 iu/l. In 97 % of cycles in which a subclinical pregnancy is demonstrated, trophoblastic hCG is detected within 14 days of ovulation (Edmonds *et al.*, 1982).

Table 7.7 Evaluation of pregnancy tests on 978 urine samples*

Test	*Sensitivity* (iu/l)	*Positive urines* +	±	−	*Negative urines* +	±	−
Pregnosticon all-in	1000	342	1†	3†	0†	0†	621
Neo-Pregnosticon	50	348	0	0	0	0	630
SPIA (colorimetry)	600‡	348	0	0	1	0	629
SPIA (eye)	500	345	3	0	0	1	629

* van Weeman *et al.*, 1982.

† Not all samples available for testing

‡ Arbitrary threshold; lower concentrations are detected

The pattern of hCG detection, presumably reflecting the time of implantation, is different in occult pregnancies, compared with normal pregnancies. Pregnancy tests with a sensitivity of 50 iu/l can be expected to give positive results even before the day of expected menses. The assay technique of hCG has been modified to increase the assay sensitivity (Louvet *et al.*, 1975) and to decrease non-specific interference (Wehmann *et al.*, 1981; Orloff *et al.*, 1979). Since several non-trophoblastic tissues show hCG activity (Orloff *et al.*, 1979; Yoshimoto *et al.*, 1977), the percentage of false-positive predictions should be minimized in estimates of embryonic mortality. Serial blood samples for evaluation of β-hCG, hPL, progesterone (P), 17-hydroxyprogesterone (17-OHP), estradiol (E_2), and estriol (E_3) using RIA (Gerhard and Runnebaum, 1982). To compare the diagnostic significance of these tests, the sensitivity specificity predictive value and relative risk were calculated. The sensitivity was 82 % for E_2, 75 % for β-hCG, 65 % for E_3 and 63 % for P. Progesterone shows the highest specificity (95 %), followed by hCG (94 %), E_3 (93 %) and E_2 (92 %). The predictive value is above 90 % for these four hormones, while the determination of hPL and 17-OHP is less sensitive, specific and predictive.

Early embryonic loss may adversely affect the interpretation of pregnancy tests in which pregnancy confirmation is based on the presence of hormones produced by the placenta. Resorptions and other forms of embryonic loss could hypothetically give a positive result for pregnancy with the hemagglutination test. Results of these tests are interpreted as false positive.

References

ACOG (1982). Prenatal detection of neural tube defects. *Tech. Bull.* No. 67. ACOG, 600 Maryland Ave SW, Washington DC 20024

Benirschke, K. and Driscoll, S. G. (1967) *The Pathology of the Human Placenta.* (Berlin: Springer)

Bishop, M. W. H. (1964). Paternal contribution to embryonic death. *J. Reprod. Fertil.*, **7,** 383

Bloch, S. K. (1976). Occult pregnancy. *Obstet. Gynecol.*, **48,** 365

Boyd, J. D. and Hamilton, W. J. (1970). *The Human Placenta.* (Cambridge: Heffer)

Braunstein, G. D., Karrow, W. G. and Wade, M. E. (1977). Subclinical spontaneous abortion. *Obstet. Gynecol.* (Suppl. 1)

Byrd, J. R., Askew, D. E., and McDonough, P. G. (1977). *Fertil. Steril.*, **28,** 246

Chartier, M., Roger, M., Barrat, J. and Michelon, B. (1979). Measurement of plasma human chorionic gonadotropin (hCG) and hCG activities in the late luteal phase: Evidence of occurrence of spontaneous menstrual abortion in infertile women. *Fertil. Steril.*, **31,** 134

Corker, C. S., Michie, E., Hobson, B. and Parboosingh, J. (1976). Hormonal patterns in conceptual cycles and early pregnancy. *Br. J. Obstet. Gynaecol.*, **83,** 489

Corner, G. W. and Bartelmez, G. W. (1954). *Contributions to Embryology,* No. 231, 1. (Washington: Carnegie Institution)

Crow, J. F. and Kimura, M. (1970). *An Introduction to Population Genetics Theory.* (New York: Harper & Row)

Edmonds, K., Lindsay, K. S., Miller, J. F., Williamson, E. and Wood, P. (1982). Early embryonic mortality in women. *Fertil. Steril.*, **38,** 447

Exalto, N., Schermers, J. P., Rolland, R. and Eskes, T. K. A. B. (1982). Morphological approach to early pregnancy. *Contracept. Deliv. Syst.*, **3,** Abstr. 355

French, F. E. and Bierman, J. M. (1962). Probabilities of fetal mortality. *Public Health Rep.*, **77,** 835

Gerhard, I. and Runnebaum, B. (1982). Hormone patterns in early pregnancy disorders. *Contracept. Deliv. Syst.*, **3,** Abstr. 359

Hendrickx, A. G. and Binkerd, P. E. (1980). Fetal deaths in nonhuman primates. In Porter, I. H. and Hook, E. B. (eds.) *Human Embryonic and Fetal Death,* pp. 45–69. (New York: Academic Press)

Henry, L. (1965). French statistical research in natural fertility. In *Public Health and Population Change,* p. 86. (Pittsburgh: University of Pittsburgh Press)

Hertig, A. T., Rock, J., Adams, E. C. and Menkin, M. C. (1952). Thirty-four fertilized human ova, good, bad and indifferent, recovered from 210 women of known fertility. *Pediatrics,* **23,** 202

Jacobs, P. A. and Hassold, T. J. (1980). The origin of chromosome abnormalities in spontaneous abortion. In Porter, I. H. and Hook, E. B. (eds.) *Human Embryonic and Fetal Death,* pp. 289–209. (New York: Academic Press)

Kajii, T. and Ferrier, A. (1978). Cytogenetics of aborters and abortuses. *Am. J. Obstet. Gynecol.*, **131,** 33

Louvet, J. P., Nisula, B. C. and Ross, G. T. (1975). Methods for extraction of glycoprotein hormones from plasma for use in radioimmunoassay. *J. Lab. Clin. Med.*, **86,** 883

MacCluer, J. W. (1980). Inbreeding and human fetal death. In Porter, I. H. and Hook, E. B. (eds.) *Human Embryonic and Fetal Death,* pp. 241–260. (New York: Academic Press)

Mennuti, M. T., Jingeleski, S., Schwarz, R. H. and Mellman, W. J. (1978). *Obstet. Gynecol.*, **52,** 308

Mishell, D. R., Nakamura, R. M., Barberia, J. M. and Thorneycrott, I. H. (1974). Initial detection of human chorionic gonadotropin in normal gestation. *Am. J. Obstet. Gynecol.*, **118.** 990

Odell, W. D., Hertz, R., Lipsett, M. B., Ross, G. T. and Hammond, L. H. (1967). Endocrine aspects of trophoblastic neoplasms. *Clin. Obstet. Gynecol.*, **10,** 290

Orloff, V. S., Yamato, S., Greenwood, F. C. and Bryant-Greenwood, G. D. (1979). Human chorionic gonadotropin subunit-like immunoreactive material in the plasma of women wearing an intra-uterine progesterone contraceptive system. *Am. J. Obstet. Gynecol.*, **134,** 632

Papp, Z., Gardo, S. and Dolhay, B. (1974). Chromosome study of couples with repeated spontaneous abortion. *Fertil. Steril.*, **25,** 713

Pernoll, M. (1980). Maternal and perinatal statistics. In Benson, R. C. (ed.) *Current Obstetric and*

Gynecologic Diagnosis and Treatment, Chap. 43. (Los Altos, CA: Lange)

Roberts, C. J. and Lowe, D. B. (1975). Where have all the conceptions gone? *Lancet*, **1**, 498

Roger, M., Feinstein, M. S. and Jondet, M. (1982). Early detection of pregnancy and prediction of abortion. *Contracept. Deliv. Syst.*, **3**, Abstr. 357

Rolfe, B. E., Cavanagh, C. A. C. and Morton, H. (1982). The use of 'EPF' for detection of fetal wastage. *Contracept. Deliv. Syst.*, **3**, Abstr. S23

Roth, D. B. (1963). The frequency of spontaneous abortion. *Int. J. Fertil.*, **8**, 431

Shepard, T. H. and Fantel, A. G. (1979). Embryonic and early fetal loss. *Clin. Perinatol.*, **6**, 219

Sheps, M. C. (1965). An analysis of reproductive patterns in an American isolate. *Pop. Stud.*, **21**, 65

Sinet, P. M., Dutrillaux, B., Prieur, M. and Lejeune, J. (1973). *Rev. Fr. Gynec.*, **68**, 655

Strobino, B. R., Kline, J., Shrout, P., Stein, Z., Susser, M. and Warburton, D. (1980). Recurrent spontaneous abortion: Definition of a syndrome. In Porter, I. H. and Hook, E. B. (eds.) *Human Embryonic and Fetal Death*, pp. 315–329. (New York: Academic Press)

van Weemen, B., Goverde, B., van Hell, H., Leuvering, J. and Schuurs, A. (1982). New developments in pregnancy testing. *Contracept. Deliv. Syst.*, **3**, Abstr. 358

Vessey, M., Doll, R., Petro, R., Johnson, R. and Wiggins, P. (1964). A long term follow-up study of women using different methods of contraception, an interim report. *J. Biosoc. Sci.*, **8**, 373

Warburton, D. and Fraser, F. C. (1964). Spontaneous abortion risks in man; data from reproductive histories collected in medical genetics unit. *Am. J. Hum. Genet.*, **16**, 1

Warburton, D., Stein, Z., Kline, J. and Susser, M. (1980). Chromosome abnormalities in spontaneous abortion: Data from the New York City study. In Porter, I. H. and Hook, E. B. (eds.) *Human Embryonic and Fetal Death*, pp. 261–287. (New York: Academic Press)

Wehmann, R. E., Harman, S. M., Birken, S., Canfield, R. E. and Nisula, B. (1981). Convenient radioimmunoassay for urinary human chorionic gonadotropin without interference by urinary human lutropin. *Clin. Chem.*, **27**, 1997

Yoshimoto, Y., Wolfsen, A. R. and Odell, W. D. (1977). Human chorionic gonadotropin-like substances in non-endocrine tissues of normal subjects. *Science*, **197**, 575

8
Early embryonic death – pathology and associated factors

H. NISHIMURA and K. SHIOTA

A large number of implanted human conceptuses are lost almost exclusively during early stage (Miller *et al.*, 1980). Chromosomal abnormalities have been accepted among the most important causes of such early prenatal loss (Boué *et al.*, 1976). Because the majority of chromosomal and other lethal disorders occur spontaneously, effective methods to avoid the embryonic death cannot be advised. Examination of a large number of specimens of intact empty chorionic sacs (ECSs) was conducted in this study.

About 500 empty embryonic sacs were singled out from the Human Embryo Collection in Kyoto University, arising mainly from induced abortion (D & C) conducted at the second and third month of pregnancy (Nishimura, 1975). These included not only the cases without the symptom of threatened abortion, but also those with such symptom. The specimens correspond to groups II (villi and chorion only) and III (villi, chorion and amnion only) according to the classification by Mall and Meyer (1921). For comparison, a number of chorionic sacs retaining the normal embryos at various developmental stages were used.

The present study is characterized first by using the products of presumably very early postimplantation death as well as their attached medical records and secondly, their good quality for examination, since such specimens retained *in utero* show little postmortem changes and allow their precise observation. Both morphological (stereomicroscopic and histological) and epidemiologic studies pertaining to the occurrence of early embryonic death were carried out.

PATHOLOGY OF EMPTY CHORIONIC SACS (ECSs)

Size of ECSs

Normal growth of the chorionic sacs was studied by using well preserved intact sacs. Figure 8.1 represents sizes of the normal sacs at various developmental stages. O'Rahilly has published data dealing with the growth of maximum diameters of the chorions in the Carnegie Collection (O'Rahilly,

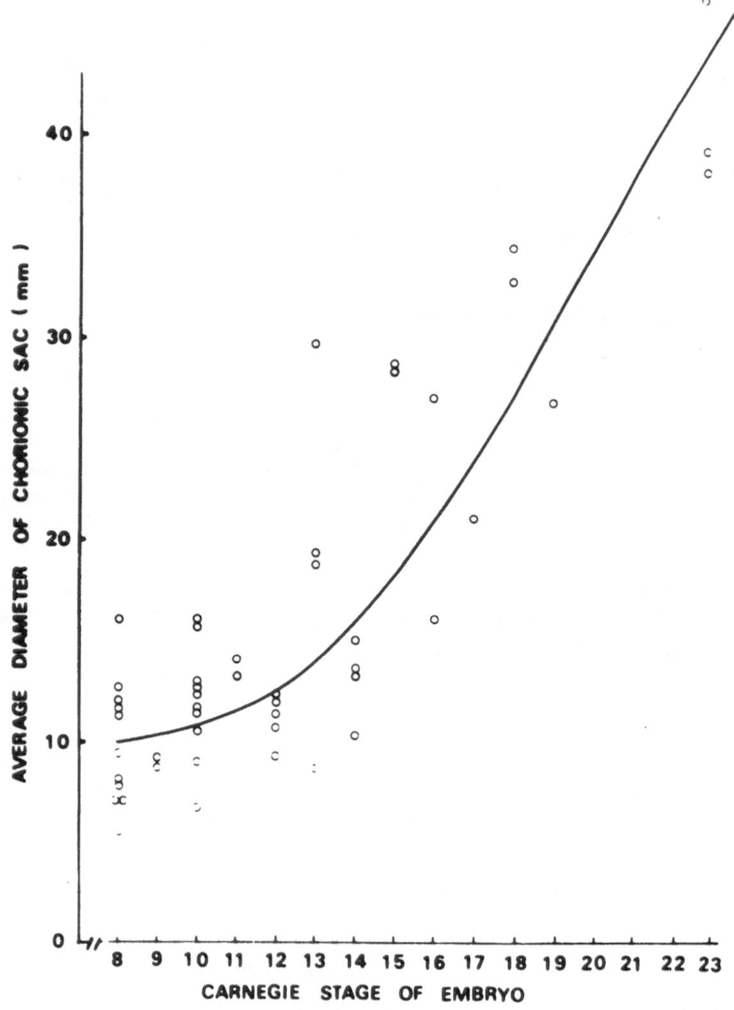

Figure 8.1 Size of chorionic sac in relation to embryonic development.

1973, p. 147). However, our data in Figure 8.1 are concerned with average diameters so that comparison of our data with O'Rahilly's is inappropriate.

Sizes of the ECSs were compared with normal sacs as shown in Figure 8.2. In this figure, the solid line indicates the approximate trend of normal growth on the basis of embryonic age and this was obtained from the data in Figure 8.1 by using the table in the paper by O'Rahilly (O'Rahilly, 1973, p. 3). It is clear that almost all solid circles representing the sizes of ECSs are located below the normal standard. This means that the suppression of chorionic sac growth takes place with appreciable individual variability when death of the embryo and its resorption occur.

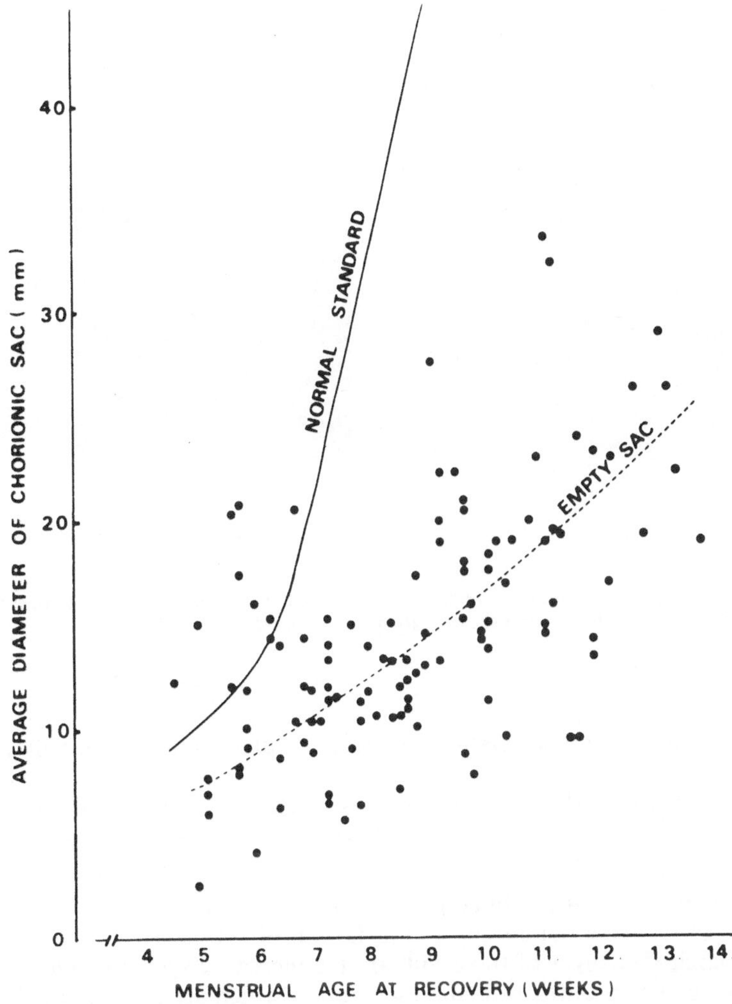

Figure 8.2 Size of empty chorionic sac (113 specimens) compared with normal standard.

Stereomicroscopic and histological observations

Figures 8.3–8.8 represent the examples of stereomicroscopic features with normal chorionic sacs and embryos at various developmental stages. Figures 8.3–8.5 show that primary as well as secondary chorionic villi cover the entire surface of the chorion. In Figure 8.6, formation of the smooth chorion laeve is visualized.

As for the characteristic pathological findings of the ECSs, the following can be summarized.

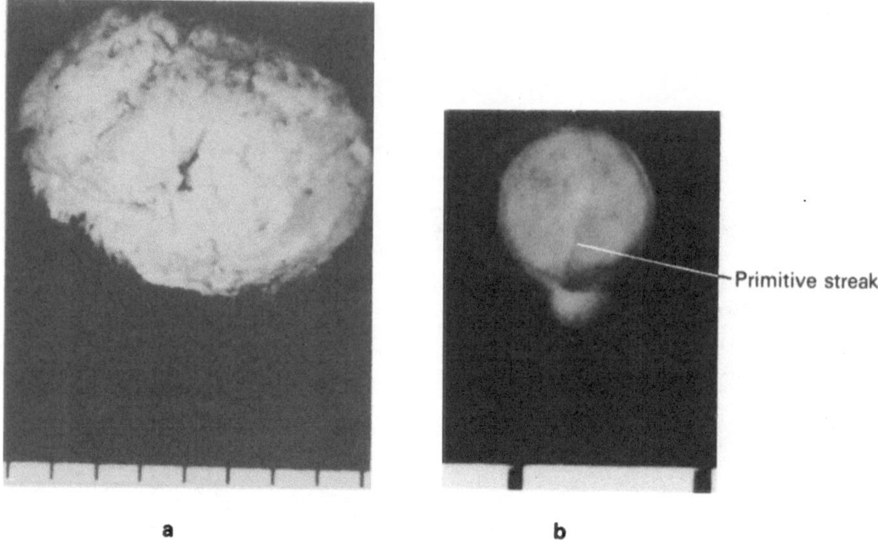

Figure 8.3 Normal chorionic sac retaining the embryo at Carnegie stage 8 (#50123). **a**, Surface of the chorionic sac. **b**, Embryo showing the primitive streak.

(1) Presence of the spot(s) showing the sparse distribution of the villi (Figure 8.9).
These were shown in the majority of ECS specimens (at *ca.* 90 %) and unlike the region of the normal chorion laeve, the loss of the villi appears somewhat irregular.

(2) Hydropic swollen villi (Figure 8.10).
These were commonly found (at *ca.* 80 %). The characteristic histological changes of those villi are the increased syncytial and cytotrophoblastic proliferation and the stromas which are often avascular and hyalinized (Figure 8.11).

(3) Hydatidiform moles (Figure 8.12).
The case with typical hydatidiform mole was found rarely (at *ca.* 2 %).

(4) Slender atrophic villi (Figure 8.13).
These were seen occasionally (at *ca.* 9 %).

(5) Abnormalities of the amnion.
Presence of the amnion was recognized only occasionally (at *ca.* 20 %) and rarely the amniotic cyst was found (Figure 8.14).

These pathological changes found in the ECSs are almost common with those reported on the spontaneous abortuses by previous investigators (Potter and Craig, 1975; Wilkin, 1977; Fantel and Shepard, 1981). The problem is the interpretation of each of the pathological findings in the present study with

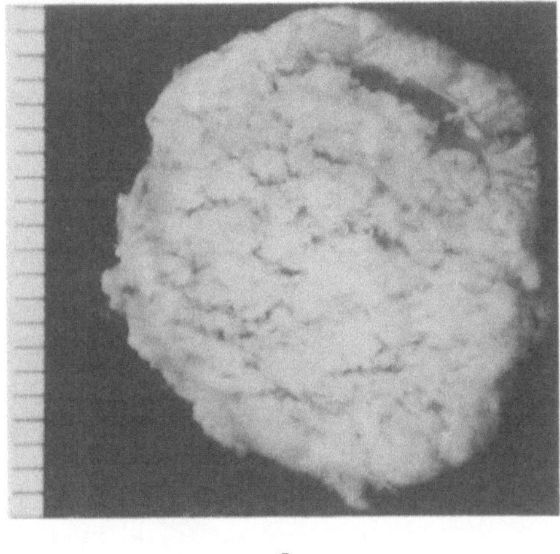

a

b

Figure 8.4 Normal chorionic sac retaining the embryo at Carnegie stage 10 (# 50823). **a**, Surface of the chorionic sac. **b**, Embryo showing several pairs of somites and the neural tube.

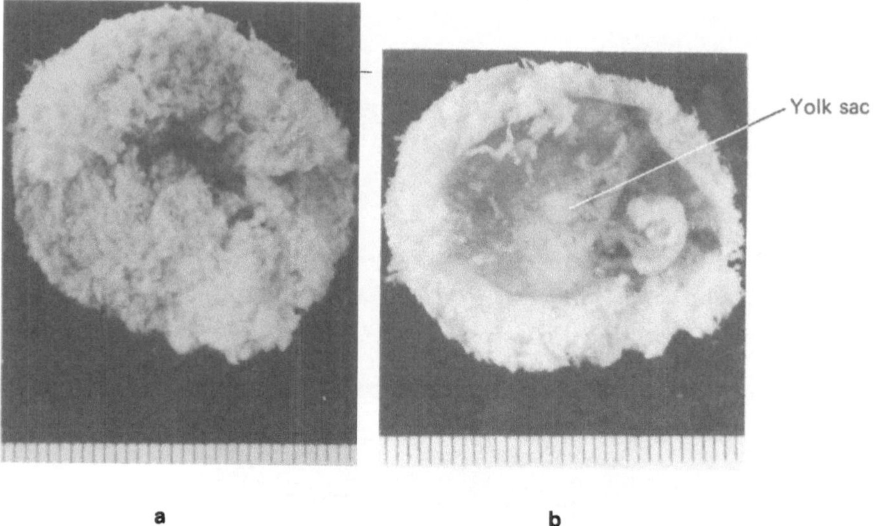

Figure 8.5 Normal chorionic sac retaining the embryo at Carnegie stage 15 (#29632). **a**, Surface of the chorionic sac. **b**, Embryo and yolk sac seen through the partially opened chorionic sac.

reference to causation of embryonic death. A plausible estimation is that all of such pathological placental changes are the consequence of the embryonic death with no bearing on causes of death. However, attention should be paid to the noteworthy reports stating that morphological examination of the placenta obtained from spontaneous abortion may have etiological significance, that is, its morphology may permit tentative identification of chromosomal anomalies (Boué *et al.*, 1976; Honore *et al.*, 1976). If such association between the abnormal placental morphology and the certain chromosomal anomalies exists in our ECS specimens, it can be presumed that a certain number of the cases showing the findings similar to the descriptions by the above mentioned investigators arose from karyotypic anomalies.

Epidemiologic analysis

Table 8.1 shows the distribution of ECSs by gestational stage at abortion. Eighty percent of the cases were aborted between the 4th and 10th weeks of estimated ovulation age, i.e., by the end of the 3rd month.

Certain parental factors associated with the occurrence of ECSs were sought and the significant or suggestive results revealed are shown in Tables 8.2–8.6.

Previous miscarriages in case women were significantly more frequent than in controls (Table 8.2). As for some other studies, reproductive histories of women interviewed in a medical genetics unit were examined with the

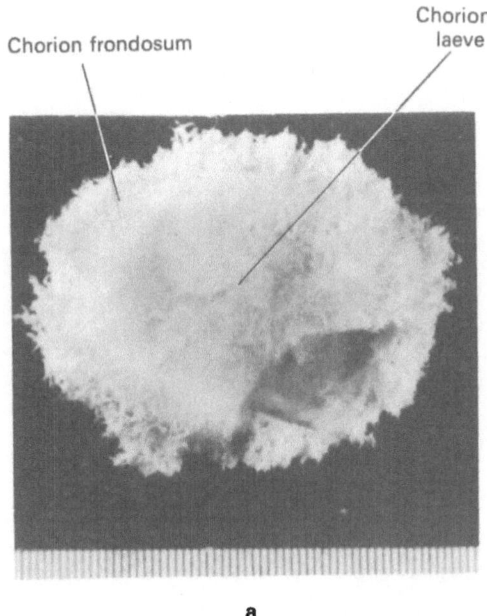

a

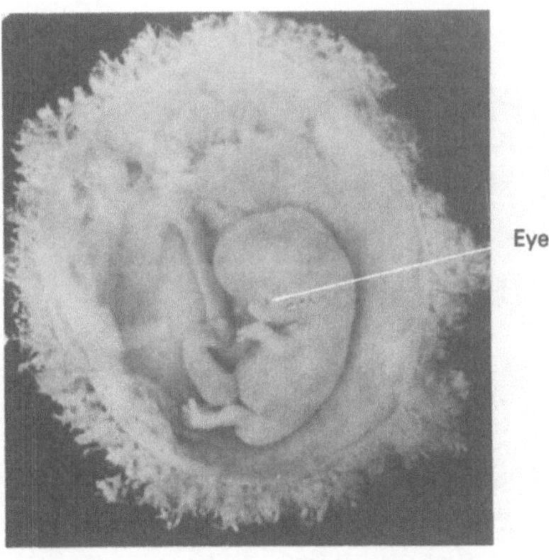

b

Figure 8.6 Normal chorionic sac (cut partially) retaining the embryo at Carnegie stage 23 (#17278). **a**, Surface of the chorionic sac showing presence of chorion laeve. **b**, Embryo seen through opened chorionic sac. *Note* opened eyelids.

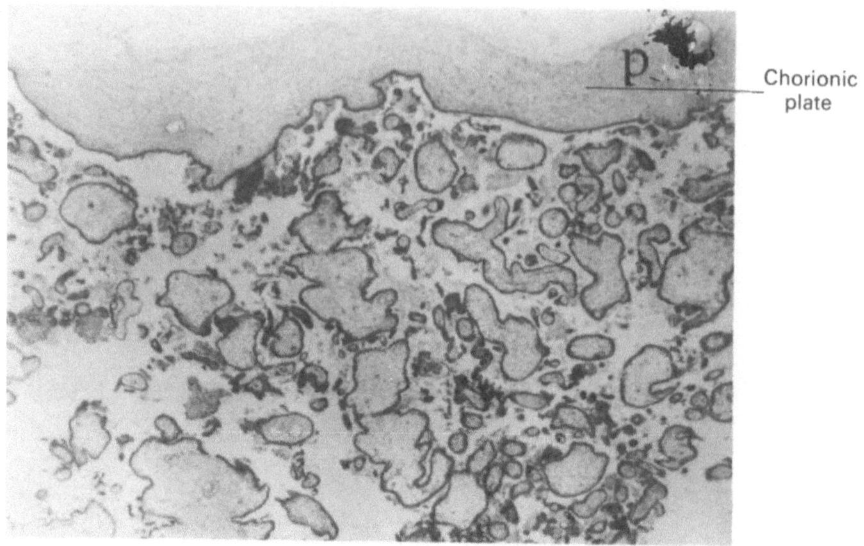

Figure 8.7 Microphotograph of normal villi of the chorion frondosum at 10 weeks (#30925, × 30).

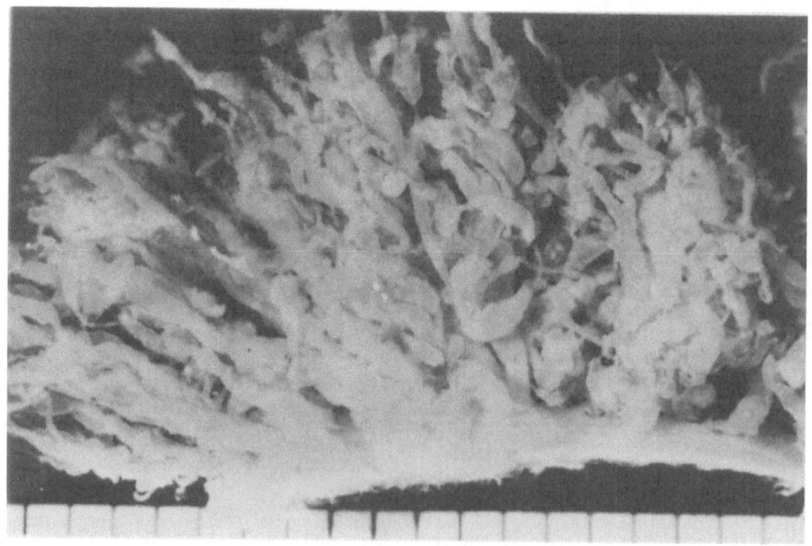

a

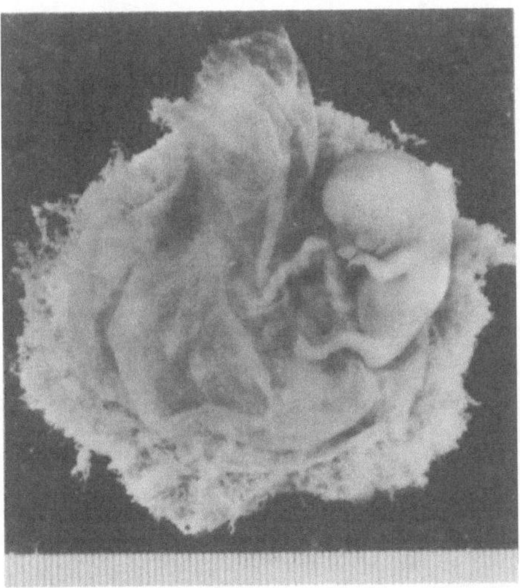

b

Figure 8.8 Normal chorion and embryo at 32 mm CRL (#52060). **a**, A part of the chorion frondosum. **b**, Embryo seen through opened chorionic sac. *Note* fused eyelids.

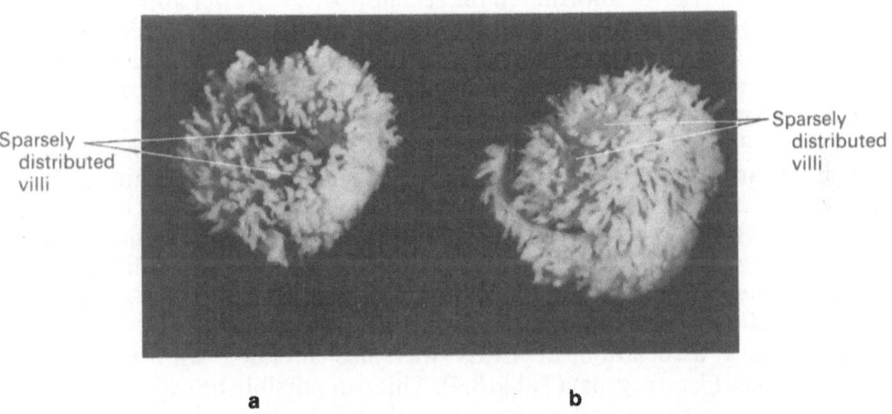

Figure 8.9 Surfaces of empty chorionic sac at 6 weeks (#51289). **a**, Front surface. *Note* presence of the spot where sparse distribution of villi is seen. **b**, Back surface. *Note* similar spot is seen.

conclusion that a woman who has had one abortion has a 25–30% risk of aborting in each successive pregnancy while the overall frequency of abortion in all the women investigated was about 15% (Warburton and Fraser, 1964). Next, the risk of repeated pregnancy loss was investigated in 3185 pregnancies in France (Leridon, 1973) and it was revealed that after an abortion in the first

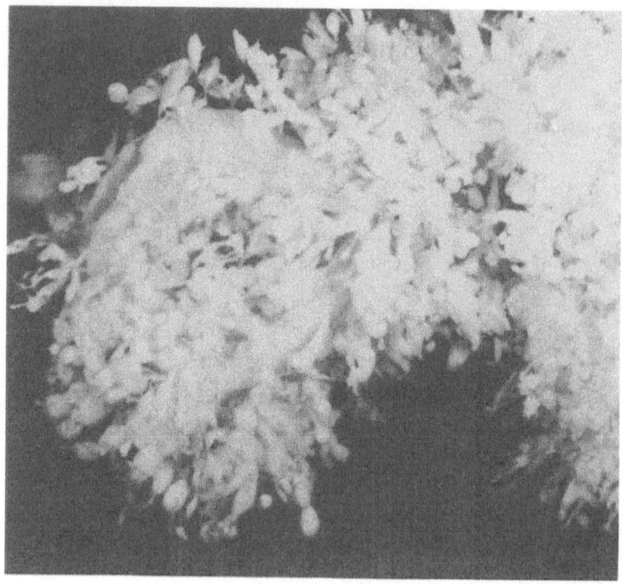

Figure 8.10 Empty chorionic sac at 12 weeks showing hydropic swollen villi (#21925).

pregnancy, the risk of abortion in the second was 28 %; after abortions in the first two pregnancies, the risk of abortion in the third was 38 %; after abortions in the first three pregnancies, the risk of abortion in the fourth was 50 %. Parental genotypes and/or environmental factors may be at work chronically or repeatedly in those abortion-prone women.

Table 8.3 shows that maternal vaginal bleeding during terminated pregnancy occurred more frequently in the ECS group. Based on the same embryo collection as in the present study, Nishimura (1970) showed that malformation or pregnancy wastage occurs more often in women with vaginal bleeding early in pregnancy. Matsunaga and Shiota (1979) examined the clinical course of the women and concluded that maternal vaginal bleeding is not a cause but a consequence of the conception of an abnormal embryo.

A positive association of ECSs was also revealed with the use of progestogens (± estrogens) (Table 8.4). This can possibly be explained by the fact that obstetricians often use progestogens to treat abnormal vaginal bleeding. An earlier epidemiologic study (Matsunaga and Shiota, 1979) showed no indication that exogenous female sex hormones could produce major malformations recognizable at embryonic stage.

Table 8.5 is concerned with the role of maternal cigarette smoking. The incidence of maternal smoking in the ECS group is significantly higher than the incidence among overall cases with alive embryos, although the difference between the ECS group and the gravidity-matched controls did not reach statistical significance. Data from the United States and Scandinavia have shown a positive association between maternal cigarette smoking and

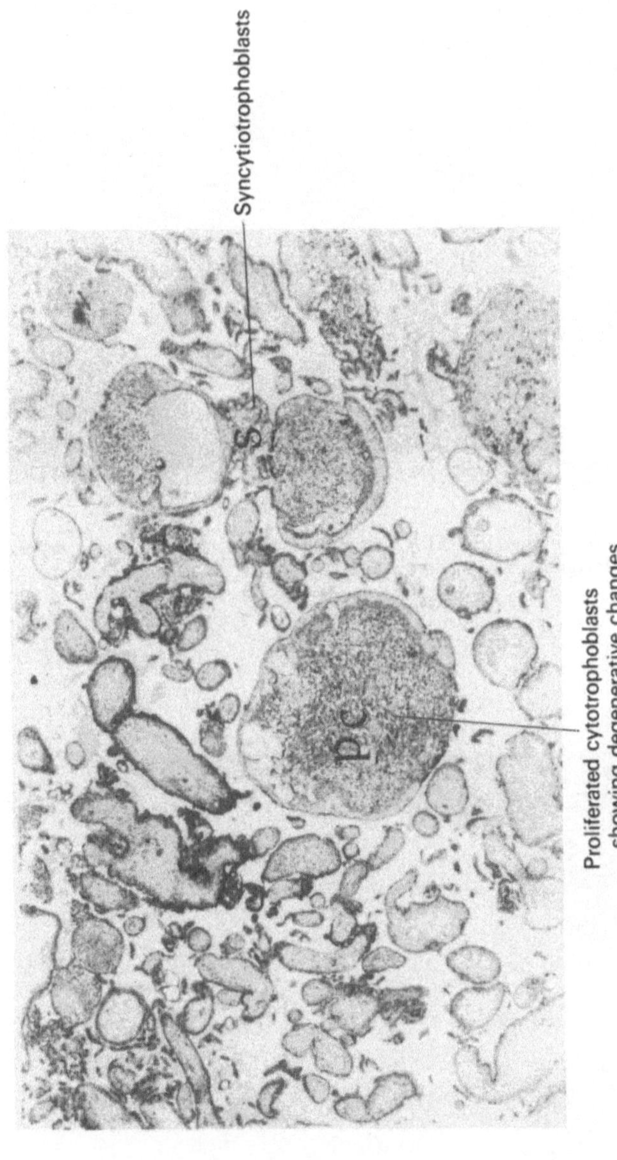

Figure 8.11 Microphotograph of the hydropic swollen villi of an empty chorionic specimen at 10 weeks (#50091, × 35). *Note* that in contrast to Figure 8.7, the syncytical and cytotrophoblastic proliferation is increased and the stroma is often avascular and hyalinized.

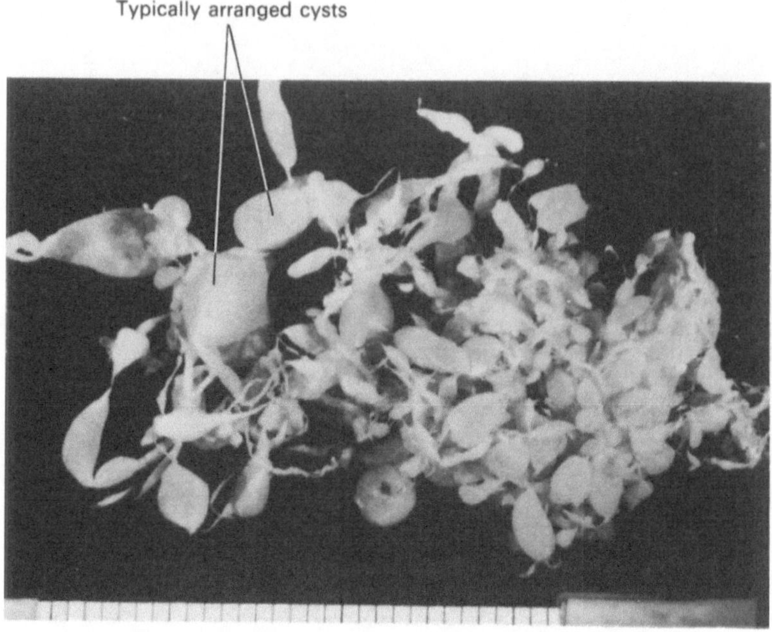

Figure 8.12 Hydatidiform moles found in an empty sac specimen at presumably 3rd month of pregnancy (#52056). Diagnosis was made by their large diameters (2 mm or more).

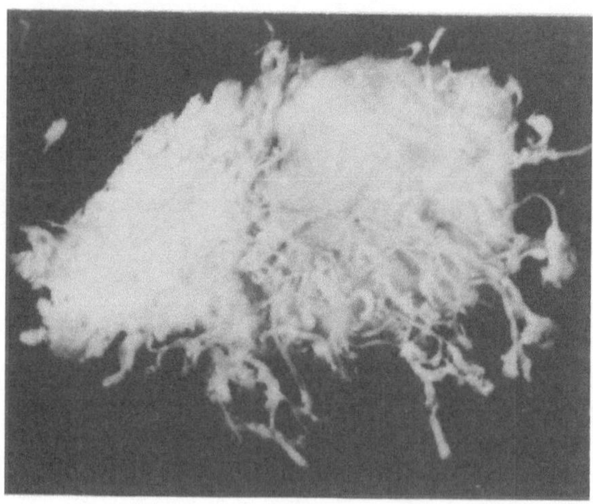

Figure 8.13 Abnormally slender villi of an embryo sac specimen at 7 weeks (#26651).

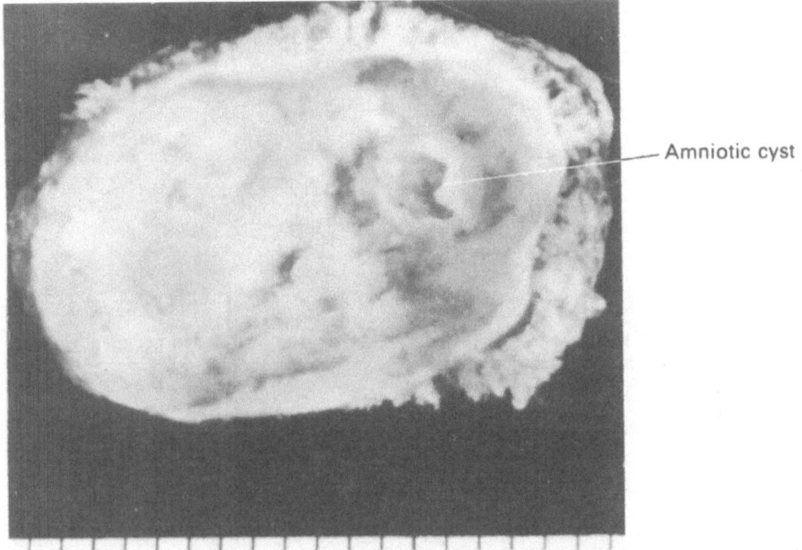

Figure 8.14 Empty chorionic sac containing an amniotic cyst at 12 weeks (#34890).

Table 8.1 Distribution of empty chorionic sacs by gestational age (estimated ovulation age)

Est. ovulation age (days)	*No. of cases* (%)
–21	13 (2·5)
22–28	51 (10·0)
29–35	71 (13·9)
36–42	72 (14·1)
43–49	63 (12·4)
50–56	64 (12·5)
57–63	49 (9·6)
64–70	45 (8·8)
71–77	29 (5·7)
78–84	11 (2·2)
85–	9 (1·8)
unknown	33 (6·5)
Total	510 (100·0)

Table 8.2 Previous miscarriage and empty chorionic sac

Group	*Frequency of previous miscarriages (spontaneous abortions/total conceptions)*
Empty chorionic sac	194/741 (26.1 %)*
Normal control†	89/741 (12.0 %)

* $\chi^2 = 4.72$; $p < 0.001$
† Matched for gravidity

Table 8.3 Maternal vaginal bleeding and empty chorionic sac

Vaginal bleeding	*Empty chorionic sac*	*Normal control**
+	292/452 (64.6%)†	89/452 (19.7%)

† $\chi^2 = 185.1$; $p < 0.001$
* Matched for gravidity

Table 8.4 Intake of progestogens (± estrogens) during the terminated pregnancy

Progestogens (± estrogens)	*Empty chorionic sac*	*Normal control**
+	98/428 (22.9%)	25/428 (5.8%)

$\chi^2 = 49.3$; $p < 0.001$
* Matched for gravidity

Table 8.5 Maternal smoking and empty chorionic sac

*Smoking**	*Empty chorionic sac*	*No. of cases (%)* Gravidity-matched control	*Background*
+	70/363 (19.3%)	110/726 (15.2%)	419/2772 (15.1%)

Empty chorionic sac vs. gravidity-matched control: $\chi^2 = 2.70$; $p \approx 0.1$

Empty chorionic sac vs. background: $\chi^2 = 3.93$; $p < 0.05$

* No significant difference in the number of consumed cigarettes per day is found between the case group and the control group

spontaneous abortion (Zabriskie, 1963; Underwood *et al.*, 1965; Kullander and Källen, 1971; Kline *et al.*, 1977). A recent study on 12 914 pregnancies and 10 523 livebirths (Himmelberger *et al.*, 1978) revealed a statistically significant increase in the risk of spontaneous abortion in women who smoked, after controlling confounding variables. The risk of abortion for the heavy smoker was as much as 1.7 times that of the non-smoker. In another study (Harlap and Shiono, 1980), however, the association was less strong, and the relative risks of abortion were 1.01 and 1.21 times in the first and second trimesters, compared with non-smokers.

The role of maternal alcoholic drinking can be considered suggestive since a borderline figure is shown (Table 8.6). Recently two studies were reported

Table 8.6 Maternal alcohol drinking and empty chorionic sac

Alcohol	*Empty chorionic sac*	*Normal control**
+	36/110 (32.7%)	51/220 (23.2%)

$\chi^2 = 2.97$; $0.05 < p < 0.1$
* Matched for gravidity

from the United States concerning the effect of maternal alcohol intake on spontaneous abortion (Harlap and Shiono, 1980; Kline *et al.*, 1980). They both revealed that alcohol consumption during pregnancy is a risk factor for, and may be a cause of, spontaneous abortion not only when alcohol is abused but also when taken in moderation.

Negative association of ECSs was shown with parental consanguinity, paternal and maternal ages, pregnancy order, pregnancy interval, the number of prior induced abortions, irradiation and drugs other than female sex hormones. It can be pointed out that because of the limited number of cases, the sensitivity of the present analysis was not sufficiently high.

CONCLUDING REMARKS

The phenomenon of very early postimplantation death of human embryos was studied. The materials were 500 cases of intact empty chorionic sacs (ECSs) as well as the normal controls, which arose from induced abortion (D & C) conducted in early pregnancy.

Examination of the growth of chorionic sacs was conducted and revealed its suppression with individual variability after embryonic death. Pathological changes of the villi of ECSs were their sparse distribution, hydropic swelling, hydatidiform moles, slenderness and amniotic abnormalities including amniotic cysts. These findings can be concluded to be almost common with those reported on the spontaneous abortuses by previous investigators.

Epidemiologic analysis was done concerning the effects of various parental factors on the occurrence of ECSs. The group of ECSs was compared with that of matched controls consisting of normal embryos. Prior miscarriages were significantly more frequent in the case women than in controls. A positive association of ECSs was also revealed with maternal vaginal bleeding during the terminated pregnancy and the use of progestogenic hormones, but these were considered to be a symptom of abnormal pregnancy and its treatment, respectively. Suggestive data were obtained regarding the role of maternal cigarette smoking and alcohol drinking. No association of ECSs was verified with parental consanguinity, paternal and maternal ages, pregnancy order, pregnancy interval, prior induced abortions, irradiation and intake of drugs other than female sex hormones.

Acknowledgements

We gratefully acknowledge the continuing help of numerous collaborating obstetricians in providing embryonic specimens. Also, we wish to express our gratitude to Ms C. Uwabe (Central Institute for Experimental Animals, Japan), Mr K. Arishima (Azabu University, Japan) and Mr M. Matsuura (Shionogi Research Laboratory in Toyonaka, Japan). This work was supported in part by the fund from Central Institute for Experimental Animals (Kawasaki, Japan).

References

Boué, J., Philippe, E., Giroud, A. and Boué, A. (1976). Phenotypic expression of lethal chromosomal anomalies in human abortuses. *Teratology*, **14**, 3

Fantel, A. G. and Shepard, T. H. (1981). Basic aspects of early (first trimester) abortion. In Iffy, L. and Kaminetzky, H. A. (eds.) *Principles and Practice of Obstetrics and Perinatology*. Vol. 1, pp. 553–563. (New York: Wiley)

Harlap, S. and Shiono, P. H. (1980). Alcohol, smoking, and incidence of spontaneous abortions in the first and second trimester. *Lancet*, **2**, 173

Himmelberger, D. U., Brown, B. W. Jr. and Cohen, E. N. (1978). Cigarette smoking during pregnancy and the occurrence of spontaneous abortion and congenital abnormality. *Am. J. Epidemiol.*, **108**, 470

Honoré, L. H., Dill, F. J. and Poland, B. J. (1976). Placental morphology in spontaneous human abortuses with normal and abnormal karyotypes. *Teratology*, **14**, 151

Kline, J., Stein, Z. A., Susser, M. and Warburton, D. (1977). Smoking: A risk factor for spontaneous abortion. *N. Engl. J. Med.*, **297**, 793

Kline, J., Shrout, P., Stein, Z., Susser, M. and Warburton, D. (1980). Drinking during pregnancy and spontaneous abortion. *Lancet*, **2**, 176

Kullander, S. and Källen, B. (1971). A prospective study of smoking and pregnancy. *Acta Obstet. Gynecol. Scand.*, **50**, 83

Leridon, H. (1973). Démographie des échecs de la reproduction. In Boué, A. and Thibault, C. (eds.) *Les Accidents Chromosomiques de la Reproduction*, pp. 13–27. (Paris: INSERM)

Mall, F. P. and Meyer, A. W. (1921). Studies on abortuses: a survey of pathologic ova in the Carnegie embryological collection. *Contr. Embryol. Carnegie Inst.* No. 56, 1

Matsunaga, E. and Shiota, K. (1979). Threatened abortion, hormone therapy and malformed embryos. *Teratology*, **20**, 469

Miller, J. F., Williamson, E., Glue, J., Gordon, Y. B., Grudzinskas, J. G. and Sykes, A. (1980). Fetal loss after implantation. A prospective study. *Lancet*, **2**, 554

Nishimura, H. (1970). Incidence of malformation in abortions. In Fraser, F. C. and McKusick, V. A. (eds.) *Congenital Malformations* (Excerpta Medica International Congress Series, No. 204), pp. 275–283. (Amsterdam and New York: Excerpta Medica)

Nishimura, H. (1975). Prenatal versus postnatal malformations based on the Japanese experience on induced abortions in the human being. In Blandau, R. J. (ed.) *Aging Gametes – Their Biology and Pathology*, pp. 349–368. (Basel: Karger)

O'Rahilly, R. (1973). *Developmental Stages in Human Embryos. Including a Survey of the Carnegie Collection. Part A: Embryos of the First Three Weeks (Stages 1 to 9)*, p. 3, p. 147. Carnegie Institution of Washington Publication 631, Washington, DC

Potter, E. L. and Craig, J. M. (1975) *Pathology of the Fetus and the Infant*. 3rd Edn., pp. 62–71. (Chicago: Year Book Medical)

Underwood, P., Hester, L. L., Laffitte, T. Jr. and Gregg, K. V. (1965). The relationship of smoking to the outcome of pregnancy. *Am. J. Obstet. Gynecol.*, **91**, 270

Warburton, D. and Fraser, F. C. (1964). Spontaneous abortion risks in man: Data from reproductive histories collected in a medical genetics unit. *Am. J. Human Genet.*, **16**, 1

Wilkin, P. (1977). The placenta, umbilical cord, and amniotic sac. In Gompel, C. and Silverberg, S. G. (eds.) *Pathology in Gynecology and Obstetrics*. 2nd Edn., pp. 374–449. (Philadelphia and Toronto: Lippincott)

Zabriskie, J. R. (1963). Effects of cigarette smoking during pregnancy. Study of 2000 cases. *Obstet. Gynecol.*, **21**, 405

9
Abnormality of the ovum and abortion

K. SATO, M. MIZUNO and S. SAKAMOTO

Current concepts of spontaneous abortion have been established by cytogenetic studies and ultrasonographic examinations. Almost all spontaneous abortions are the result of embryonic death, the major cause of embryonic death being chromosome anomalies. Because chromosome anomalies are still not amenable to treatment, the cause of chromosome anomalies must be discovered before their occurrence can be avoided. Here fertilization defects will be discussed as a cause of ovum abnormality and spontaneous abortion.

SPONTANEOUS ABORTION AND EMBRYONIC ABNORMALITIES: CLINICAL STUDIES

The first sign of threatened abortion is usually uterine bleeding. The fate of a pregnancy can be determined at the onset of uterine bleeding by means of ultrasonography. Cases with positive fetal heart beat despite severe bleeding seldom result in abortion, while those with negative fetal heart beat invariably result in fetal loss. Usually no fetal heart beat is detected during the course of pregnancies resulting in abortion. This is one of the major findings indicating that abortion is only the result of embryonic death and that embryonic death is caused by abnormality of the embryo itself. Fetal heart beat is detected in 20% of normal pregnancies at 6 weeks, 70% at 7 weeks, and 100% at 8 weeks.

Chromosome anomalies are found in about 50% of spontaneous abortions (Boué *et al.*, 1975; Creasy *et al.*, 1976; Kajii and Ferrier, 1978). As abortuses with chromosome anomalies may not provide sufficient tissue culture for chromosome analysis, the frequency of chromosome anomalies probably depends on the detection rate of chromosome examinations: higher detection rates correspond to higher incidences of chromosome anomalies. Since no study has yet been conducted with a 100% detection rate, it is reasonable to suppose that the frequency of chromosome anomalies is higher than that already reported. These cytogenetic observations of spontaneous abortion were confirmed by those of induced abortion. Yamamoto *et al.* (1975) report a 6.8% rate of chromosome anomaly in 500 induced abortions. If one assumes that 15% of pregnancies result in abortions, this 6.8% incidence is about half that for spontaneous abortions.

Trisomy accounts for about 50% of the chromosome anomalies found in spontaneous abortions. Monosomy X is found in 15–30% of chromosomally abnormal abortuses. Trisomy as well as monosomy are caused by errors in meiotic division of gametogenesis or in early cleavage of zygotes. Chromosome heteromorphisms have been used to reveal that the additional chromosome in trisomy is almost always maternal in origin, especially from an error in the first meiotic division (Jacobs and Hassold, 1980). Monosomy of autosomal chromosomes is rarely found in spontaneous abortions, while monosomy X is, as mentioned above, common. As X chromosomes have no special heteromorphisms that identify the origin of the defect, so far no information is available on the origin of monosomy X in spontaneous abortuses.

Polyploidy is also a common chromosome anomaly found in spontaneous abortion, although only a few cases have been reported in liveborn infants. It occurs in 15–25% of chromosomally abnormal abortuses. Chromosome heteromorphisms are also useful in determining the origin of additional haploid sets and about 80% in triploidy are thought to be paternally derived (Jacobs and Hassold, 1980). The defect thus occurs either during spermatogenesis, causing diploid spermatozoon, or in the fertilization process, resulting in polyspermic fertilization. Polyspermic fertilization is probably the main cause of triploidy (Schindler and Mikamo, 1970). Tetraploidy is also noted in spontaneous abortuses and the incidence is almost half that of triploidy. Studies employing chromosome heteromorphisms indicate that tetrapolidy results from a defect in early cleavage division of a diploid zygote. Thus the origin of additional chromosomes is known in some chromosomally abnormal abortuses, although the causes are not well understood. Even in couples with repeated spontaneous abortions, the incidence of balanced chromosome anomalies – the clearest cause of chromosome anomalies in abortuses – is reported to be 3–10% (Byrd *et al.*, 1977; Ward *et al.*, 1980; Sant-Cassia and Cooke, 1981). In a study on 82 couples with repeated spontaneous abortions, we detected chromosomal abnormalities in five of them (6.1 %) (one father and four mothers). Three of these were Robertsonian translocations, one a balanced-reciprocal translocation and one a mosaic with a chromosome composition 46,XX/47,XXX (unpublished data). These results indicate that the cause of chromosome anomalies leading embryos to abort remains unexplained.

RISK FACTORS FOR ABNORMALITY OF THE OVA AS A CAUSE OF SPONTANEOUS ABORTION: CLINICAL STUDIES

Although numerous risk factors have been reported for spontaneous abortions (Table 9.1), only a few have revealed how these work to bring about spontaneous abortions. As almost all spontaneous abortions occur some time after death of the embryo and, in the majority of cases, are the result of abnormalities in the embryo, the factors leading to these abnormalities must be elucidated. The influence of many of the factors mentioned in Table 9.1 remains unclear.

Table 9.1 Risk factors for spontaneous abortion

Genetic
1. Parental chromosome translocation
2. Some recessive genes, dominant genes
3. Incompatibility of ABO and other blood groups

Maternal
1. Age
2. Birth order, gravidity
   Previous pregnancy outcome
   Interval between last pregnancy and LMP
   Ovulation induction
3. Endocrine defects
   Some wasting diseases
   Peritonitis
   Operation (pelvic surgery)
   Uterine anomalies
   Uterine myomas
4. Social class, race
   Infection
   Radiation
   Smoking
   Alcohol
   Drugs

Although endocrine defects during pregnancy have long been singled out as a major factor in spontaneous abortion and progesterone or hCG have been prescribed to control endocrine defects for almost all of first trimester threatened abortions, it is obvious that these drugs cannot save the life of dead embryos. However, so far as very early abortion is concerned, this might not be true. The incidence of chromosome abnormalities is much lower in abortuses before 8 weeks' gestation age than in those between 8 and 11 weeks. Subclinical pregnancies ending in abortion are known to exist in luteal phase defects (Cline, 1979), and the plasma progesterone levels at the midluteal phase in recurrent aborters are sometimes lower than in controls (Yip and Sung, 1977). Inadequate corpus luteum function might therefore interfere with the normal implantation and maintenance of very early human embryos. Administration of progesterone or hCG might then be effective. However, it is not clear whether luteal phase defects are of only one kind or more. Recent progress in ovulation detection by ultrasonography has revealed that luteal phase defects are sometimes preceded by abnormal ovulation such as anovulation or 'immature' ovulation (unpublished data). 'Immature' ovulation occurs even when the follicle size is under 15 mm in diameter, whereas normal ovulation occurs when follicles are 22–23 mm in diameter. We do not know whether 'immature' ova are fertilizable. Another possibility is that the 'immature' ovum might end in very early abortion not because of progesterone defects but because of lethal abnormalities in the ovum itself.

Maternal age is well-known as a risk factor for spontaneous abortions and abnormalities of fertilized ova. The increased incidence of trisomic conceptions with maternal age is known for spontaneous abortuses (Hassold *et al.*,

1980) and neonates (Lubs and Ruddle, 1970), although there is also an increased risk of spontaneous abortion in the case of euploid conceptions with maternal age (Stein *et al.*, 1980). In most trisomic abortuses the defect occurs at the first maternal meiotic division. In *in vitro* fertilized eggs of aged female mice, a higher incidence of aneuploidy was also observed (Maudlin and Fraser, 1978). Maternal age is thus a risk factor closely related to ovum abnormalities and embryonic death. A decline in chiasma frequency and increase in univalent formation during oogenesis in aged mice have also been tentatively linked to the relationship between age and aneuploidy (Luthardt *et al.*, 1973).

Ovulation induction with gonadotropins or clomiphene is known to be one of the risk factors closely related to spontaneous abortions (Adashi *et al.*, 1979; Schwartz and Jewelewicz, 1981). There are several explanations for the higher abortion rate (Schwartz and Jewelewicz, 1981): (1) close monitoring of the patients detects every pregnancy, including very early abortions that are missed in spontaneous conceptions, (2) there is a high rate of multiple pregnancies, which result in a high second-trimester abortion rate and (3) treatment with human menopausal gonadotropin (HMG) for less than 9 days during the conception cycle often results in inadequate maturation of the follicle and consequently an inadequate corpus luteum. A higher incidence of chromosome abnormality, especially trisomy and triploidy, has been noted in abortuses after therapy in the cycle during which fertilization occurred and in those after therapy administered in the cycle before fertilization (Boué *et al.*, 1975). Ovulation stimulation is another factor which may be closely related to ovum abnormalities and embryonic death.

Thus, some of the risk factors for spontaneous abortions are likely to involve inherent abnormalities in the ovum leading to spontaneous abortion (Table 9.1). However, the bearing on ovum abnormality of other factors such as uterine anomalies, myomas, social class, smoking and alcohol is unclear. Several other potentially complex variables associated with these risk factors might play an important role in producing lethal abnormalities in the ovum. A normal ovum may be rejected resulting in spontaneous abortion directly due to intrauterine environmental factors, but this is probably rare.

ABNORMALITY OF THE OVUM AND ABORTION: EXPERIMENTAL STUDIES

Intrafollicular overripeness of ova and embryonic development

Increased incidence of abnormal zygotes is reported in rats following ovulation delayed by pentobarbital sodium (Fugo and Butcher, 1966; Butcher and Fugo, 1967; Butcher *et al.*, 1969; Toyoda and Chang, 1969). These abnormal zygotes include polyploids caused by polyspermic fertilization and aneuploids caused by abnormal meiotic chromosomal behavior (Mikamo and Hamaguchi, 1975). When 6-day cycle groups treated with pentobarbital sodium were compared with the 4-day control groups, the loss of zygotes prior to implantation as well as the abnormal development of embryos after implantation increased significantly. The abnormal development of embryos included small embryos, degenerating sites, and embryos with gross anomalies resulting in loss of the embryo. Thus, intrafollicular overripeness of ova induced by blockage of ovulation with pentobarbital sodium was revealed to cause abnormal ova and, as a result, embryonic loss and abortion.

In women ovulation sometimes takes place after the 14th day of the cycle. If delay of the time of ovulation itself can cause ovum abnormalities, this is of major importance. To test how delayed ovulation is related to reproductive loss, the possibility and causes of teratologic development of fertilized ova were studied using mature virgin Wistar rats with regular 4-day cycles. In group 1 of rats, pentobarbital sodium was injected to delay ovulation for 2 days, starting at proestrus. In group 2 estradiol benzoate was used at estrus to induce prolonged diestrus. Group 3 served as controls. About half of the rats in each group were sacrificed on day 2 of gestation to recover zygotes which were studied under a phase-contrast microscope. The other half were killed near term and fetuses were examined using Wilson's freehand section method. Supplementary sperm were observed at a significantly higher rate in group 1, which also showed less implantation sites and viable fetuses, as well as slightly more malformations in internal organs compared with the controls. Group 2, however, showed almost no difference from group 3. These findings suggest that mere prolongation of the cycle without overripeness of ova produces no teratogenicity in the following pregnancy. Intrafollicular overripeness of ova might occur due to ovulation delay when the follicle has developed enough for ovulation. They also suggest that intrafollicular overripeness of ova does not occur in all ovulations which take place after the 14th day of the cycle in women.

Ovulation induction, ovum abnormality and abortion

Ovulation induction in experimental animals can also be used to study the relationship between ovum abnormality and abortion.

Ovulation induction in animals increases the risk of preimplantation loss of zygotes as well as postimplantation loss of embryos (Beaumont and Smith, 1975). Although the effect of intrauterine environment changed by superovulation on the development of embryos is still a problem requiring further discussion, increased incidence of chromosome abnormalities in treated embryos has been noted in animals (Fujimoto *et al.*, 1974; Maudlin and Fraser, 1977) and in man (Boué *et al.*, 1975). The chromosome abnormalities included both polyploidy and aneuploidy.

The origins of polyploidy in men and animals are of great interest. The origin of polyploidy, especially triploidy, may depend on the animals used for the experiments. In some strains of mice, triploidy was produced by digyny (Takagi and Sasaki, 1976); in another strain equally by dispermy and digyny; in another mainly by dispermy (Maudlin and Fraser, 1977). The origin of polyploidy may not be altered by the mode of ovulation, i.e. spontaneous ovulation or superovulation, or dose of gonadotropins used for superovulation. By continuous observation of fertilization under a microscope (Sato and Blandau, 1979), polyploids caused by polyspermic fertilization were found in about 10% of eggs obtained from superovulated Swiss-Albino mice and fertilized *in vitro*, whereas only two digynic polyploids out of 2648 fertilized eggs were found (unpublished data).

As for polyspermic polyploidy, the proportion of polyploids depends on the dose of pregnant mare's serum (PMS) (Maudlin and Fraser, 1977). How it acts on polyspermic fertilization is, however, not well known. We studied intrafollicular overripeness of ova and effects in the ova in PMS- and hCG-induced ovulation using adult hypophysectomized female rats. Ovulation was induced with 100 iu of PMS and 100 iu of hCG administered at various intervals between 2 and 6 days. After the hCG injection, rats were placed with fertile males and ova were recovered on the day when sperm were found in vaginal smears. The relationship between the interval of injection and developmental abnormalities of ova was studied. The highest fertilization rate was observed with a 3-day interval; extensions to 4 or more days significantly reduced the incidence of fertilization; the number of ova containing supernumerary sperm increased, however (Table 9.2). Chromosomal analysis of the fertilized ova at metaphase, one-cell stage, revealed that polyploidy gradually increased as the injection of hCG was delayed (Table 9.3). Thus intrafollicular overripeness of ova occurs and has some teratological effects on the ova when the injection of hCG is delayed during PMS- and hCG-induced ovulation. Besides delay in the injection of hCG, high dosages of PMS can induce intrafollicular overripeness of ova. This presumption is consistent with the observation that intrafollicular overripeness of ova also can cause polyspermic fertilization. The eggs protect themselves against polyspermic fertilization by the so-called 'zona reaction' and 'vitelline block' which are known to take place in less than 1 minute following sperm fusion with the vitellus in mice (Sato, 1979). Intrafollcular overripeness of ova caused by the high dosages of PMS and the delay in the injection of hCG might affect the properties of the zona pellucida and vitelline surface to block polyspermic fertilization.

Increased incidence of aneuploidy was also found in the ova of aged and superovulated mice (Maudlin and Fraser, 1978) and hamsters (Mizoguchi and Dukelow, 1981). To study the effect of superovulation on chromosome segregation during the first meiotic division in adult Chinese hamsters, superovulation was induced by intraperitoneal injections of 6 iu of PMS on the day of estrus and 6 iu of hCG 48 hours after the injection of PMS. Ova were collected from oviducts the morning of the day of ovulation and subjected to chromosome analysis in metaphase II. No significant difference in the incidence of chromosome aberrations was observed between the treated and control groups (Table 9.4). Mizoguchi and Dukelow (1981) obtained almost identical results: no significant difference in the incidence of chromosome aberrations of metaphase II oocytes in young superovulated golden hamsters, whereas increased chromosomal abnormalities were found in oocytes superovulated from aged golden hamsters. Ovarian occytes which are abnormal not as a result of superovulation but as a result of the age of the animals might have been made to ovulate through gonadotropin treatment. These abnormal oocytes might have degenerated in atretic follicles if the gonadotropins had not been injected. Besides intrafollicular overripeness of

Table 9.2 The effects of the intervals between injections of PMS and hCG on fertilization

Interval between PMS and hCG (Days)	*Total no. of rats*	*No. of ovulated rats*	%* *Rats ovulated and mated*	*No. of oocytes examined*	%† *Ova fertilized*	%‡ *Fertilized ova with supplementary sperm*
2	5	0	0	0	0	0
3	8	8	87	131	74	23
4	13	13	61	143	43‖	58§
5	8	8	37	65	43§	50
6	3	2	50	16	0‖	0

* Based on ovulated rats
† Based on examined oocytes
‡ Based on fertilized ova
§ Significant difference from the 3-day interval group ($p < 0.05$)
‖ Highly significant difference from the 3-day interval group ($p < 0.01$)

Table 9.3 The relation between the incidence of polyploidy and the interval of PMS and hCG injection

Interval between PMS and hCG (days)	*No. of ova fertilized*	*No. of ova studied*	*Diploid*		*Polyploid*			
			No.	%*	*Triploid*	*Tetraploid*	*Total*	%*
3	97	70	67	95.7	2†	1	3	4.3
4	62	38	35	92.1	3†	0	3	7.9
5	28	17	15	88.2	1†	1	2	11.8

* Based on studied ova
† Polyspermic

Table 9.4 Superovulation and chromosome aberrations in metaphase II (Chinese hamsters)

	No. of litters	*No. of ova collected (mean)*	*No. of ova karyotyped (%*)*	*No. of chromosomes*					*No. of chromosome aberrations (%†)*
				≤ 9	*10*	*11*	*12*	*22*	
Control	10	76 (7.6)	67 (88.2)	1	2	61	2	1	6 (9.0)
Superovulation	8	129 (16.1)	86 (66.7)	1	3	81	1	0	5 (5.8)

* Based on ova collected
† Based on ova karyotyped

ova, the number of oocytes forced to ovulate might also be one of the factors causing abnormality of fertilized ova in superovulated animals. However, this hypothesis does not rule out the possibility of the gonadotropin having a direct detrimental effect on the meiotic division of oocytes.

Ovum abnormality seems therefore to be at least partly responsible for the increased incidence of abortion in superovulated animals. Further studies must investigate the role of maternal environmental factors in abortion, since some hormone levels are known to be affected by superovulation and to influence the cleavage and development of ova (Allen and McLaren, 1971; Greenwald, 1976).

CONCLUDING REMARKS

Abortion is the result of embryonic death. Embryonic death is caused by abnormality of the embryo itself. Chromosome abnormality is the major abnormality of the embryo. Even in couples with repeated spontaneous abortions, the incidence of balanced chromosome anomalies, the clearest cause of chromosome anomalies in abortuses, is only 3–10%. Advanced maternal age and ovulation induction are important risk factors leading embryos to abort. Intrafollicular ovum overripeness has some teratological effects on the ova when the injection of hCG is delayed during PMS- and hCG-induced ovulation. The number of oocytes forced to ovulate may be another factor causing abnormality of fertilized ova in superovulation. Superovulation has no detrimental effect on the first meiotic division of Chinese hamster.

References

Adashi, E. Y., Rock, J. A., Sapp, K. C., Martin, E. J., Wentz, A. C. and Jones, G. S. (1979). Gestational outcome of clomiphene–related conceptions. *Fertil. Steril.*, **31,** 620

Allen, J. and McLaren, A. (1971). Cleavage rate of mouse eggs from induced and spontaneous ovulation. *J. Reprod. Fertil.*, **27,** 137

Beaumont, H. M. and Smith, A. F. (1975). Embryonic mortality during the pre- and post-implantation periods of pregnancy in mature mice after superovulation. *J. Reprod. Fertil.*, **45,** 437

Boué, J., Boué, A. and Lazer, P. (1975). Retrospective and prospective epidemiological studies of 1500 karyotyped spontaneous human abortions. *Teratology*, **12,** 11

Butcher, R. L. and Fugo, N. W.(1967). Overripeness and the mammalian ova. II. Delayed ovulation and chromosome anomalies. *Fertil. Steril.*, **18,** 297

Butcher, R. L., Blue, J. D. and Fugo, N. W. (1969). Overripeness and the mammalian ova. III. Fetal development at midgestation and at term. *Fertil. Steril.*, **20,** 223

Byrd, J. R., Askew, D. E. and McDonough, P. G. (1977). Cytogenetic findings in fifty-five couples with recurrent fetal wastage. *Fertil. Steril.*, **28,** 246

Cline, D. L. (1979). Unsuspected subclinical pregnancies in patients with luteal phase defects. *Am. J. Obstet. Gynecol.*, **134,** 438

Creasy, M. R., Crolla, J. A. and Alberman, E. D. (1976). A cytogenetic study of human spontaneous abortions using banding techniques. *Hum. Genet.*, **31,** 177

Fugo, N. W. and Butcher, R. L. (1966). Overripeness and the mammalian ova. I. overripeness and early embryonic development. *Fertil. Steril.*, **17,** 804

Fujimoto, S., Pahlavan, N. and Dukelow, W. R. (1974). Chromosome abnormalities in rabbit preimplantation blastocysts induced by superovulation. *J. Reprod. Fertil.*, **40,** 177

Greenwald, G. S. (1976). Effects of superovulation on fetal development and hormone levels in the pregnant hamster. *J. Reprod. Fertil.*, **48**, 313

Hassold, T., Jacobs, P., Kline, J., Stein, Z. and Warburton, D. (1980). Effect of maternal age on autosomal trisomies. *Ann. Hum. Genet.*, **44**, 29

Jacobs, P. A. and Hassold, T. J. (1980). The origin of chromosome abnormalities in spontaneous abortion. In Porter, I. H. and Hook, E. B. (eds.) *Human Embryonic and Fetal Death*, pp. 289–298. (New York: Academic Press)

Kajii, T. and Ferrier, A. (1978). Cytogenetics of aborters and abortuses. *Am. J. Obstet. Gynecol.*, **131**, 33

Lubs, H. A. and Ruddle, F. A. (1970). Chromosomal abnormalities in the human population: Estimation of rates based on New Haven newborn study. *Science*, **169**, 495

Luthardt, F. W., Palmer, C. G. and Yu P.-L. (1973). Chiasma and univalent frequencies in aging female mice. *Cytogenet. Cell Genet.*, **12**, 68

Maudlin, I. and Fraser, L. R. (1977). The effect of PMSG dose on the incidence of chromosomal anomalies in mouse embryos fertilized in vitro. *J. Reprod. Fertil.*, **50**, 275

Maudlin, I. and Fraser, L. R. (1978). Maternal age and the incidence of aneuploidy in first-cleavage mouse embryos. *J. Reprod. Fertil.*, **54**, 423

Mikamo, K. and Hamaguchi, H. (1975). Chromosomal disorder by preovulatory overripeness of oocytes. In Blandau, R. J. (ed.) *Aging Gametes – Their Biology and Pathology*, pp. 72–97. (Basel: Karger)

Mizoguchi, H. and Dukelow, W. R. (1981). Fertilizability of ova from young or old hamsters after spontaneous or induced ovulation. *Fertil. Steril.*, **35**, 79

Sant-Cassia, L. J. and Cooke, P. (1981). Chromosomal analysis of couples with repeated spontaneous abortions. *Br. J. Obstet. Gynecol.*, **88**, 52

Sato, K. (1979). Polyspermy-preventing mechanisms in mouse eggs fertilized in vitro. *J. Exp. Zool.*, **210**, 353

Sato, K. and Blandau, R. J. (1979). Time and process of sperm penetration into cumulus-free mouse eggs fertilized in vitro. *Gamete Res.*, **2**, 295

Schindler, A. and Mikamo, K. (1970). Triploidy in man – report of a case and a discussion on etiology. *Cytogenet.*, **9**, 116

Schwartz, M. and Jewelewicz, R. (1981). The use of gonadotropins for induction of ovulation. *Fertil. Steril.*, **35**, 3

Stein, Z., Kline, J., Susser, E., Shrout, P., Warburton, D. and Susser, M. (1980). Maternal age and spontaneous abortion. In Porter, I. H. and Hook, E. B. (eds.) *Human Embryonic and Fetal Death*, pp. 107–127. (New York: Academic Press)

Takagi, N. and Sasaki, M. (1976). Digynic triploidy after superovulation in mice. *Nature (Lond.)*, **264**, 278

Toyoda, Y. and Chang, M. C. (1969). Delayed ovulation and embryonic development in the rat treated with pentobarbital sodium. *Endocrinology*, **84**, 1456

Ward, B. E., Henry, G. P. and Robinson, A. (1980). Cytogenetic studies in 100 couples with recurrent spontaneous abortions. *Am. J. Hum. Genet.*, **32**, 549

Yamamoto, M., Fujimori, R., Ito, T., Kamimura, K. and Watanabe, G. (1975). Chromosome studies in 500 induced abortions. *Humangenetik*, **29**, 9

Yip, S. K. and Sung, M. L. (1977). Plasma progesterone in women with a history of recurrent early abortion. *Fertil. Steril.*, **28**, 151

10
Repeated abortions and chromosome analysis

J. KLEINHOUT and K. MADAN

INTRODUCTION

Morphological abnormalities in preimplanted and early implanted embryos were reported as early as 1943 (Hertig and Sheldow, 1943). A proportion of embryonic losses occurred even prior to clinically recognized pregnancies (Hertig and Rock, 1949). The principal etiological factor in spontaneous abortion was an intrinsic abnormality in the fertilized ovum. There have been numerous reports of abnormalities which cause fetal wastage (Carr, 1970; Boué and Boué, 1973; Creasy *et al.*, 1976; Lauritsen, 1976). Sixty percent of detectable first trimester abortions are chromosomally abnormal (Boué and Boué, 1975; Lauritsen, 1976).

Three main groups of chromosome abnormalities were discovered. *Aneuploids* form the largest proportion (70 %) of chromosomally abnormal abortions (Boué and Boué, 1975). Aneuploidy is caused by failure of chromosomes to separate (non-disjunction) during the meiotic cell division in the gonad of one of the parents. Thus one chromosome too many (trisomy) or too few (monosomy) results. Non-disjunction during mitosis in the zygote may cause a mosaic with more than one cell line. Whereas trisomies for certain human chromosomes (e.g. 2, 14, 15, 16, 21 and 22) are very common in spontaneous abortions, trisomies for other chromosomes (e.g. 1, 3, 4, 5, 7, 10, 11, 12, 17, 19 and 20) have been rarely reported (Creasy *et al.*, 1976). Monosomy X is very frequent (15 %). However, autosomal monosomies have rarely been reported in spontaneous abortions. In theory monosomy must arise as frequently as trisomy. This is true in mice (Gropp, 1974) but monosomic mouse embryos are lost before they become implanted or in early pregnancy. In man the rare trisomies and autosomal monosomies appear to be compatible with only minimal embryonic development and are expelled before the pregnancy is clinically recognized. Trisomy for chromosome 13, 18 and 21 and rarely 8, 9, 20 and 22 may survive to term and are reported in liveborns.

The second group of chromosome abnormalities (about 26 %) in spontaneous abortions is *polyploidy* (triploidy or tetraploidy) which have three or four haploid sets of chromosomes. Polyploidy is caused by the presence of two sets of chromosomes of paternal and/or maternal origin. This may occur by double fertilization or inclusion of the second polar body into the zygote (Jacobs *et al.*, 1978; Boué *et al.*, 1980).

The third group of chromosomally abnormal abortions (4%) has duplications or deletions of chromosome segments as a result of *chromosomal rearrangements*. In a proportion of cases the anomaly is transmitted by one of the parents who is a carrier of a balanced chromosomal rearrangement.

More chromosomal rearrangements are expected in couples with repeated abortions than in the general population. Results from 23 reports in the literature and from our own laboratory of chromosome studies in couples with repeated abortions are shown in Table 10.1. Chromosome analyses in all cases have been performed using banding techniques. Sex chromosomes mosaics and aneuploids have been excluded from the table. There is no difference in the sex chromosome mosaicism between couples with and without repeated fetal wastage (Reinisch *et al.*, 1981). The frequency of balanced chromosome rearrangements in 5474 individuals is 2.7% (Table 10.1). Analysis of 43 518 consecutive newborns accumulated from six different surveys (Evans, 1977) shows a frequency of 0.19% balanced chromosome rearrangements. This accounts for a 14-fold increase among individuals with repeated abortions.

A carrier of a balanced chromosome rearrangement is phenotypically normal. There is no gain or loss of chromosome material. However he or she may have an increased risk of producing gametes with an unbalanced chromosome constitution. The zygotes produced by these gametes may end in an early abortion or in rare cases in a birth of an abnormal child. The imbalance is caused by the malsegregation during meiosis of chromosomes involved in the rearrangement.

Chromosome inversions (inversions of a segment within the chromosome) are the least frequent of the chromosome rearrangements (Table 10.1). Some inversions, particularly those involving a heterochromatic segment of the chromosome, (e.g. chromosome 9) are found in a high frequency in the population (Madan and Bobrow, 1974). These inversions carry no ill effects and are considered as polymorphic variants (de la Chapelle *et al.*, 1974; Vine *et al.*, 1976; Winsor *et al.*, 1978). Carriers of other inversions have a high risk of producing recombinant gametes with duplication and deficiency of chromosome segments (Ferguson-Smith, 1966). Inversions of very small segments rarely result in chromosomally unbalanced gametes. However, in families in which a child with a recombinant chromosome has been identified, the risk for an inversion carrier of having an abnormal child is 5–10% (Sutherland *et al.*, 1976).

Robertsonian translocations are 'centric fusions' of two acrocentric chromosomes belonging to the D (13, 14 and 15) and the G (21 and 22) group of human chromosomes. The risk of a carrier having a spontaneous abortion or an abnormal child ranges from a few percent to 100% depending on the chromosomes involved (Hamerton, 1970; Duttrilaux and Lejeune, 1970; de Grouchy *et al.*, 1970; Evans *et al.*, 1978).

Reciprocal translocations are the most common form of chromosome

Table 10.1 Chromosome abnormalities in patients with repeated abortions

References	*No. of subjects studied*		*No. of subjects with balanced chromosome rearrangement*			
	female	*male*	*Reciprocal transloc.*	*Robertsonian transloc.*	*Inversion*	*Total*
Tsenghi *et al.*, 1976	77	77	4	1		5
Kim *et al.*, 1975	50	50	3			3
Schmidt *et al.*, 1976	22	18	1			1
Byrd *et al.*, 1977	55	55	4	2		6
Heritage *et al.*, 1978	37	37		2		2
Kajii & Ferrier, 1978	425	358	3	3		6
Mennuti *et al.*, 1978	34	34	5	2		7
Turleau *et al.*, 1979	413	413	9	5	4	18
Neu *et al.*, 1979	32	30		1		1
Tho *et al.*, 1979	100	100	8	3		11
Antich *et al.*, 1980	32	32	3	2	1	6
Ballesta *et al.*, 1980	34	34	2			2
Bortotto *et al.*, 1980	145	145	4	4	4	12
Matton *et al.*, 1980	96	96	6	2		8
Schmid, 1980	96	96	4	2		6
Stoll *et al.*, 1980	217	217	4			4
Kardon *et al.*, 1980	40	40				–
Ward *et al.*, 1980	100	100				–
Subrt, 1980	115	115	9			9
Simpson *et al.*, 1981	120	104	1		1	2
Sant-Cassia & Cooke, 1981	182	182	13	2		15
Husslein *et al.*, 1982	150	150	4	1	1	6
Davis *et al.*, 1982	100	100	5	3		8
Madan (unpublished)	114	105	5	1	2	8
Total	2786	2688	97	36	13	146
	5474					
Percent chromosome rearrangements			1.77%	0.66%	0.24%	2.67%

rearrangement among individuals with repeated abortions (Table 10.1). A balanced reciprocal translocation is a reciprocal exchange of chromosome segments between two chromosomes. Frequency of balanced and unbalanced gametes produced by a translocation carrier depends on the particular chromosomes involved and the length of the segments exchanged in the translocation (Ford, 1969; Ford and Clegg, 1969). Since the chromosome breakpoints are largely, randomly distributed over the whole chromosome complement, each translocation is likely to be unique. The frequency of different types of gametes is, therefore, unique to each translocation. The frequency of unbalanced zygotes that may result in a spontaneous abortion or survive to birth depends also on the genetic content of the particular chromosome segments involved. Various predictions have been made about the segregation of chromosomes involved in a reciprocal translocation, based on the position of the breakpoints, on the formation of a particular translocation complex during meiosis, on the likelihood of occurrence of chiasmata in the various segments of the chromosome complex and on accumulated family data (Ford and Clegg, 1969; Hamerton, 1971; Lindenbaum and Bobrow, 1975; Chandley *et al.*, 1976; Jalbert *et al.*, 1980). The risk of malsegregation resulting in a livebirth in most translocation carriers ranges from 5 to 20% (Lejeune *et al.*, 1970). The actual assessment of risk of an abortion or an abnormal child for a carrier of a particular translocation must be based on the reproductive history of the family in which that translocation is segregating.

This will be illustrated in a large family in which several members suffered from an unusually high rate of spontaneous abortion and in which a reciprocal translocation was segregating.

Case report

Patient with three abortions.

Investigation after three abortions:
- Diabetes: negative
- Thyroid function: normal
- Lues, listeria brucella, toxoplasma: negative
- Menstrual cycle: ovulatory
- Hysterosalpingography: normal, except occluded left tube
- Laparoscopy: tiny spots of endometriosis in the cul de sac
- Semenanalyses: $13 \times 10^9/1$
- Sims Hühner-test: slightly positive

Investigation pregnancy 4:
- Ultrasound: empty sac at 11 weeks amenorrhea
- D & C: no fetal parts

Investigation pregnancy 5:
- Ultrasound: normal pregnancy with positive heartaction at 10 weeks
- 18 weeks amenorrhea admission for vaginal bleeding
- Pregnancy uneventful
- 40 weeks amenorrhea. Cesarean section due to cephalic pelvic dysproportion. Healthy boy of 3700 g

Twelve family members had had two or more first trimester abortions. Fetal parts had never been seen in any of the cases.

Cytogenetic investigations

Initial chromosome studies using conventional staining techniques done in 1974 showed both the proposita and her husband to have a normal karyotype. The chromosome investigation was repeated using the banding techniques after the fourth abortion in 1977. The patient was a carrier of a balanced reciprocal translocation between the short arm of chromosome 1 and the short arm of chromosome 20, the breakpoints being in bands 1p36 and 20p11. The karyotype of the patient was 46,XX,t(1;20) (p36;p11) (ISCN, 1978). The size of the segments exchanged between the two chromosomes is so similar that this translocation could not have been detected without the aid of banding techniques. Although both the chromosomes involved in the translocation could be clearly distinguished from their normal partners using G-banding (Figure 10.1), it was not always possible to distinguish the

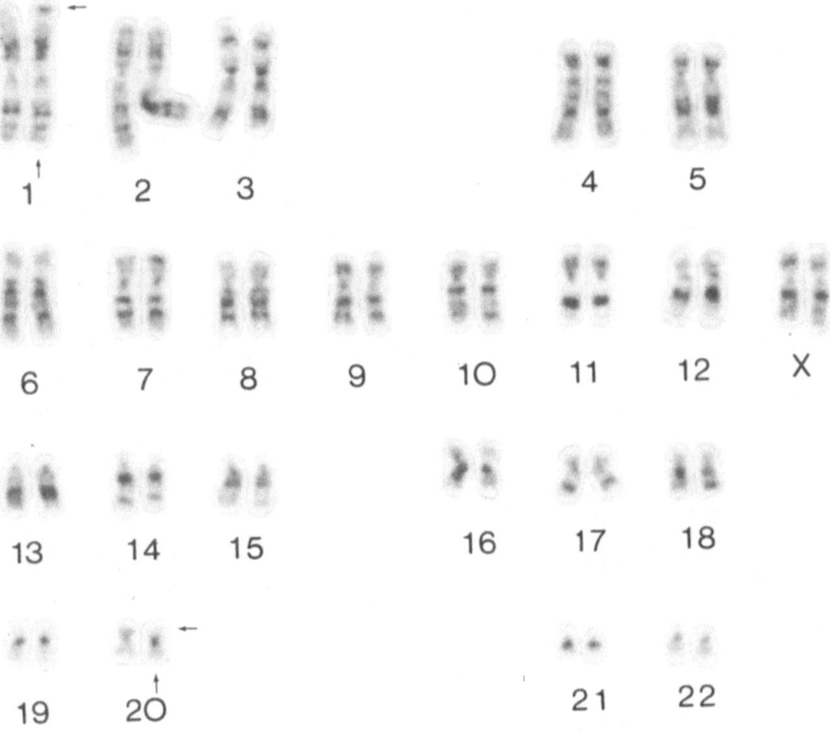

Figure 10.1 G-banded karyotype of the proposita showing a balanced reciprocal translocation between chromosome 1 and 20 46,XX,t(1;20) (p36;p11).

derivative 20 from its normal partner using Q-banding.

Amniocentesis for chromosome analysis was not performed because the patient decided against it. The reason for this was the possible difficulty in detecting a fetus with an unbalanced karyotype that included a derivative 20 in a laboratory that routinely used Q-banding for amniotic cell cultures.

Chromosome analysis on the child after birth revealed the balanced translocation, karyotype: 46,XY,t(1;20) (p36;p11). Chromosome analyses were done on a total of 61 family members including the parents, brothers and sisters and relatives of the mother of the patient (Figure 10.2). All 61 individuals were phenotypically normal. Of these, 29 had a normal karyo-

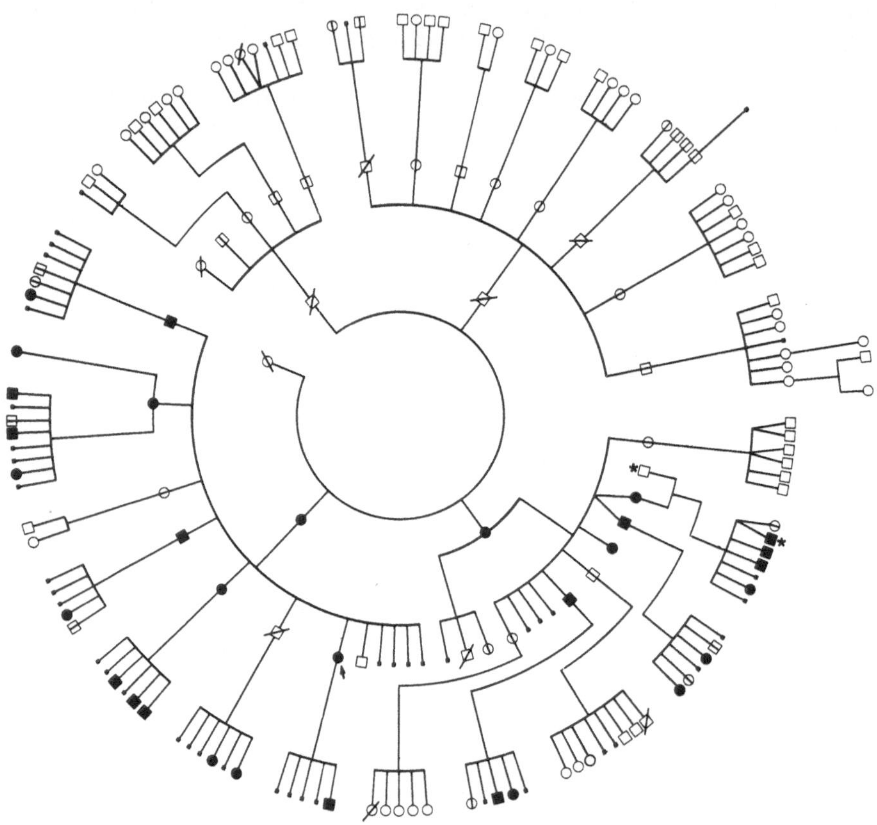

Figure 10.2 Pedigree of the family in which the translocation t(1;20) is segregating. The proposita is indicated by an arrow. Lines ending in a dot denote spontaneous abortions.

type and 31 were carriers of the balanced translocation t(1;20) (p36;p11). One male had a second balanced translocation t(8;22) (q34;q11) inherited from his father in addition to the t(1;20) (p36;p11) inherited from his mother. Chromosome investigation of the father's family is in progress.

Discussion

There appears to be a clear positive correlation between the occurrence of miscarriages and the presence of the translocation in this family. Only one of the 12 couples that had had two or more abortions had a normal karyotype. One of the partners in the other 11 cases was a translocation carrier.

For this particular translocation with exchange of equal segments, with breakpoints close to the end of the chromosomes and with a high chance of chiasma formation in the interstitial segment (between the breakpoint and the centromere) of one of the chromosomes, one would expect a ratio of balanced to unbalanced gametes to be one. Assuming that in this family the abortions were caused by the presence of an unbalanced translocation, the ratio of abortions to liveborns (36:45) is not significantly different from the expected one.

Among the phenotypically normal offspring of translocation heterozygotes the ratio of individuals with a normal karyotype to translocation carriers is expected to be one (Ford and Clegg, 1969; Lejeune *et al.*, 1970). Thus there are more translocation carriers (30) than members with a normal karyotype (13). Although there is an excess of translocation heterozygotes in accumulated data from many different translocation families there is no difference between the progeny of male and female heterozygotes (Ford and Clegg, 1969; Hamerton, 1971).

The ratio of translocation to normal karyotype among progeny of males is 8:6 whereas for females it is 22:7. There is no explanation for this apparent selection of heterozygotes in the female translocation carriers in this family.

Partial monosomy for the terminal segment of 1p36 (Prescott *et al.*, 1975), partial monosomy 20p (Kogame *et al.*, 1978) and partial trisomy 20p (Cohen *et al.*, 1975) are known in liveborn children. However, the combinations of duplication and deficiency arising from this particular translocation appear to be incompatible with life beyond about 12 weeks. None of the 81 pregnancies of translocation carriers has ended in a birth of a child with an unbalanced karyotype. Whereas the risk of abortion appears to be 50 %, the probability of a birth of a child with an unbalanced karyotype for a translocation carrier is very low.

Some individuals have two balanced reciprocal translocations (Bijlsma *et al.*, 1978; Tabor *et al.*, 1981). For the carrier of the double translocation (see Figure 10.2) there is a risk of 75 % for a spontaneous abortion or an abnormal child. However the final risk assessment must await the investigation of chromosomes and of the reproductive history of the family with the second translocation.

CONCLUDING REMARKS

Chromosome studies using banding techniques should be done in couples with fetal wastage. Investigation of chromosomes and reproductive history of the family should be done after a chromosome rearrangement has been found in one of the partners. Carriers of chromosome rearrangements should be offered the option of having any subsequent pregnancies monitored by amniocentesis.

Acknowledgements

We are very grateful to the family members for their willingness and cooperation, to Ms E. Namavar, Ms Y. Heins, Ms G. Favié and Ms E. de Vries for their expert technical assistance and to Mr F. van Oorschot for the collection of material and information during the family study. We thank Mr G. J. Lijnzaad for the careful drawing of the pedigree and Ms H. C. de Jonge for sorting out the references.

References

Antich, J., Clusellas, N., Twose, A. and Godó, R. M. (1980). Chromosomal abnormalities in parents in cases of reproductive failure. *Clin. Genet.*, **17**, 52

Ballesta, F., Fernandez, E. and Mila, M. (1980). Infertility and chromosomal variations. *Clin. Genet.*, **17**, 54

Bijlsma, J. B., de France, H. F., Bleeker-Wagemakers, L. M. and Dijkstra, P. F. (1978). Double translocation t(7;12),t(2;6) heterozygosity in one family: a contribution to the trisomy 12p syndrome. *Hum. Genet.*, **40**, 135

Bortotto, L., Baccichetti, C., Lenzini, E., Tenconi, R., Delendi, N. and Caufin, D. (1980). Cytogenetic survey of couples with habitual abortion and other reproductive wastage. *Clin. Genet.*, **17**, 56

Boué, J. and Boué, A. (1973). Chromosomal analysis of two consecutive abortuses in each of 43 women. *Humangenetik*, **19**, 275

Boué, A. and Boué, J. (1975). Reproductive failure secondary to chromosome abnormalities. *Acta Europ. Fertil.*, **6**, 39

Boué, J., Couillin, P. and Boué, A. (1980). Mechanisms of triploidy. *Clin. Genet.*, **19**, 493

Byrd, J. R., Askew, D. E. and McDonough, P. G. (1977). Cytogenetic findings in fifty-five couples with recurrent fetal wastage. *Fertil. Steril.*, **28**, 246

Carr, D. H. (1970). Chromosome abnormalities and spontaneous abortions. In Jacobs, P. A., Price, W. H. and Law, P. (eds.) *Human Population Cytogenetics*, pp. 103–117. (Edinburgh: Edinburgh University Press)

Chandley, A. C., Seuanez, H. and Fletcher, J. M. (1976). Meiotic behavior of five human reciprocal translocations. *Cytogenet. Cell Genet.*, **17**, 98–111

Chapelle de la, A., Schröder, J., Stenstrand, K., Fellman, J., Herva, R., Saarni, M., Anttolainen, I., Tallila, I., Tervilä, L., Husa, L., Tallqvist, G., Robson, E. B., Cook, P. J. L. and Sanger, R. (1974). Pericentric Inversions of Human Chromosomes 9 and 10. *Am. J. Hum. Genet.*, **26**, 746–766

Cohen, M. M., Davidson, R. G. and Brown, J. A. (1975). A familial F/G translocation [t(20p−;22q+)] observed in three generations. *Clinical Genetics*. **7**, 120–127

Creasy, M. R., Crolla, J. A. and Alberman, E. D. (1976). A Cytogenetic Study of Human Spontaneous Abortions Using Banding Techniques. *Hum. Genet.*, **31**, 177–196

Davis, J. R., Weinstein, L., Veomett, I. C., Shenker, L., Giles, H. R. and Hauck, L. (1982). Balanced translocation karyotypes in patients with repetitive abortion. *Am. J. Obstet. Gynecol.*, Vol. 144, nr. 2, pp. 229–233

Dutrillaux, B. and Lejeune, J. (1970). Etude de la descendance des individus porteurs d'une translocation t(DqDq). *Anales de Génétique*. vol. 13, nr. 1, pp. 11–18
Evans, H. J. (1977). Chromosome anomalies among livebirths. *Journal of Medical Genetics*. **14,** 309–312
Evans, J. A., Canning, N., Hunter, A. G. W., Martsolf, J. T., Ray, M., Thompson, D. R. and Hamerton, J. L. (1978). A cytogenetic survey of 14,069 newborn infants. *Cytogenet. Cell Genet.*, **20,** 96–123
Ferguson-Smith, M. A. (1966). Clinical cytogenetics. In Crow, J. F. and v. Neel, J. (eds.) *Proceedings of the Third International Congress of Human Genetics*, pp. 91–106. (Baltimore: Johns Hopkins UP)
Ford, C. E. (1969). Meiosis in mammals. In Benirschke, K. (ed.) *Comparative Mammalian Cytogenetics*, pp. 91–106. (New York: Springer)
Ford, C. E. and Clegg, H. M. (1969). Reciprocal translocations. *Br. Med. Bull.*, **25,** 110
Gropp, A. (1974). Fetal mortality due to aneuploidy and irregular meiotic segregation in the mouse. In Boué, A. and Thibault, C. (eds.) *Chromosomal Errors in Relation to Reproductive Failure*, pp. 255–269. (Paris: INSERM)
de Grouchy, J., Crippa, L. and German, J. (1970). Etudes autoradiographiques des chromosomes humains. VII. Cinq observations de t (DqDq) familiales. *Ann. Genet.*, **13,** 19
Hamerton, L. J. (1970). Robertsonian translocations. Evidence on segregation from family studies. In Jacobs, P. A., Price, W. H. and Law, P. (eds.) *Human Population Cytogenetics*, pp. 63–80. (Edinburgh: Edinburgh University Press)
Hamerton, J. L. (1971). *Human Cytogenetics*. Vol. 1, pp 254–272. (New York and London: Academic Press)
Heritage, D. W., English, S. C., Young, R. B. and Chen, A. T. L. (1978). Cytogenetics of recurrent abortions. *Fertil. Steril.*, **29,** 414
Hertig, A. T. and Rock, J. (1949). A series of potentially abortive ova recovered from fertile women prior to the first missed menstrual period. *Am. J. Obstet. Gynecol.*, **58,** 968
Hertig, A. T. and Sheldow, W. H. (1943). Minimal criteria required to prove prima facie case of traumatic abortion and miscarriage: an analysis of 1000 spontaneous abortions. *Ann. Surg.*, **117,** 596
Husslein, P., Huber, J., Wagenbichler, P. and Schnedl, W. (1982). Chromosome abnormalities in 150 couples with multiple spontaneous abortions. *Fertil. Steril.*, **37,** 379
ISCN (1978). An International System for Human Cytogenetics Nomenclature. *Cytogenet. Cell Genet.*, **21,** 311
Jacobs, P. A., Angell, R. R., Buchanan, I. M., Hassold, T. J., Matsuyama, A. M. and Manuel, B. (1978). The origin of human triploids. *Ann. Hum. Genet.*, **42,** 49
Jalbert, P., Sele, B. and Jalbert, H. (1980). Reciprocal translocations: a way to predict the mode of imbalanced segregation by pachytene-diagram drawing. *Hum. Genet.*, **55,** 209
Kajii, T. and Ferrier, A. (1978). Cytogenetics of aborters and abortuses. *Am. J. Obstet. Gynecol.*, **131,** 33
Kardon, N. B., Davis, J. G., Berger, A. L. and Broekman, A. (1980). Incidence of chromosomal rearrangements in couples with reproductive loss. *Hum. Genet.*, **53,** 161
Kim, H. J., Hsu, L. Y. F., Paciuc, S., Cristian, S., Quintana, A. and Hirschhorn, K. (1975). Cytogenetics of fetal wastage. *N. Engl. J. Med.*, **293,** 844
Kogame, K., Fukuhara, T., Maeda, A. and Kudo, Y. (1978). A partial short arm deletion of chromosome 20:46,XY,del (20) (p11). *Jpn. J. Human Genet.*, **23,** 153
Lauritsen, J. G. (1976). Aetiology of spontaneous abortion. A cytogenetic and epidemiological study of 288 abortuses and their parents. *Acta Obstet. Gynaecol. Scand. Suppl.* 52
Lejeune, J., Dutrillaux, B. and de Grouchy, J. (1970). Reciprocal translocations in human populations. A preliminary analysis. In Jacobs, P. A., Price, W. H. and Law, P. (eds.) *Human Population Cytogenetics*, pp. 81–87. (Edinburgh: Edinburgh University Press)
Lindenbaum, P. H. and Bobrow, M. (1975). Review article: reciprocal translocations in man. 3 : 1 meiotic disjunction resulting in 47- or 45-chromosome offspring. *J. Med. Genet.*, **12,** 29
Madan, K. and Bobrow, M. (1974). Structural variation in chromosome no. 9. *Ann. Genet.*, **17,** 81
Matton, M., Verschraegen-Spae, M. R., de Bie, S. and van den Wijngaert, J. (1980). Incidence of T carriers amongst couples with repetitive abortion, after exclusion of any other etiology. *Clin. Gen.*, **17.** 78
Mennuti, M. T., Jingeleski, S., Schwarz, R. H. and Mellman, W. J. (1978). An evaluation of

cytogenetic analysis as a primary tool in the assessment of recurrent pregnancy wastage. *Obstet. Gynecol.*, **52,** 308

Neu, R. L., Entes, K. and Bannerman, R. M. (1979). Chromosome analysis in cases with repeated spontaneous abortions. *Obstet. Gynecol.*, **53,** 373

Prescott, G. H., McCaw, B. K., Tolby, B. E., Hecht, F., Miller, R. C., Greene, A. E. and Coriell, L. L. (1975). A (1;15) translocation, balanced, 46 chromosomes. Repository identification No GM-126. *Cytogenet. Cell Genet.*, **14,** 84

Reinisch, L. C., Silvey, K. L. and Dumars, K. W. (1981). Sex chromosome mosaicism in couples with repeated fetal loss. *Am. J. Hum. Genet.*, **33,** 117A

Sant-Cassia, L. J. and Cooke, P. (1981). Chromosomal analysis of couples with repeated spontaneous abortions. *Br. J. Obstet. Gynaecol.*, **88,** 52

Schmid, W. (1980). Cytogenetic results in 96 couples with repeated abortions. *Clin. Genet.*, **17,** 85

Schmidt, R., Nitowsky, H. M. and Dar, H. (1976). Cytogenetic studies in reproductive loss. *J. Am. Med. Assoc.*, **236,** 369

Simpson, J. L., Elias, S. and Martin, A. O. (1981). Parental chromosomal rearrangements associated with repetitive spontaneous abortions. *Fertil. Steril.*, **36,** 584

Stoll, C., Flori, E., Rumpler, Y. and Warter, S. (1980). Cytogenetic findings in 217 couples with recurrent fetal wastage. *Clin. Genet.*, **17,** 88

Subrt, I. (1980). Reciprocal translocation with special reference to reproductive failure. *Hum. Genet.*, **55,** 303

Sutherland, G. R., Gardiner, S. J. and Carter, R. F. (1976). Familial pericentric inversion of chromosome 19, inv(19) (p13q13) with a note on genetic counselling of pericentric inversion carriers. *Clin. Genet.*, **10,** 54

Tabor, A., Jensen, L. K., Lundsteen, C. and Niebuhr, E. (1981). A 5;7, 5:12 double reciprocal translocation in a normal mother and a 5;7 translocation with a recombinant chromosome 5 in her normal child. *J. Med. Genet.*, **18,** 307

Tho, P. T., Byrd, J. R. and McDonough, P. G. (1979). Etiologies and subsequent reproductive performance of 100 couples with recurrent abortion. *Fertil. Steril.*, **32,** 389

Tsenghi, C., Metaxotou-Stavridaki, C., Strataki-Benetou, M., Kalpini-Mavrou, A. and Matsaniotis, N. (1976). Chromosome studies in couples with repeated spontaneous abortions. *Obstet. Gynecol.*, **47,** 463

Turleau, C., Chavin-Colin, F. and de Grouchy, J. (1979). Cytogenetic investigation in 413 couples with spontaneous abortions. *Europ. J. Obstet. Gynec. Reprod. Biol.*, **9,** 65

Vine, D. T., Yarkoni, S. and Cohen, M. M. (1976). Inversion homozygosity of chromosome no. 9 in highly inbred kindred. *Am. J. Hum. Genet.*, **28,** 203

Ward, B. E., Henry, G. P. and Robinson, A. (1980). Cytogenetic studies in 100 couples with recurrent spontaneous abortions. *Am. J. Hum. Genet.*, **32,** 549

Winsor, E. J. T., Palmer, C. G., Ellis, P. M., Hunter, J. L. P. and Ferguson-Smith, M. (1978). Meiotic analysis of a pericentric inversion, inv(7) (p22q32), in the father of a child with a duplication-deletation of chromosome 7. *Cytogenet. Cell Genet.*, **29,** 169

11
Chromosome mutations and fetal wastage

P. HUSSLEIN, W. SCHNEDL and P. WAGENBICHLER

About one in five fertilizations ends as a spontaneous abortion (Poland *et al.*, 1977). The most common cause for fetal wastage could be identified in numeric and structural chromosome aberrations and in polyploid (mostly triploid and tetraploid) embryos (Boué *et al.*, 1975; Kajii *et al.*, 1973). About 50% of all spontaneous abortions are caused by such a chromosomal abnormality (Byrd *et al.*, 1977; Breuker *et al.*, 1978; Tsenghi *et al.*, 1976; Kim *et al.*, 1975; Turleau *et al.*, 1979), whereas the others have miscellaneous origins, e.g. lethal dominant mutations deficiencies in the endocrine system of the mother, infections or immunological factors (Lauritsen, 1976; Lucas *et al.*, 1972).

Not all fetuses with chromosome aberrations are aborted. Few chromosomally aberrant fetuses are born full term. Since only few types of aberrations are compatible with survival, only certain typical syndromes are liveborn. The most frequent liveborn aberration is the trisomy 21, the Down syndrome. Some of these viable aberrations are also frequently noted in spontaneous abortion. For example in Turner syndrome about 95% of the fetuses are aborted; the remaining cases are born alive and can be expected to have a passable life.

ORIGIN OF CHROMOSOMALLY ABERRANT EMBRYOS

Chromosome aberrations occur in all dividing cells, and in everybody's cells they will occur at a small rate. To give rise to an embryo composed at least in a large proportion of aberrant cells, the chromosome error (chromosome mutation) must have taken place in a 'bottleneck' of cell development. Thus only aberrations that are occurring during gametogenesis (meiosis or the preceding mitotic divisions) or in the very early embryonic stages will result in an embryo with a generalized chromosome aberration. Moreover, meiosis is a mode of chromosome division permitting the origination of structural chromosome aberrations, which can hardly ever be produced in mitosis. Theoretically triploid zygotes may arise not only by mitotic and meiotic failures, but also from dispermy.

Three types of errors in cell division may be involved in the production of an aberrant embryo: (1) non-disjunction, (2) chromosome mutation and (3) failure of haploidization during meiosis.

Non-disjunction

Non-disjunction may take place either in mitosis or meiosis. It consists in a failure of sister chromatids in mitosis, or of the paired chromosomes in meiosis, to be distributed regularly during division. In both cases the division products will show a complementary numerical chromosome aberration. What is missing in one cell will be supernumerary in the other.

Chromosome mutations

In contrast to gene mutation, genes are not affected by chromosome mutations, but the proportion of a great number of the genes within the cell

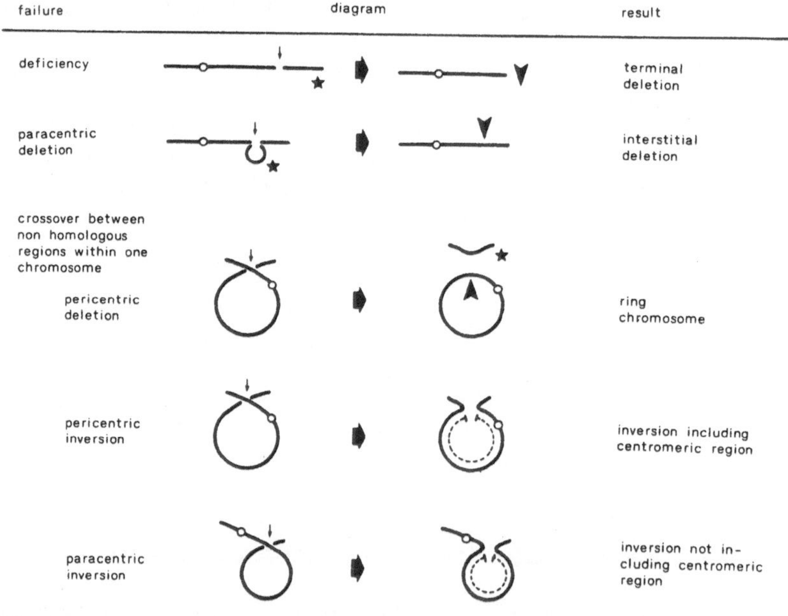

Figure 11.1 Origin of chromosome aberrations due to meiotic failures within one chromosome. In *terminal deletion* a terminal chromosome segment is lost due to a break. This fragment cannot be transported in the following divisions since it does not contain a centromere. Interstitial deletion is the result of two paracentric breaks and fusion of the distal parts of the chromosome and loss of the interstitial (acentric) fragment. *Ring chromosomes* arise by cross-over within the same chromosome. Fusion of the distal ends results in an acentric fragment, which is lost. By fusion of the pericentric segments the ring is formed. *Pericentric inversions* have a similar origin. The fusion of the segments involved, however, does not result in loss of chromosomal material, but in the formation of a chromosome, where a region including the centromere is inserted upside down in the chromosome. *Paracentric inversions* are comparable events occurring in the distal segments of chromosomes not including the centromere.

will be shifted, as in chromosome non-disjunction. Chromosome mutations can be explained by chromosome breaks and by irregular pairing of homologues during meiosis including cross-over-like events in the regions involved. Various types of chromosome mutations are illustrated in Figures 11.1 and 11.2.

Some events in chromosome mutations are harmful to the embryo arising from the damaged gamete. Usually the loss of genetic material (terminal or interstitial deletions, ring chromosomes) is not compatible with life. Only in the case of the Robertsonian translocation, the loss of the small segment containing the short arms of the fusing chromosomes does not have harmful effects to the individual.

Balanced structural mutations (reciprocal translocations, paracentric and pericentric inversions) may result in a genome with the normal diploid number of each gene. Some apparently balanced aberrations, as for instance in the short arm of chromosome No. 5, may have severe effects on the carrier.

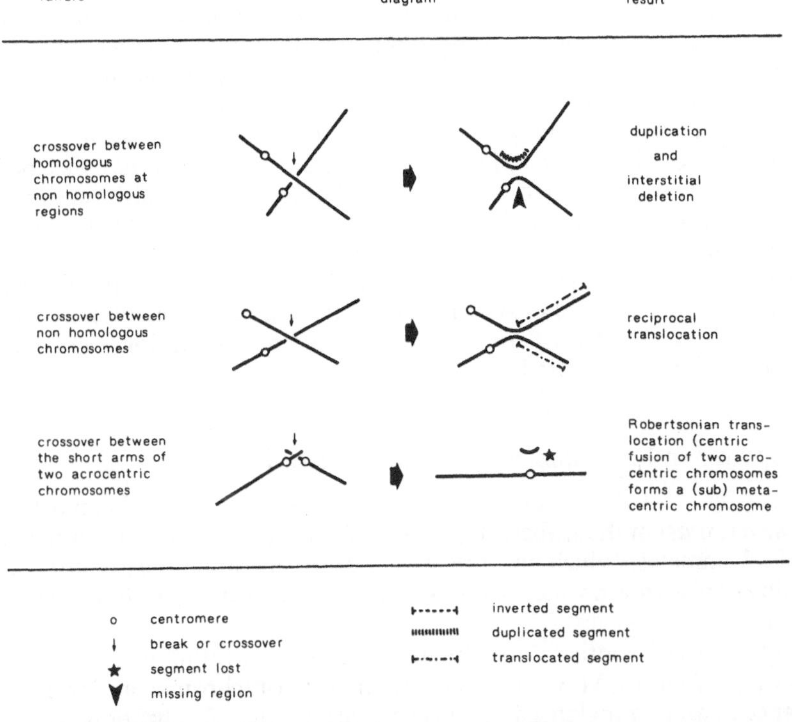

Figure 11.2 Origin of chromosome aberrations due to meiotic failures involving two chromosomes (either homologous or non-homologous chromosomes). *Duplication* and *interstitial deletions* may result by cross-over between homologous chromosomes at non-homologous regions. The segment lost by one chromosome is inserted into the other homologue, resulting in duplication of the segment involved. *Reciprocal translocation* is due to exchange of chromosome segments between non-homologous chromosomes after an irregular cross-over event. In *Robertsonian translocation* two acrocentric chromosomes fuse by loss of the small short arms. Only one of the centromeres remains active.

Failure of haploidization during meiosis

Triploidy is found in about 20% of chromosomally abnormal abortuses (Carr, 1971). The majority of these cases has a 69,XXY chromosome set. The supernumerary haploid chromosome set may cause failure in the first or second meiotic division. These and other possibilities of origin are under discussion (Niebuhr, 1974).

Tetraploidy is more likely the result of a failure in mitosis of very early embryonic cells. Embryonic cells tend to polyploidization as can be frequently observed in cell culture for prenatal chromosome analysis.

TYPES AND FATE OF CHROMOSOMALLY ABNORMAL EMBRYOS

The majority of chromosomally abnormal abortuses is the result of a *de novo* aberration. In these cases no abnormality is found in the somatic cells of the parents. Only in few cases is the chromosome aberration of the embryo caused by a generalized balanced chromosome mutation is one parent.

The fate of a chromosomally abnormal fetus depends on the type of the chromosome mutation. Balanced aberrations will be compatible with survival, but a small percentage will show abnormalities after birth.

Unbalanced aberrations will be aborted in the majority of the cases, but the few fetuses coming to birth will show more or less severe malformations and psychomotoric retardation depending on the type and extent of chromosome aberration.

There is no direct correlation between the length and the genetic importance of chromosome segment. A very short unbalanced segment may be not compatible with life, whereas in other regions rather long unbalanced segments may be tolerated.

Offspring in balanced aberration carriers

The carrier of a balanced chromosome mutation is not affected in most cases. However, most of these aberrations may result in chromosomally unbalanced haploid gametes, which in turn give rise to an abnormal embryo after fertilization with a normal haploid gamete of the other parent (Sinet *et al.*, 1973).

Examples of meiotic failure due to balanced aberration in the carrier are shown in Figures 11.3–11.5. The frequency of chromosomally normal, balanced and unbalanced embryos within the fertilization products of a balanced translocation carrier is dependent on the chromosome involved and on the localization of the translocation points (Boué, 1981). The frequencies of meiotic failure in the same translocation may be also different in males and females. The risk depends therefore on the question of whether the carrier is the father or the mother. Still more information is required to give a definite risk evaluation in a given balanced translocation.

Some aberrations do not interfere with meiosis. For instance, the frequent

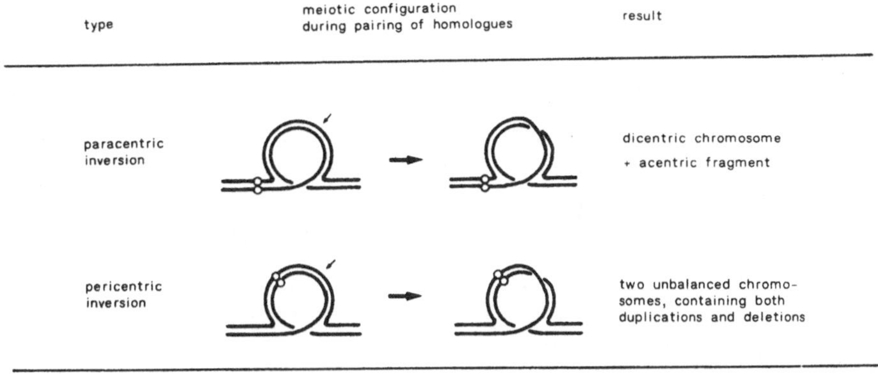

Figure 11.3 Meiotic failures due to balanced chromosome aberrations. Failures resulting from paracentric and pericentric inversions. Simplified diagram, only one chromatid of each chromosome shown. Since one of the homologues contains an inverted region, pairing with the other (normal) homologue is feasible only by formation of a loop. If crossover takes place in this loop, various unbalanced chromosomes, dicentrics and acentric fragments will be formed.

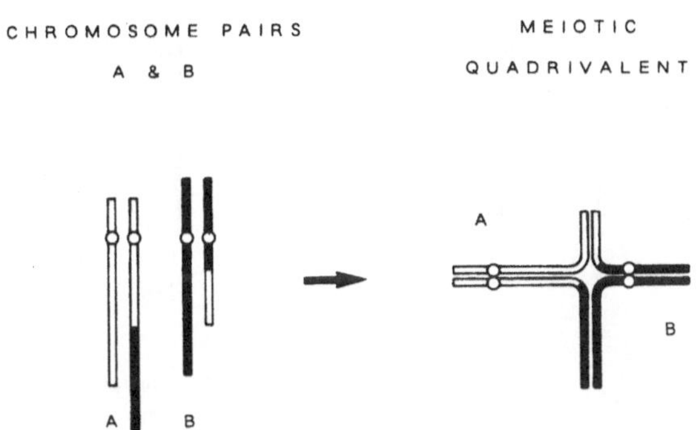

Figure 11.4 Meiotic failures due to balanced chromosome aberrations. Pairing of homologous chromosomes carrying reciprocal translocations during 1st meiotic division. Chromosome regions belonging to chromosome A white, those belonging to chromosome B black. Since all homologous regions tend to pair, a quadrivalent is formed during preparation for 1st meiotic division.

pericentric inversion of the heterochromatic segment in chromosome 9 does not give rise to aberrant fetuses. The same is true for structural mutations of the Y chromosome.

A special situation is noted in Robertsonian translocations. Fusions between different acrocentric chromosomes will result in about 10% abnormal fetuses, if the translocation is present in the maternal chromosome set. Robertsonian translocations in the father's karyotype will show only a

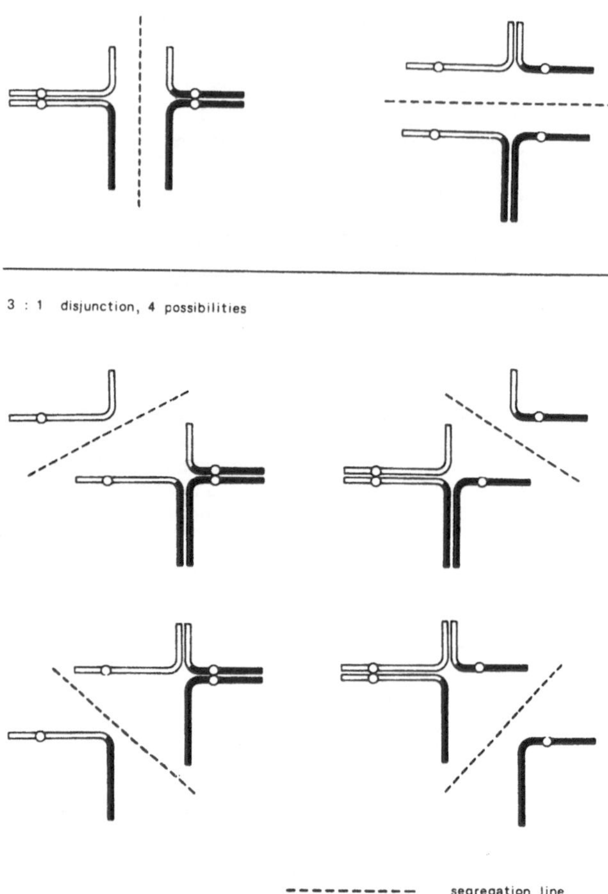

Figure 11.5 Meiotic failures due to balanced chromosome aberrations. Modes of chromosome distribution during 1st meiotic division resulting in unbalanced gametes. Both in 2:2 disjunction and 3:1 disjunction (classified by segregation of centromeres) unbalanced gametes will result. It should be kept in mind that other possibilities, resulting in balanced or even normal gametes, do exist.

very low risk for unbalanced offspring (about 1% (Murken and Stengel-Rutkowski, 1982)).

A centric fusion between homologous chromosomes is an absolute obstacle to the production of normal offspring. The gametes of a carrier may or may not contain this double chromosome. After fertilization with a normal gamete of the other sex the embryo will be either trisomic or monosomic for the chromosome affected. Most of these aberrations are fatal to the embryo. The few fetuses coming to birth alive will show the typical features of the trisomy for the chromosome involved. No normal offspring are to be expected from a parent carrying a centric fusion between two homologue acrocentric chromosomes.

CYTOGENETIC ASPECTS OF HABITUAL ABORTION

Owing to repetitive fetal wastage, 208 couples were examined in a cytogenetic laboratory. Children who had a chromosomal aberration were excluded from this report. This was done to prevent selection for causes of infertility.

In all 208 instances, peripheral blood cultures of both partners were prepared. The chromosome preparations were analysed after applying a trypsin-G-band method. In each individual, a minimum of 20 metaphase plates was counted, and at least five cells were karyotyped.

Included in the study were couples with two or more first-trimester abortions only, couples with repeated abortions and intrauterine fetal death or fetal malformation, and couples with repeated abortions and live offspring. The frequencies of chromosome abortions found in these groups are given in Table 11.1.

Among the 208 couples, 11 major chromosomal abnormalities were found (Table 11.1 and Figure 11.6). Eight aberrations were found in the females; three occurred in the male partner. In six cases balanced reciprocal translocations between non-homologous autosomes were found. One case showed centric fusion within one homologous chromosome pair, in one case a pericentric inversion was found and in four patients gonosomal mosaicism was found (one of which also had a reciprocal translocation).

Chromosome polymorphism in the form of enlarged satellites, secondary constrictions, other heterochromatic segments, or other non-systematic anomalies, such as a slightly increased frequency of chromosome breakage, are of less clinical significance.

The male partners of two aborters had pericentric inversion of the heterochromatic part of chromosome 9. Therefore, this inversion, which is usually considered a polymorphism, occurs in 0.5% of the patients.

CLINICAL CONSIDERATIONS

The finding of a balanced chromosome abnormality in course of a screening study in a random population is a very rare event. When screening couples with repetitive fetal wastage, mostly aberrations with a high risk for chromosomally inbalanced gametes will be recorded (Ward *et al.*, 1980). Therefore, only poor information is available on balanced structural aberrations with no or moderate risk of generating imbalanced offspring.

Nevertheless, different groups of balanced aberrations may be classified from the standpoint of risk magnitude.

(1) Translocations with no chance of generating a healthy offspring. This situation is found virtually only in Robertsonian translocations between homologous chromosomes.

Table 11.1 Frequencies of chromosome aberrations in 208 couples with recurrent abortions

Reason for referral	*No. of couples*	*Frequency of pathologic findings*	*Chromosome aberration of parent*
2 spontaneous abortions	53	–	–
3 spontaneous abortions	78	3(3.9%)	46,XX,t(7;22)(p21;q11) 46,XY,inv.10(p12;q21) Mosaicism 46.XX/47,XXX/45,X
4 and more spontaneous abortions	50	3(6.0%)	Mosaicism 46,XX,t(7;8)(p21;q23)/ 47,XXX,t(7;8)(p21;q23) 45,XY,t(22;22) Mosaicism 46,XX/45,X
Abortions and intrauterine fetal death or fetal malformation	14	2(14.3%)	46,XX.t(11;14)(q21;q13) 46,XX,t(13;18)(q22;p11)
Abortions and normal live offspring	13	3(23.1%)	46,XX,t(11;22)(q25;q13) 46,XX,t(6;20)(q23;p13) Mosaicism 46,XY/47,XXY
Totals	208	11(5.3%)	

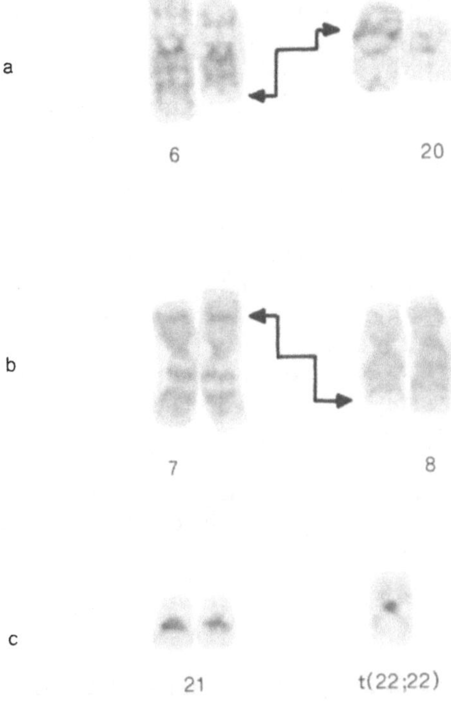

Figure 11.6 Examples of balanced structural chromosome aberrations. Trypsin–Giemsa-banding. Only chromosome pairs involved are shown. **a**, Case 5; 46,XX,t(6;20) (q23;p13). **b**, Case 6: mosaicism 46,XX,t(7;8) (p21;q23)/47,XXX,t(7;8) **c**, Case 7: 45,XX,t(22;22). For comparison, the normal chromosome pair No. 21 is shown.

(2) Translocations with high risk (up to 30%). Examples for such translocations can be found in the literature (Murken and Stengel-Rutkowski, 1982). In the 'high risk' group, it is necessary to consider whether all developing imbalanced embryos will be aborted spontaneously, or if some of them could be liveborn, showing severe malformations and psychomotoric retardation.

(3) Translocation with a moderate risk (below 5%). (For additional references see Murken and Stengel-Rutkowski, 1982).

(4) Translocations with very little or no risk. These are the cases with Robertsonian translocation in the male parent, and pericentric inversions of the heterochromatic segment in chromosome 9 and Y.

At present, a general screening for chromosome abnormalities in the population is not feasible. Therefore the search for balanced aberrations has to be limited to couples with increased probability for a chromosome mutation. After excluding cases where other causes are the likely cause for multiple fetal wastage, couples with more than two spontaneous abortions and/or stillbirths, malformed children and so on should be analysed.

Balanced chromosome mutations where only abortions or malformed children can be generated are very rare. Therefore, an apparently healthy child in addition to several spontaneous abortions and/or malformed children is no proof for the absence of a chromosome mutation in one parent. If a malformed offspring is born, the first step in evaluation of the situation should be chromosome analysis in the child affected. The absence of a chromosome aberration in the child makes the presence of a balanced aberration in one parent very unlikely. If only spontaneous abortions are observed, chromosome analysis in the abortus material can be done. Since such studies are difficult, chromosome analysis in the parents seems to be the preferable recommendation in such cases.

The consequence of a verified balanced chromosome aberration in a couple with multiple fetal wastage is twofold, depending on the type of aberration. In those cases where no normal offspring can be expected, the carrier of the aberrations should be sterilized. In the majority, however, normal children, or at least chromosomally balanced offspring, are possible. In these cases prenatal chromosome analysis should be conducted in every pregnancy.

References

Boué, A. (1981). European data collection. Presented at *6th International Congress of Human Genetics*, Jerusalem. (Abstr.)

Boué, J., Boué, A. and Lazar, P. (1975). The epidemiology of human spontaneous abortions with chromosomal anomalies. In Blandau, R. J. (ed.) *Aging Gametes – Their Biology and Pathology*, (Basel: Karger) pp. 330–348.

Breuker, K. H., Winkhaus-Schindl, I. and Citoler, P. (1978). Chromosomenanomalien bei Ehepaaren mit wiederholten Aborten. *Geburts. Frauenheilk.*, **38**, 11

Byrd, J. A., Askew, D. E. and McDonough, P. G. (1977). Cytogenetic findings in fifty-five couples with recurrent fetal wastage. *Fertil. Steril.*, **28**, 246

Carr, D. H. (1971). Chromosome studies in selected spontaneous abortions. Polyploidy in man. *J. Med. Genet.*, **8**, 164

Kajii, T., Ohama, K., Niikawa, N., Ferrier, A. and Avirachan, S. (1973). Banding analysis of normal karyotypes in spontaneous abortion. *Am. J. Hum. Genet.*, **25**, 539

Kim, H. J., Hsu, L. Y. F., Paciue, S., Christian, S., Quintana, A. and Hirschhorn, K. (1975). Cytogenetics of fetal wastage. *N. Engl. J. Med.*, **293**, 844

Lauritsen, J. G. (1976). Aetiology of spontaneous abortion: a cytogenetic study of 288 abortions and their parents. *Acta Obstet. Gynecol. Scand. Suppl.*, **52**, 1

Lucas, M., Wallace, I. and Hirschhorn, K. (1972). Recurrent abortions and chromosome abnormalities. *J. Obstet. Gynaecol. Br. Commonw.*, **79**, 1119

Murken, J. and Stengel-Rutkowski, S. (1982). Pränatale Diagnostik genetisch bedingter Defekte, 16. Informationsblatt der Deutschen Forschungsgemeinschaft, München. Abteilung für pädiatrische Genetik, Kinderklinik der Universität, Goethestraße 29, D-8000 München 2

Niebuhr, E. (1974). Triploidy in man. *Humangenetik*, **21**, 103

Poland, B., Miller, J. R., Jones, O. C. and Trimble, B. K. (1977). Reproductive counseling in patients who have had a spontaneous abortion. *Am. J. Obstet. Gynecol.*, **127**, 685

Sinet, P. M., Dutrilleaux, B., Prieur, M. and Lejeune, J. (1973). Rôle des translocations parentales en cas de fausses couches à répétitions. *Rev. Fr. Gynecol.*, **68**, 655

Tsenghi, C., Metaxotou-Stauridaki, C., Strataki-Benetou, M., Kaplin-Mavrou, A. and Matsaniotis, N. (1976). Chromosome studies in couples with repeated spontaneous abortions. *Obstet. Gynecol.*, **47**, 463

Turleau, C., Chavin-Colin, F. and de Grouchy, J. (1979). Cytogenetic investigation in 418 couples with spontaneous abortions. *Eur. J. Obstet. Gynecol. Reprod. Biol.*, **9**, 65

Ward, B. E., Henry, G. P. and Robinson, A. (1980). Cytogenetic studies in 108 couples with recurrent spontaneous abortions. *Am. J. Hum. Genet.*, **32**, 549

12
Chrosome abnormalities and advanced maternal age

K. TSUJI

The incidence of infants with congenital anomalies, perinatal deaths and spontaneous abortions increases with the advancing age of the mother. The types of congenital anomalies are Down's syndrome, congenital heart defects and hydrocephalus. In some cases of spontaneous abortions the abnormal embryos are often found when the mothers' ages are over 40. Hydatidiform moles also occur in older pregnant women. The relationship between the conceptuses of older pregnant women and chromosomal anomalies is discussed.

INDUCED ABORTION

Chromosome abnormalities in induced abortions are few compared to spontaneous abortions. When embryos were collected as materials for cytogenetic survey, without considering the maternal age, the incidence of abnormal karyotypes was 1.5% (Sasaki *et al.*, 1971; Hahnemann, 1973; Tonomura *et al.*, 1973; Ohama, 1978). However, little attention has been directed to the early stage of pregnancy, with regard to surveying the increased chromosome abnormalities in relationship to the advancing age of the mother.

Chromosome abnormalities in cases of induced abortions were studied in women, aged 35 years and older, who were considered to have oocytes of advancing age. No signs of threatened or spontaneous abortions were observed in any of these cases. The embryonic tissues were identified in all cases (Tsuji, 1978; Tsuji and Ichinoe, 1978; Tsuji and Nakano, 1978; Fujimoto *et al.*, 1978). Chromosomal anomalies were found to be 2.1% in the 35–39 year age group, 6.1% in the 40–44 year age group, and 25.0% in the 45–49 year age group (Table 12.1). All the abnormal karyotypes except one triploidy were autosomal trisomies, mainly trisomy 21 and 18. Chromosomal anomalies increase in older pregnant women, especially in premenopausal pregnancies.

Table 12.1 Karyotypes and incidence of fetal chromosomal anomalies in various maternal age groups

Maternal age (y)	*No. of cases*	*Abnormal karyotypes*	*Incidence* (%)
35–39-y group			3/145(2.1%)
35	32		
36	31	(69,XXX)	
37	25		
38	31	(47,XX,+21) (47,XX,+21)	
39	26		
40–44-y group			8/131(6.1%)
40	45	(47,XX,+21) (47,XX,+21)	
41	33	(47,XY,+18)	
42	26	(47,XY,+13) (47,XY,+21)	
43	14	(47,XY,+18) (47,XY,+21)	
44	13	(47,XX,+9)	
45–49-y group			4/16 (25.0%)
45	8	(47,XY,+18) (47,XX,+21)	
46	4	(47,XX,+15)	
47	1		
48	2	(47,XX,+18)	
49	1		
Total	292	15	15/292(5.2%)

SPONTANEOUS ABORTION

There is a positive relationship between the rate of spontaneous abortion and advanced maternal age. At the maternal age of 44 years and over the rate is 33% of pregnancies, and 80% at the age of 47 years and over (Stanton, 1956). The proportion of cases in which the fetus is normal at the time of spontaneous abortion is 3% at age 40 and over, as compared to 33% under age 25. In the case of an abnormal embryo and an empty intact chorion, the proportion increases when the mothers are 40 and over (MacMahon *et al.*, 1954).

A cytogenetic survey of 2439 abortuses (Boué and Boué, 1975; Creasy *et al.*, 1976) revealed 1208 cases (49.5%) with abnormal karyotypes, i.e., autosomal trisomy (26.2%); polyploidy (triploidy, 9.1%; tetraploidy, 2.8%); monosomy

(45,X, 8.6%); translocation and others (2.8%). The mean maternal age in abortuses with autosomal trisomy was very high in mothers at 31.3 years of age as compared to 26.8–27.6 years of age with the other karyotypes (Boué and Boué, 1975). Only autosomal trisomy seems to be influenced by the maternal age.

If the spontaneous abortuses account for 20% of all the pregnancies, 10% have chromosomal anomalies. Since the incidence of the newborn infants with abnormal chromosomes is 0.6%, 95% of all the conceptuses with chromosomal anomalies end in spontaneous abortion.

HYDATIDIFORM MOLE

Hydatidiform moles often occur in older pregnant women. The incidence of hydatidiform moles increases after the age of 40; after 45, the rate is over 10 times that at the maternal age of 20–30 (Figure 12.1, A). Hydatidiform mole (complete) is an abortus associated with an abnormal karyotype, which shows exclusively 46,XX, but in a few cases 46,XY is found. The chromosomal complement of the diploid is androgenic in origin, probably by a diploid spermatozoon or by duplication of haploid (Kajii and Ohama, 1977). It appears that the chromosome in the oocyte is absent (lost) or inactivated.

High potential for malignant changes of hydatidiform mole after the age of 40 has been described (Ichinoe *et al.*, 1979; Kawashima *et al.*, 1979). Cytogenetic studies in cases of complete hydatidiform mole were made (Tsuji *et al.*, 1981). The rate of occurrence of aneuploid cells between 2n and 4n in the 18–39 age group of mothers was 13% of the total cells; the rate in the 43–52 age group was 23% (Figure 12.2). Therefore, the hydatidiform mole is more apt to undergo malignant transformation in mothers over 40 years of age.

PRENATAL DIAGNOSIS

High frequencies of chromosomal anomalies in the fetuses of mothers 40 years old and over are evident (Table 12.2). The incidences of chromosomal anomalies in prenatal diagnosis are 2.4% in mothers 35 and over (Polani *et al.*, 1976; Goldman *et al.*, 1977; Golbus *et al.*, 1979; Daniel *et al.*, 1982), 6.2% in mothers 38 and over (Wirtz *et al.*, 1978), and 14% in those 40 and over (Meredith *et al.*, 1978). Many of the fetuses with abnormal karyotypes show trisomy 21 and 18, 47,XXY and 47,XXX. Fetuses with an extra chromosome are found predominantly in the prenatal chromosome studies of women aged 40 and over.

PERINATAL DEATH

Perinatal death increases with the advance in maternal age. Six percent of the infants dying during the perinatal period have abnormal karyotypes which show trisomy 18 (33%), translocations (18%), trisomy 21 (10%), and others

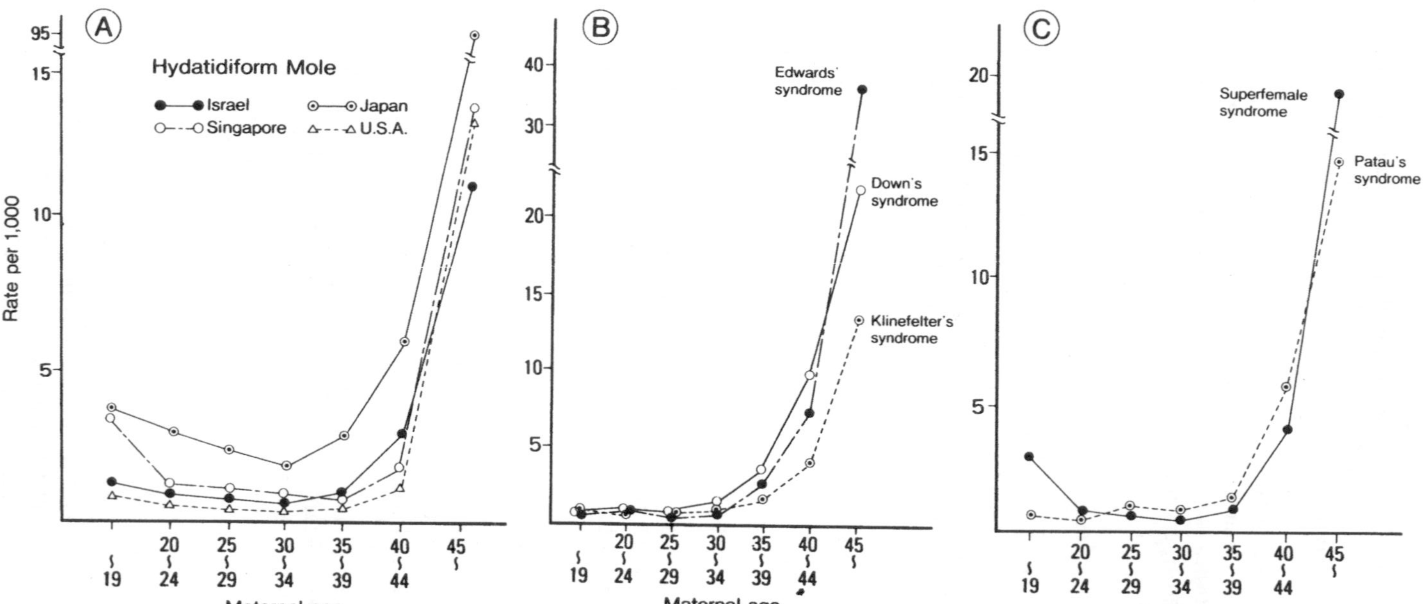

Figure 12.1 Incidence of hydatidiform mole (A) and newborn infants (B; C) with chromosome abnormalities to maternal age. A, Incidence of hydatidiform moles per 1000 livebirths increases when the pregnant women are 40 and over in Israel (Matalon and Modan, 1972), Japan (Ichinoe *et al.*, 1979), Singapore (Teoh *et al.*, 1971) and USA (Yen and MacMahon, 1968). B, Rates (per 1000) of Edwards' syndrome (Lenz *et al.*, 1966), Down's syndrome (Collmann and Stoller, 1962) and Klinefelter's syndrome (Lenz *et al.*, 1966) increase when the mother's age is 35 or over. C, rates (per 1000) of superfemale syndrome and Patau's syndrome (Lenz *et al.*, 1966) also increase when the mother's age is 40 or over.

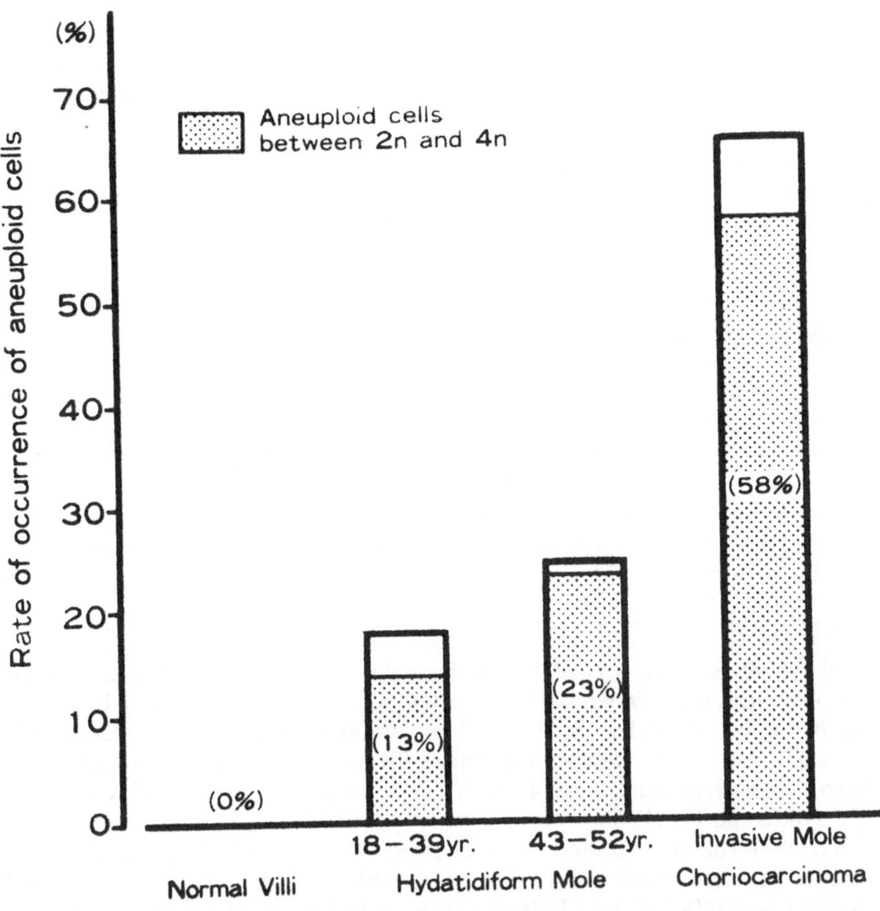

Figure 12.2 Rate of aneuploid cells of the total cells observed for chromosome count in normal villi and trophoblastic diseases.

(39 %). Chromosome abnormalities in those infants also increase with the advancing age of the pregnant women. In cases of mothers over 40 years of age one of three infants dying during this period has a chromosome abnormality, which is mainly trisomy (Table 12.2).

LIVE BIRTH

In some types of congenital malformation, i.e. Down's syndrome, congenital heart defects, cleft lip and/or palate, hydrocephalus, there is an increased incidence with advanced maternal age (Hay and Barbano, 1972). Down's syndrome, which occurs frequently when mothers are over 35, is the most dramatic. Chromosome abnormalities in newborn infants total 0.6 % (Jacobs

Table 12.2 Chromosome abnormalities in prenatal studies and in studies of infants dying in the perinatal period with advancing maternal age

Country	*Maternal age* (y)	*Incidence of abnormal karyotype* (%)
1. Infants in prenatal diagnosis		
Australia*	35–39	2
	40–42	2
	43–45	9
USA†	35–39	2
	40–44	3
	45–49	13
Netherlands‡	35–40	4
	41–43	6
	44–46	22
2. Infants dying during the perinatal period		
England§	20–29	6
	30–39	8
	40–	37

* Daniel *et al.*, 1982; † Schreinemachers *et al.*, 1982; ‡ Sachs *et al.*, 1977; § data summarized from Bauld *et al.*, 1974 and Machin and Crolla, 1974

et al., 1974; Hamerton *et al.*, 1975). Many newborn infants with autosomal abnormalities have Down's syndrome (associated with trisomy 21). Edwards' syndrome (associated with 47, + 18) and Patau's syndrome (associated with 47, + 13) also occur. Newborn infants with sex-chromosomal abnormalities have Klinefelter's syndrome (47,XXY), superfemale syndrome (47,XXX), and YY syndrome (47,XYY).

The maternal age-specific rates for these chromosome abnormalities were calculated. The incidence of Down's syndrome by 5-year maternal-age intervals was 0.06 for the 20–24 age group, 0.08 for the 25–29 age group, 0.11 for the 30–34 age group, 0.35 for the 35–39 age group, 0.99 for the 40–44 age group, and 2.2 for the 45 and up age group (Collmann and Stoller, 1962). Newborn infants with Edwards' syndrome and Klinefelter's syndrome increase remarkably when the mother is 35 or over, as in the case of Down's syndrome (Figure 12.1, B). With Patau's syndrome and superfemale syndrome, the increases are evident when the mother is 40 or over (Figure 12.1, C).

The estimated incidence rate of these five syndromes, associated with an extra chromosome, increases from 0.3 in mothers in the 20–24 age group to 0.38 at age 25–29, 0.41 at age 30–34, 0.96 at age 35–39, 3.2 at age 40–44, and 10.6 at age 45 and over. At the age of 45 and over the incidence is 35-fold or higher than in those age 20–24.

ORIGIN AND CAUSE OF THE EXTRA CHROMOSOME

The relationship between the increasing incidence of conceptuses with chromosome abnormalities and advanced maternal age has been gradually accepted as a fact in biostatistics. It seems that unlike spermatogenesis, oogenesis occurs only during the fetal period.

Thus it was found that chromosome abnormalities, especially trisomy, were remarkably high in older pregnant women, particularly in premenopausal women. This suggests that oocytes remaining in the ovary at the dictyotene stage – for up to 50 years from birth until the time of ovulation – have increased opportunities for contact with factors inducing chromosome nondisjunction. However, the most probable cause of the chromosome abnormalities may be related to the aging process of the oocyte itself. This was determined from the finding that the incidence of chromosome abnormalities increases sharply in a relatively few years once the maternal age advances past 40. This is the case especially before menopause when the reproduction potential diminishes. The abnormal karyotype of conceptus in older pregnant women has an extra chromosome, as in the cases described above. The origin of the extra chromosome in spontaneous abortions (Niikawa *et al.*, 1977), Down's syndrome (Magenis *et al.*, 1977; Manning and Goodman, 1981), and Klinefelter's syndrome (Race and Sanger, 1969), is mainly caused by nondisjunction of maternal first meiosis.

Acknowledgement

Gratitude is due to M. Ohara of Kyushu University for helping me to prepare this article.

References

Bauld, R., Sutherland, G. R. and Bain, A. D. (1974). Chromosome studies in investigation of stillbirths and neonatal deaths. *Arch. Dis. Child.*, **49**, 782

Boué, A. and Boué, J. (1975). Chromosome abnormalities and abortion. In Coutinho, E. M. and Fuchs, F. (eds.) *Physiology and Genetics of Reproduction. Part B*, pp. 317–339. (New York: Plenum)

Collmann, R. D. and Stoller, A. (1962). A survey of mongoloid births in Victoria, Australia, 1942–1957. *Am. J. Public Health*, **52**, 813

Creasy, M. R., Colla, J. A. and Alberman, E. D. (1976). A cytogenetic study of human spontaneous abortions using banding techniques. *Hum. Genet.*, **31**, 177

Daniel, A., Stewart, L., Saville, T., Brookwell, R., Paull, H., Purvis-Smith, S. and Lam-Po-Tang, P.R.L.C. (1982). Prenatal diagnosis in 3000 women for chromosome, X-linked, and metabolic disorders. *Am. J. Med. Genet.*, **11**, 61

Fujimoto, S., Tsuji, K. and Ichinoe, K. (1978). Maternal age dependence of chromosome aberrations in induced abortions. *Proc. Jpn. Acad.*, **54**, 601

Golbus, M. S., Loughman, W. D., Epstein, C. J., Halbasch, G., Stephens, J. D. and Hall, B. D. (1979). Prenatal genetic diagnosis in 3000 amniocenteses. *N. Engl. J. Med.*, **300**, 157

Goldman, B., Mashiah, S., Serr, D. M., Brankstein, J., Chaki, R., Navon, R. and Padeh, B. (1977). A survey of amniocentesis in 925 patients at high risk of fetal genetic disorder. *Brit. J. Obstet. Gynaecol.*, **84**, 808

Hahnemann, N. (1973). Chromosome studies in induced abortions. *Clin. Genet.*, **4**, 328

Hamerton, J. L., Canning, N., Ray, M. and Smith, S. (1975). A cytogenetic survey of 14069 newborn infants: I. incidence of chromosome abnormalities. *Clin. Genet.*, **8**, 223

Hay, S. and Barbano, H. (1972). Independent effects of maternal age and birth order on the incidence of selected congenital malformations. *Teratology*, **6**, 271

Ichinoe, K., Okada, Y., Mabuchi, Y., Yokota, H. and Kanamaru, H. (1979). Incidence of hydatidiform mole and its sequent chorionic disease in reference to aging of mothers. *Acta Obst. Gynaecol. Jpn.*, **31**, 192

Jacobs, P. A., Melville, M. and Ratcliffe, S. (1974). A cytogenetic survey of 11 680 newborn infants. *Ann. Hum. Genet.*, **37**, 359

Kajii, T. and Ohama, K. (1977). Androgenetic origin of hydatidiform mole. *Nature (Lond.)*, **268**, 633

Kawashima, Y., Noto, H. and Kobayashi, T. (1979). Prognosis of hydatidiform mole – Follow-up study on 2918 cases in special reference to aging. *Acta Obstet. Gynaecol. Jpn.*, **31**, 2229

Lenz, W., Pfeiffer, A. and Tunte, W. (1966). Chromosomenanomalien durch Uberzahl (Trisomien) und alter der Mutter. *Dtsch. Med. Wochenschr.*, **91**, 1262

Machin, G. A. and Crolla, J. A. (1974). Chromosome constitution of 500 infants dying during the perinatal period. *Humangenetik*, **23**, 183

MacMahon, B., Hertig, A. and Ingalls, T. (1954). Association between maternal age and pathologic diagnosis in abortion. *Obstet. Gynecol.*, **4**, 477

Magenis, R. E., Overton, K. M., Chamberlin, J., Brady, T. and Lovrien, E. (1977). Parental origin of the extra chromosome in Down's syndrome. *Hum. Genet.*, **37**, 7

Manning, C. H. and Goodman, H. O. (1981). Parental origin of chromosomes in Down's syndrome. *Hum. Genet.*, **59**, 101

Matalon, M. and Modan, B. (1972). Epidemiologic aspects of hydatidiform mole in Israel. *Am. J. Obstet. Gynecol.*, **112**, 107

Meredith, R., Taylor, A. I. and Ansl, F. M. (1978). High risk of Down's syndrome at advanced maternal age. *Lancet*, **1**, 564

Niikawa, N., Merotto, E. and Kajii, T. (1977). Origin of acrocentric trisomies in spontaneous abortuses. *Hum. Genet.*, **40**, 73

Ohama, K. (1978). Chromosomal anomalies and sex ratio of induced abortuses in early embryogenesis. *Acta Obstet. Gynaecol. Jpn.*, **30**, 1687

Polani, P. E., Alberman, E., Berry, A. C., Blunt, S. and Singer, J. D. (1976). Chromosome abnormalities and maternal age. *Lancet*, **2**, 516

Race, R. R. and Sanger, R. (1969). Xg and sex-chromosome abnormalities. *Br. Med. Bull.*, **25**, 99

Sachs, E. S., Jahoda, M. C. J., Niermeijer, M. F. and Galjaard, H. (1977). An unexpected high frequency of trisomic fetuses in 229 pregnancies; Monitored for advanced maternal age. *Hum. Genet.*, **36**, 43

Sasaki, M., Ikeuchi, T., Obara, Y., Hayata, I., Mori, M. and Kohno, S. (1971). Chromosome studies in early embryogenesis. *Am. J. Obstet. Gynecol.*, **111**, 8

Schreinemachers, D. M., Cross, P. K. and Hook, E. B. (1982). Rates of trisomies 21, 18, 13 and other chromosome abnormalities in about 20 000 prenatal studies compared with estimated rates in live births. *Hum. Genet.*, **61**, 318

Stanton, E. F. (1956). Pregnancy after forty-four. *Am. J. Obstet. Gynecol.*, **71**, 270

Teoh, E. S., Dawood, M. Y. and Ratnam, S. S. (1971). Epidemiology of hydatidiform mole in Singapore. *Am. J. Obstet. Gynecol.*, **110**, 415

Tonomura, A., Sasaki, M., Yamada, K. and Aoki, H. (1973). Cytogenetic studies in induced abortions. *Jpn. J. Hum. Genet.*, **18**, 120

Tsuji, K. (1978). Chromosome studies in induced abortion of older pregnant women. *J. Wakayama Med. Soc.*, **29**, 1

Tsuji, K. and Ichinoe, K. (1978). Chromosome studies in induced abortions of older pregnant women. *Acta Obstet. Gynaecol. Jpn.*, **30**, 435

Tsuji, K. and Nakano, R. (1978). Chromosome studies of embryos from induced abortions in pregnant women aged 35 and over. *Obstet. Gynecol.*, **52**, 542

Tsuji, K., Yagi, S. and Nakano, R. (1981). Increased risk of malignant transformation of hydatidiform moles in older gravidas: A cytogenetic study. *Obstet. Gynecol.*, **58**, 351

Wirtz, A., Haas, B., Krauss, C., Stengel-Rutkowski, S. and Murken, J. D. (1978). Pränatale Diagnostik bei erhöhtem gebäralter. *Geburtsh. Frauenheilk.*, **38**, 422

Yen, S. and MacMahon, B. (1968). Epidemiologic features of trophoblastic disease. *Am. J. Obstet. Gynecol.*, **101**, 126

13
Spontaneous abortion: a screening device for abnormal conceptuses

K. SHIOTA

INTRODUCTION

Major congenital defects are found in approximately 3 % of newborn infants (Holmes, 1979). The prevalence is much higher in prenatal human populations and a considerably large proportion of spontaneous abortuses are morphologically and/or karyotypically abnormal (Fantel *et al.*, 1980; Hook, 1981; Poland *et al.*, 1981). Thus spontaneous abortion is an important screening process which reduces the incidence of congenital malformations prenatally by elimination of abnormal embryos and fetuses. In other words, the malformations recognized in newborn infants are only a part of the total anomalies that are produced at organogenesis. This chapter reviews the morphology and cytogenetics of early human abortuses and portrays the effects of prenatal natural screening on the incidence of birth defects.

INCIDENCE OF PRENATAL REPRODUCTIVE LOSS

It has been estimated that 15–20 % of recognized human pregnancies end in spontaneous abortion, mostly during the first trimester (Warburton and Fraser, 1964; Boué *et al.*, 1976). A broad epidemiologic approach to the investigation of the outcome of all pregnancies occurring in an entire community was made on the Hawaiian island of Kauai (French and Bierman, 1962; Bierman *et al.*, 1965). During the period 1953–1956, they followed over 3000 pregnancies from 4 weeks' gestation throughout pregnancy, and found that about 24 % of the pregnancies resulted in loss or death of the conceptus. This means that, for each 1000 livebirths there were an estimated 1311 pregnancies which had advanced to 4 weeks; 286 had ended in embryonic or fetal deaths before 20 weeks and 25 more after that time. There was a decreasing curve in the monthly risk of reproductive loss from a high of 11 % in weeks 4–7 to 3 % in weeks 32–35.

Although the rates of spontaneous abortion reported by many investigators have been fairly consistent and between 15 % and 25 %, these incidence figures certainly underestimate the true frequency because most of the studies have considered only recognized pregnancies that survived the first missed menstrual period. A series of gravid uteri of less than 4 weeks' gestation were examined following hysterectomy and an impressive rate of pathological ova in the uteri was found (Hertig, 1967; Hertig *et al.*, 1956, 1959). Their results can be formulated as follows: about 16% of human ova exposed to sperm do not cleave; another 15% of the ova are lost during the first week at preimplantation stages; and some 27% of the ova are aborted spontaneously during the second week. Accordingly, only about 42% of the ova in the starting group survive the first 2 weeks and succeed in causing a missed menstrual period. Since about one-fourth of human ova that survive the first missed menstrual period are aborted spontaneously (French and Bierman, 1962), the total reproductive loss rate in the human would be as high as 68% ($58 + (42 \times 1/4)$).

More recently, a postimplantation loss rate was detected directly by human chorionic gonadotropin (hCG) (Miller *et al.*, 1980). Of the 153 conceptions confirmed by urinary hCG, 14 ended in clinically recognized spontaneous abortions before 20 weeks, but the 50 cases (33%) with elevated urinary hCG were recognized neither as pregnancies nor as abortions. Thus the total postimplantation loss rate before 20 weeks was at least 43% including both recognized and unrecognized abortions, while the apparent spontaneous abortion rate among recognized pregnancies was 14% (14/103).

GROSS ANATOMICAL ABNORMALITIES IN SPONTANEOUS ABORTUSES

In the studies of structural abnormalities found in human abortions, the prevalence of abnormalities was reported very high, ranging from 40% to 70% (Mall and Meyer, 1921; Fujikura *et al.*, 1966; Stratford, 1970). In their studies, the frequency of localized anomalies in the embryo or fetus varied from 2% to 28%. These variations are largely a function of the method of ascertainment and of the segment of the specimens examined. From 4% to 20% of the abortuses were growth retarded, often referred to as stunted or cylindrical. These specimens are severely macerated or autolyzed because they were retained in the uterus for several weeks following conceptual death.

Fantel *et al.* (1980) summarized their study for 7½ years of the 748 spontaneous abortuses received from a hospital in Seattle area. The prevalence of specific anomalies was nearly 5% in the specimens from the first 2 months, whereas it increased to about 15% in the subsequent gestational groups. The most common anomalies were neural tube defects, anencephaly and spina bifida most frequent. Cleft lip (± cleft palate), cardiovascular defects and eye anomalies were also encountered frequently. Growth retarded specimens made up 14% of their total collection. About 13% were empty, intact chorionic sacs. An empty sac may result from very early developmental arrest, and its pathology and epidemiology are discussed in a separate paper (Nishimura and Shiota, 1984).

In another study of over 2000 spontaneously aborted products from British Columbia, the frequency of abnormalities was 84% in embryos and 26% in fetuses, including specific defects and 'growth disorganization' (Poland *et al.*, 1981). Of the 943 morphologically abnormal embryos, 865 (92 %) had general defects and 78 (8 %) had defects of specific systems. Of the latter 30 (39 %) had defects in more than one system. Of the 210 abnormal fetuses, 109 (52 %) had a defect in only one system and 101 (48 %) had defects in more than one. Defects of the cardiovascular system were the most prevalent of the local defects.

All the studies cited above showed that defects occurring in any given system are far more frequent in spontaneous abortuses than in newborns. According to the systematic study of induced abortions in Japan (Nishimura, 1974, 1975), the incidence rates of specific anomalies in the early intrauterine population are at least several times higher than the corresponding values for newborn infants. (Table 13.1). It is interesting that not only embryos or fetuses with lethal malformations such as neural tube defects but those with less severe anomalies which may not be in themselves lethal, e.g. cleft lip and polydactyly, seem more likely to abort than morphologically normal conceptuses. A mechanism possibly exists which favors good over faulty conceptions and causes selective abortion of defective embryos and fetuses.

Table 13.1 Incidence rates of specific malformations in Japanese induced abortuses and newborns

Malformation	*Incidence* (× 1000) *in* *Embroys**	*Newborns†*	*Ratio*
Exencephaly	2.7	0.6	5:1
Holoprosencephaly	7.3	0.1	73:1
Cleft lip	4.3	1.7	2.5:1
Polydactyly	14.1	0.9	16:1

* Nishimura (1975)
† Mitani and Kitamura (1968)

CHROMOSOME ABNORMALITIES IN SPONTANEOUS ABORTUSES

The frequency of chromosome abnormalities in liveborn babies has been reported to be approximately six per 1000 (Jacobs, 1977; Takahara *et al.*, 1977). It has long been known that the frequency is much greater in spontaneously aborted conceptuses. Abnormal chromosomes were found in about 60 % of all aborted embryos and fetuses and cytogenetic anomalies are often associated with morphologically abnormal conceptuses (Boué and Boué, 1973; Poland *et al.*, 1981). An 80 % incidence of abnormalities was noted in embryos whose development stopped at 2 weeks (Boué and Boué, 1973).

Recently excellent calculations were provided on the frequency of cytogenetic abnormalities in intrauterine populations at various gestational intervals up to 28 weeks (Hook, 1981). His summed data for all gestational intervals indicated that an estimated 5 % of all recognizable human conceptuses have a chromosome abnormality. According to his estimation, the proportion of chromosomally affected conceptuses drops to 4.2% at age 8 weeks, 2.4% at 12 weeks, 1.1% at 16 weeks, 0.8% at 20 weeks and 0.6% in livebirths. This clearly shows the selective death of chromosomally abnormal embryos and fetuses during gestation.

A relationship between maternal age and chromosome anomalies in spontaneous abortuses has been recognized (Leridon, 1973). He estimated that at maternal age 20 the ratio of spontaneously aborted embryos with and without a chromosome defect is about 2:3 and that at age 40 or older the ratio is 6:1. This is interesting because about one-half of early abortuses are trisomic (Alberman and Creasy, 1977) and because the occurrence of at least several trisomies found in newborns (e.g., 13, 18 and 21) is dependent on maternal age.

Pertinent to the question of the outcome of subsequent pregnancies in women who have had spontaneous abortion with a chromosome defect is a report by Jacobs (1977). She showed that those who have had one chromosomally abnormal abortion tend to have another chromosomally abnormal abortion and that conversely, those who have had a chromosomally normal abortion tend to have another abortion with a normal chromosome constitution.

MATERNAL REPRODUCTIVE LOSS AND ABNORMAL CONCEPTUSES

From the discussion above, it is evident that a large proportion of embryos or fetuses that are morphologically and/or karyotypically abnormal are eliminated prenatally and end in spontaneous abortion. Data on the reproductive histories of the women who conceived a malformed embryo are presented in Tables 13.2–13.4. The index conceptuses are 337 embryos with specific malformations (neural tube defects, holoprosencephaly, cleft lip and polydactyly) and 424 empty chorionic sacs from the human embryo collection of Kyoto (Figure 13.1). The average number of miscarriages in prior pregnancies is 0.51 for the case women and is twice as large as 0.24 for the mothers of normal embryos matched for gravidity (Table 13.2). Thirty-three percent of the mothers of abnormal conceptuses had at least one previous abortion, whereas only 17% of the mothers of normal embryos had a prior miscarriage. The difference is statistically significant ($p < 0.001$). The proportion of prior recognized pregnancies which resulted in spontaneous abortion is 25% in the case women and is twice as large as that in normal controls (Table 13.3). If the index case under study is included, the reproductive loss rate in the case women would be even higher because many malformed embryos would die *in utero* and abort sooner or later.

The average number of prior recognized pregnancies is lower in the mothers of abnormal conceptuses than in normal controls matched for maternal age (Table 13.4). Twenty six percent (19/72) of the mothers of embryos with neural tube defects are primigravidae, and this is significantly greater than the corresponding incidence for normal controls (8/72 = 11%). This result is consistent with the previous reports that neural tube defects are most frequent

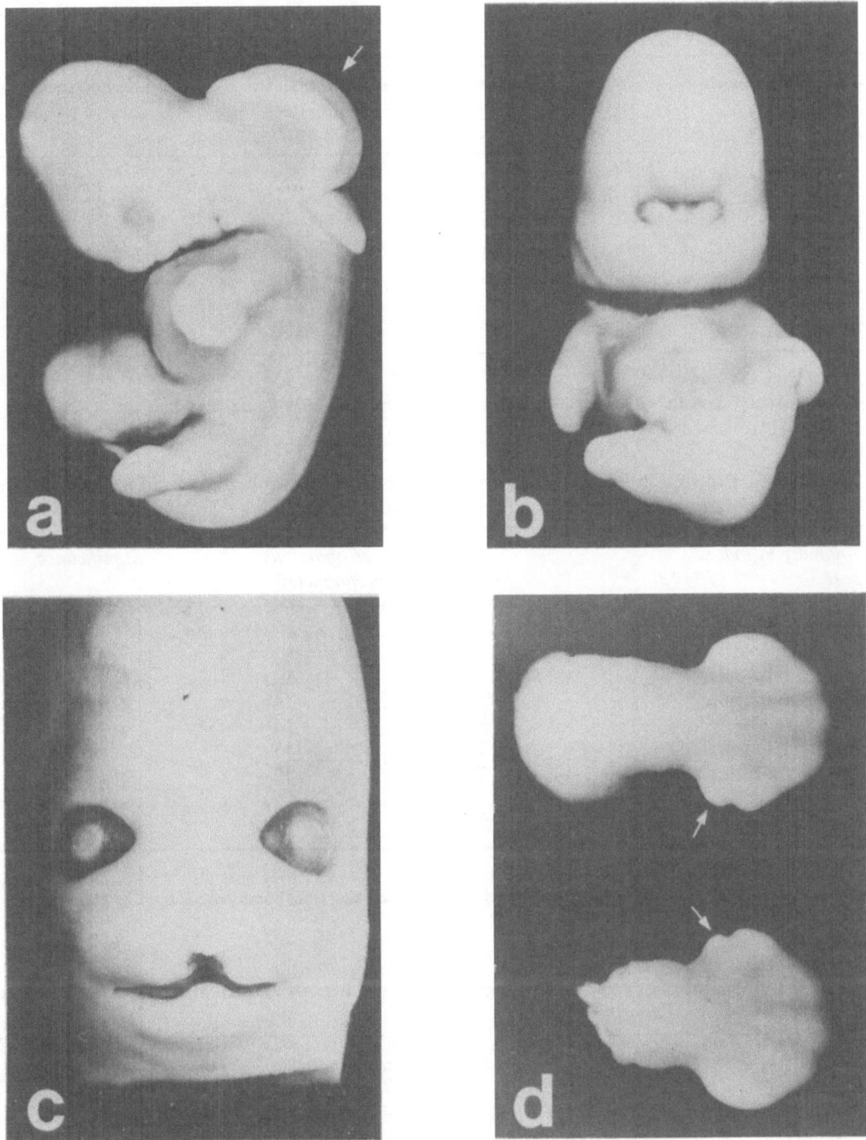

Figure 13.1 Examples of malformed human embryos. **a**, Open neural tube (arrow) in a 6-week embryo (#32337, Carnegie stage 18). **b**, Cyclopia (holoprosencephaly) in a $5\frac{1}{2}$-week embryo (#15936, Carnegie stage 17). **c**, Cleft lip in a 7-week embryo (#14153, Carnegie stage unknown). **d**, Preaxial polydactyly of the hand (arrows) in a 6-week embryo (#26955, Carnegie stage 19).

in first-borns (Horowitz and McDonald, 1969; Czeizel and Révész, 1970; Elwood and McBride, 1979). The gravidity of the case women may underestimate the true number because maternal age is adjusted between the case and control women. Such underestimated gravidity in the mothers of

Table 13.2 Frequency of recognized spontaneous abortions in multigravid mothers of abnormal embroys and normal controls

Anomaly in index case	*Mean number of prior abortions**		*Significance*
	Case	*Control*†	
Neural tube defects	0.47	0.25	NS
Holoprosencephaly	0.46	0.27	NS
Cleft lip	0.65	0.28	$p < 0.05$
Polydactyly	0.31	0.24	NS
Empty chorionic sac	0.54	0.22	$p < 0.01$
Totals	0.51	0.24	

* Excluding index case
† Normal controls matched for gravidity (excluding induced abortions) and gestational age at abortion

Table 13.3 Proportion of spontaneous abortions among prior recognized pregnancies in mothers of abnormal embryos and normal controls

Anomaly in index case	*% Spontaneous abortions in previous pregnancies**		*Significance*
	Case	*Control*†	
Neural tube defects	25	13	$p < 0.05$
Holoprosencephaly	23	14	$p < 0.05$
Cleft lip	34	14	$p < 0.01$
Polydactyly	17	13	NS
Empty chorionic sac	26	12	$p < 0.01$
Total	25	13	

* Previous pregnancies exclude induced abortions
† Normal controls matched for gravidity (excluding induced abortions) and gestational age at abortion

Table 13.4 Number of recognized pregnancies in mothers of abnormal embryos and normal controls

Anomaly in index case	*Mean number of recognized pregnancies**		*Significance*
	Case	*Control*†	
Neural tube defects	1.9	2.6	$p < 0.05$
Holoprosencephaly	2.7	2.8	NS
Cleft lip	2.4	2.5	NS
Polydactyly	2.3	2.8	NS
Empty chorionic sac	2.9	3.0	NS
Total	2.7	2.8	

* Excluding index case
† Normal controls matched for maternal age

abnormal embryos could possibly be accounted for by the increase in unrecognized abortions in their previous pregnancies.

Thus it became clear that both recognized and unrecognized abortions occur more frequently in the mothers of abnormal embryos than in those of normally developing embryos. Since a substantially large proportion of spontaneously aborted embryos are morphologically abnormal, many mothers of malformed embryos seem to conceive abnormal conceptuses repeatedly. Parental genotypes and/or environmental factors may be at work chronically or repeatedly in such cases of recurrent pathological conceptions. Most of the abnormal conceptuses, however, seem to be eliminated from a sufficiently early stage of development to escape detection.

CONCLUDING REMARKS

Mankind as well as other mammals suffers from a remarkably high risk of reproductive loss. However, since many spontaneous abortuses are phenotypically and/or karyotypically abnormal, spontaneous abortion is an important screening process that reduces the births of malformed infants. The prenatal elimination rate could be as high as over 90 % for some malformations (Table 13.1). Similarly, about 90 % of chromosomally affected conceptuses are known to be eliminated before birth (Polani, 1970; Hook, 1981). A relation between spontaneous abortion rate and the prevalence of neural tube defects at birth was reported from South Wales (Roberts and Lloyd, 1973). They found that the spontaneous abortion rates were lower in mothers living in the coalmining valleys which are known for high birth prevalence of neural tube defects than in mothers living in the rest of South Wales. This means that the difference in area prevalence of neural tube defects at birth may be controlled by area differences in mortality of malformed embryos. Warkany (1978, 1980) coined the name *terathanasia* for such a selective mechanism and suggested that if the screening mechanism could be enhanced properly, this would result in the abortion of an even larger proportion of abnormal conceptuses than is now aborted spontaneously.

Although many human malformations are apparently of sporadic occurrence, they must be only a part of the total anomalies that are produced in the early intrauterine population. The recurrence risk of abnormal conceptions seems high in the mothers of a malformed embryo and needs to be assessed in future. Reproductive histories of the mother should be considered in genetic counseling especially when she has had repeated abortions or her gravidity is unexpectedly low. Knowledge of the characteristics of aborted conceptuses, if available, would provide a basis for prognosis of her pregnancy and also a prospect of prevention of further anomalies. Such knowledge could provide a criteria for selecting patients for amniocentesis and other prenatal diagnostic measures.

Acknowledgements

I gratefully acknowledge the collaboration of several hundred physicians and of the members of the Congenital Anomaly Research Center and the

Department of Anatomy, Kyoto University Faculty of Medicine. Thanks are also due to Dr Thomas H. Shepard and Dr Alan G. Fantel for very helpful discussions, and to Miss Yuko Taniguchi for secretarial assistance.

References

Alberman, E. D. and Creasy, M. R. (1977). Frequency of chromosomal abnormalities in miscarriages and perinatal deaths. *J. Med. Genet.*, **14,** 313

Bierman, J. M., Siegel, E., French, F. E. and Simonian, K. (1965). Analysis of the outcome of all pregnancies in a community. Kauai pregnancy study. *Am. J. Obstet. Gynecol.*, **91,** 37

Boué, J. and Boué, A. (1973). Anomalies chromosomiques dans les avortements spontanés. In Boué, A. and Thibault, C. (eds.) *Les Accidents chromosomiques de la reproduction*, pp. 29–56. (Paris: INSERM)

Boué, J., Philippe, E., Giroud, A. and Boué, A. (1976). Phenotypic expression of lethal chromosomal anomalies in human abortuses. *Teratology*, **14,** 3

Czeizel, A. and Révész, C. (1970). Major malformations of the central nervous system in Hungary. *Br. J. Prev. Soc. Med.*, **24,** 205

Elwood, J. M. and McBride, M. L. (1979). Contrasting effects of maternal fertility and birth rank on the occurrence of neural tube defects. *J. Epidemiol. Community Health*, **33,** 78

Fantel, A. G., Shepard, T. H., Vadheim-Roth, C., Stephens, T. D. and Coleman, C. (1980). Embryonic and fetal phenotypes: Prevalence and other associated factors in a large study of spontaneous abortion. In Porter, I. H. and Hook, E. B. (eds.) *Human Embryonic and Fetal Death*, pp. 71–87. (New York: Academic Press)

French, F. E. and Bierman, J. E. (1962). Probabilities of fetal mortality. *Public Health Rep.*, **77,** 835

Fujikura, T., Frohlich, L. A. and Driscoll, S. G. (1966). A simplified anatomic classification of abortions. *Am. J. Obstet. Gynecol.*, **95,** 902

Hertig, A. T. (1967). The overall problem in man. In Benirschke, K. (ed.) *Comparative Aspects of Reproductive Failure*, pp. 11–41. (Berlin, Heidelberg, New York: Springer)

Hertig, A. T., Rock, J. and Adams, E. C. (1956). A description of 34 human ova within the first 17 days of development. *Am. J. Anat.*, **98,** 435

Hertig, A. T., Rock, J., Adams, E. C. and Menkin, M. (1959). Thirty-four fertilized human ova, good, bad and indifferent, recovered from 210 women of known fertility. A study of biological wastage in early human pregnancy. *Pediatrics*, **23,** 202

Holmes, L. B. (1979). Congenital malformations. In Vaughan, V. C. III, McKay, R. J. Jr. and Behrman, R. E. (eds.) *Nelson's Textbook of Pediatrics*, pp. 370–371. (Philadelphia, London, Toronto: Saunders)

Hook, E. B. (1981). Prevalence of chromosome abnormalities during human gestation and implications for studies of environmental mutagens. *Lancet*, **2,** 169

Horowitz, I. and McDonald, A. D. (1969). Anencephaly and spina bifida in the Province of Quebec. *Can. Med. Assoc. J.*, **100,** 748

Jacobs, P. A. (1977). Epidemiology of chromosome abnormalities in man. *Am. J. Epidemiol.*, **105,** 180

Leridon, H. (1973). Démographie des échecs de la reproduction. In Boué, A. and Thibault, C. (eds.) *Les Accidents chromosomiques de la reproduction*, pp. 13–27. (Paris: INSERM)

Mall, F. P. and Meyer, A. W. (1921). Studies on abortuses: A survey of pathologic ova in the Carnegie Embryological Collection. *Contrib. Embryol. Carnegie Inst.*, **12,** 3

Miller, J. F., Williamson, E., Glue, J., Gordon, Y. B., Grudzinskas, J. G. and Sykes, A. (1980). Fetal loss after implantation. A prospective study. *Lancet*, **2,** 554

Mitani, S. and Kitamura, Y. (1968). Malformations and their classification. *Obstet. Gynecol. Ther. (Tokyo)*, **17,** 265. (In Japanese)

Nishimura, H. (1974). Detection of early developmental anomalies in human abortuses. In Gianantonio, C. A. and Berri, G. G. (eds.) *Pediatria XIV*, pp. 159–170. (Buenos Aires: Editorial Medica Panamericana)

Nishimura, H. (1975). Prenatal versus postnatal malformations based on the Japanese experience on induced abortions in the human being. In Blandau, R. J. (ed.) *Aging Gametes – Their Biology and Pathology*, pp. 349–368. (Basel: Karger)

Nishimura, H. and Shiota, K. (1984). Early embryonic death: Pathology and associated factors. This volume, Chapter 8

Poland, B. J., Miller, J. R., Harris, M. and Livingston, J. (1981). Spontaneous abortion. A study of 1961 women and their conceptuses. *Acta Obstet. Gynecol. Scand. Suppl.*, **102,** 1

Polani, P. E. (1970). The incidence of chromosomal malformations. *Proc. R. Soc. Med.*, **63,** 14

Roberts, C. J. and Lloyd, S. (1973). Area differences in spontaneous abortion rates in South Wales and their relation to neural tube defect incidence. *Br. Med. J.*, **4,** 20

Stratford, B. F. (1970). Abnormalities of early human development. *Am. J. Obstet. Gynecol.*, **107,** 1223

Takahara, H., Ohama, K. and Fujiwara, A. (1977). Cytogenetic study in early spontaneous abortion. *Hiroshima J. Med. Sci.*, **26,** 291

Warburton, D. and Fraser, F. C. (1964). Spontaneous abortion risks in man: Data from reproductive histories collected in a medical genetics unit. *Am. J. Human Genet.*, **16,** 1

Warkany, J. (1978). Terathanasia. *Teratology*, **17,** 187

Warkany, J. (1980). Teratology in perspective. Explanations and recommendations for prevention. In Porter, I. H. and Hook, E. B. (eds.) *Human Embryonic and Fetal Death*, pp. 355–363. (New York: Academic Press)

14
Pregnancy wastage in DES-exposed female progeny

N. P. VERIDIANO, I. DELKE and M. L. TANCER

Diethylstilbestrol (DES) was first synthesized in 1938 by Sir Charles Dodds. It exhibits significant effectiveness when administered orally. Its main advantage is that it is easy to prepare in its pure form at very low cost.

In the years between 1945 and 1955, DES was frequently prescribed for complications of pregnancy, premature labor, diabetes, toxemia, Rh incompatibility. A history of previous miscarriage, infertility, advanced age of the mother, stillbirth, are indications for DES therapy. In 1953 Dieckman *et al.* published a study which cast serious doubt on the efficacy of DES in preventing abortion. In 1958 Goldzieher and Benigno concluded that there was no statistical evidence that DES therapy is effective in preventing pregnancy loss. The use of DES began to decline after 1955. The first case of adenocarcinoma of the vagina in adolescents was reported by Herbst and Scully, (1970). In 1971, Herbst and colleagues pointed out the relationship between clear vaginal cell adenocarcinoma in young women and maternal stilbestrol ingestion (Herbst *et al.*, 1971). As more and more cases of malignancy were reported, other related information became available.

STRUCTURAL AND MICROSCOPIC GENITAL TRACT ANOMALIES RESULTING FROM *IN UTERO* EXPOSURE

Adenosis of the vagina is a well-recognized problem associated with prenatal exposure to DES. The incidence ranges from 40% to 91% (O'Brien *et al.*, 1979). The frequency of occurrence correlates with the gestational age at which the fetus was exposed to the hormone. The overall risk it may carry is as yet largely unknown.

Cervical and vaginal structural deformities such as cockscomb, erythroplasia, pseudopolyp formation, circumvaginal hood, have been found in association with adenosis.

The first report of uterine and tubal anomalies in the DES-exposed group of women was published in 1977 (Kaufman *et al.*, 1977). These anomalies consisted of T-shaped appearance of the uterus, constricting bands in the uterine cavity, a hypoplastic uterus, and in some cases synecchiae. The incidence of uterine anomaly correlated with the presence or absence of gross defects in the cervix or vagina.

REPRODUCTIVE PERFORMANCE

A DES-exposed patient with cervical hypoplasia who sustained two midtrimester (22 weeks' gestation) fetal losses as a result of cervical incompetence was reported in 1978 (Singer and Hochman, 1978). Several papers since then reported on the use of cerclage to accomplish fetal salvage (Goldstein, 1978). A comparison of pregnancy experience in DES-exposed and unexposed daughters carried out at the University of Chicago (Herbst *et al.*, 1980) showed some very interesting differences between the two groups. The fertility and outcome of pregnancy in women exposed *in utero* to DES were examined in women participating in the cooperative Diethylstilbestrol Adenosis (DESAD) Project (Barnes *et al.*, 1980). An increased risk of unfavorable outcome of pregnancy was associated with DES exposure (Barnes *et al.*, 1980) (Table 14.1). Two hundred and sixty-seven DES-exposed patients who got pregnant had high fetal wastage (Veridiano *et al.*, 1982).

The study correlating hysterosalpingogram (HSG) findings and pregnancy outcome showed that out of a total of 119 pregnancies in 93 women, only 54 (45%) resulted in term births (Kaufman *et al.*, 1980). In the group with abnormal X-ray films, a consistently poor outcome was seen more often than in those women with normal X-ray films. A direct relationship exists between the presence of gross and microscopic vaginal epithelial changes and abnormal hysterographic findings.

Table 14.1 Numbers and percentages of women exposed to DES and of control subjects who had unfavourable outcomes of pregnancy and relative risks of unfavourable outcomes with DES exposure

Outcome	*Exposed to DES (220)**	*Controls (224)**	*Relative risk*	p *value*	*95% confidence limits on relative risk*
Any unfavorable outcome	83(37.7)	50(22.3)	1.69	<0.001	1.20–2.18
Miscarriage	57(25.9)	36(16.1)	1.61	0.008	1.11–2.34
Ectopic pregnancy	8(3.6)	3(1.3)	2.77	NS†	0.73–10.46
Stillbirth	8(3.6)	3(1.3)	2.77	NS	0.73–10.46
Premature birth	17(7.7)	10(4.5)	1.7	NS	0.80–3.65
Never had a full-term livebirth	42(19.1)	11(4.9)	3.90	<0.001	2.06–7.37

* Figures in parentheses denote percentages
† Not significant ($p \geqslant 0.10$)
From Barnes *et al.* 1980. Used by permission

ECTOPIC PREGNANCY

The incidence of ectopic pregnancy varies in different population groups and could range between 9.5 % and 2 %. In a group of 220 DES-exposed patients, eight (3.6 %) had ectopic pregnancy as compared to three out of 224 (1.3 %) control women (Barnes *et al.*, 1980). The outcome of first pregnancy in 89 exposed women in another series (Herbst *et al.*, 1980) showed an incidence of four (4.5 %) ectopic gestations as compared to no ectopic outcome in 118 unexposed controls. An analysis of 261 first pregnancies in another series showed seven ectopic pregnancies for an incidence of 2.6 % (Veridiano *et al.*, 1982). There was no control population in this last series.

Ninety-three DES-exposed women in another study (Kaufman *et al.*, 1980) who underwent hysterosalpingogram had a total of 144 pregnancies. Ectopic gestation occurred as a first pregnancy in six of the 93 women. Four (7 %) occurred in women with abnormal X-ray films and two (4 %) occurred in women with normal X-ray films. Even though women with abnormal HSG had a higher frequency of ectopic pregnancy, there was no significant difference between the two groups. Another series reported four ectopic pregnancies out of 97 evaluable first pregnancies (Sandberg *et al.*, 1981). The number of women who experienced ectopic pregnancy among the exposed and unexposed control was analysed by Sandberg and his group (Table 14.2). It was apparent that one in every 24 exposed patients who became pregnant had at least one ectopic pregnancy as compared to one in every 141 unexposed controls.

SPONTANEOUS ABORTION

For the purpose of uniformity, definitions used by the majority of investigators are used in this article. Spontaneous abortion is a pregnancy ending spontaneously before the 20th week of gestation. A preterm delivery is that which resulted in the birth of an infant weighing between 500 and 2500 g. A term birth is that which results in the birth of an infant weighing more than 2500 g. An evaluable pregnancy is any pregnancy having an outcome other than elective abortion.

The incidence of spontaneous abortion in the DES-exposed population ranges from 19 to 48 %. The incidence of the same outcome in the unexposed controls ranges from 8 to 21 % (Sandberg *et al.*, 1981). The few reports which separated spontaneous abortion into first and second trimester terminations showed that DES-exposed females have a higher chance of having midtrimester miscarriages (12 %) than the general population (2.3 %) (Kaufman *et al.*, 1981). Spontaneous abortion occurs more often (37 %) in women with abnormal HSG than in women with normal HSG (23 %) (Table 14.3).

PRETERM BIRTHS

The incidence of preterm births is 22 % in the DES exposed females compared to 7 % among control subjects. There is no significant difference in the

Table 14.2 Ratio of women with ectopic pregnancy to all women with pregnancies among DES-exposed patients and unexposed control women

	Herbst et al.		*Barnes* et al.		*Kaufman* et al. *(exposed)*	*This study (exposed)*	*All studies combined*	
	Exposed	*Unexposed*	*Exposed*	*Unexposed*			*Exposed*	*Unexposed*
Women with ectopic pregnancies	4	0	8	3	7	7	26	3
Women with pregnancies	82	112	289	310	93*	167	631	422
Ratio	1:21	0	1:36	1:103	1:13	1:24	1:24	1:141

* Includes only women 'who agreed to undergo' hysterosalpingographic evaluation
From Sandberg *et al.*, 1981. Used by permission

Table 14.3 Outcome of 144 pregnancies in 93 women exposed to DES in utero

HSG	*Total no. of pregnancies*	*Elective abortion*	*Ectopic pregnancies*	*Spontaneous abortions* — *Trimester* *First*	*Second*	*Total*	*Premature deliveries*	*Term deliveries*	*Total no. of live-births*
Abnormal	78	12	5(8%)	16(26%)	8(13%)	24(39%)	14(38%)*	23(34%)	37
Normal	66	13	2(4%)	6(12%)	6(12%)	12(23%)	8(20%)*	31(58%)	39
Total	144	25	7(6%)	22(20%)	14(12%)	36(32%)	22(29%)*	54(45%)	76

* Percent of livebirths.
(From Kaufman *et al.*, 1980. Used by permission.

occurrence of premature delivery in the first pregnancy in women who had normal compared to those who had abnormal X-ray findings. Our series at the Brookdale Hospital Medical Center consists of 320 evaluable pregnancies.

CONCLUDING REMARKS

DES female progeny should be counseled concerning the possibility of future impaired reproductive performance although they should not be discouraged. Eighty-seven percent of pregnant DES women in our series had at least one living infant. The incidence of ectopic pregnancy is higher in the exposed women than in unexposed control population. Sandberg suggests that approximately one in every 30 pregnancies occurring in exposed patients will be ectopically located. The incidence of spontaneous abortion is approximately twice as great in exposed patients as in control women. There is, however, no statistical significance of the differences between the two groups. The incidence of preterm pregnancy is three times greater in exposed patients than in control population.

Routine hysterosalpingograms may not be indicated. However, in those women who did have an unfavorable outcome, a hysterosalpingogram may be of some benefit. Information concerning the anatomic changes found should be transmitted to the future obstetric attendant. In the presence of such changes, the attention of the obstetrician should focus on the possibility of early cervical effacement and appropriate steps should be taken to avoid spontaneous abortion. None of the changes in the vagina, cervix, uterine fundus or fallopian tubes, individually or in combination, have been shown to prevent the occurrence of term pregnancy.

References

Barnes, A. B., Colton, T., Gunderson *et al.* (1980). Fertility and outcome of pregnancy in women exposed in utero to diethylstilbestrol. *N. Engl. J. Med.*, **302**, 609

Diekman, W. J., Davis, M. E., Rignkiewica, L. M. and Pattinger, R. E. (1953). Does the administration of diethylstilbestrol during pregnancy have therapeutic value? *Am. J. Obstet. Gynecol.*, **66**, 1062

Goldstein, D. P. (1978). Incompetent cervix in offspring exposed to diethylstilbestrol in utero. *Obstet. Gynecol.*, **52**, 73

Goldzieher, J. W. and Benigno, B. B. (1958). The treatment of threatened and recurrent abortion. A critical review. *Am. J. Obstet. Gynecol.*, **75**, 1202

Herbst, A. L. and Scully, R. E. (1970). Adenocarcinoma of the vagina in adolescence. A report of seven cases including six clear cell carcinomas. *Cancer*, **25**, 745

Herbst, A. L., Ulfelder, H. and Poskanzer, D. C. (1971). Adenocarcinoma of the vagina: Association of maternal stilbestrol therapy with tumor appearance in young women. *N. Engl. J. Med.*, **284**, 878

Herbst, A. L., Hubby, M. M., Blough, R. R. *et al.* (1980). A comparison of pregnancy experience in DES exposed and DES unexposed daughters. *J. Reprod. Med.*, **24**, 62

Kaufman, R. H., Binder, G. L., Gray, P. M. Jr. *et al.* (1977). Upper genital tract changes associated with exposure in utero to diethylstilbestrol. *Am. J. Obstet. Gynecol.*, **128**, 51

Kaufman, R. H., Adam, E., Binder, G. L. *et al.* (1980). Upper genital tract changes and pregnancy outcome in offspring exposed in utero to diethylstilbestrol. *Am. J. Obstet. Gynecol.*, **137**, 299

O'Brien, P. C., Noller, K. L., Robboy, S. J. *et al.* (1979). Vaginal epithelial changes in young women enrolled in the national cooperative diethylstilbestrol adenosis (DESAD) project. *Obstet. Gynecol.*, **53,** 300

Sandberg, E. C., Riffle, N. L., Higdon, J. V. *et al.* (1981). Pregnancy outcome in women exposed to diethylstilbestrol in utero. *Am. J. Obstet. Gynecol.*, **140,** 194

Singer, M. S. and Hochman, M. (1978). Incompetent cervix in a hormone exposed offspring. *Obstet. Gynecol.*, **51,** 625.

Veridiano, N. P., Delke, I., Rogers, J. and Tancer, M. L. (1982). Reproductive performance of DES-exposed female progeny. Presented at *Symposium on Reproductive Health Care: Changing Concepts in Fertility Regulation,* October 10–15, Maui, Hawaii

15
Role of ureaplasma urealyticum and mycoplasma hominis in spontaneous abortion

W. FOULON and A. NAESSENS

MICROBIOLOGY

Mycoplasmas have the smallest size of all free living organisms. They lack a true cell wall and are incapable of synthesizing cell wall precursors. Cells are highly pleomorphic. Colonies on solid media are minute, their diameter ranging from 10 to 600 μm. They have a typical 'fried egg' appearance, which consists of an opaque central area (that grows down into the medium) surrounded by a translucent peripheral zone (Freundt, 1967). Mycoplasmas are neither bacteria nor viruses, as bacteria have a true cell wall or are able to produce cell wall precursors and viruses grow in cell cultures only. Mycoplasmas belong to the class of Mollicutes of which there is only one order, i.e. the Mycoplasmatales. These are divided into two families, Mycoplasmataceae and Acholeplasmataceae. Mycoplasmataceae require sterol for growth; this compound is not necessary for the growth of Acholeplasmataceae. The Mycoplasmataceae have two genera: genus *Mycoplasma* and genus *Ureaplasma* (Table 15.1).

Table 15.1 Taxonomy of the mycoplasmas (class: Mollicutes; order: Mycoplasmatales)

Family	*Genus*	*Species**
1. Mycoplasmataceae	(1) *Mycoplasma*	*M. pneumoniae*
		M. salivarium
		M. orale 1
		M. orale 2
		M. orale 3
		M. fermantans
		M. hominis
	(2) *Ureaplasma*	*U. urealyticum*
2. Acholeplasmataceae		

* Only human species were noted

Most species of the genus *Mycoplasma* utilize glucose or arginine as the major source of energy. The distinction between the two genera, *Mycoplasma* and *Ureaplasma*, is made because of the ability of *Ureaplasma* to hydrolyse urea with the accumulation of ammonia.

HISTORICAL BACKGROUND

An organism resembling mycoplasma was first isolated in 1898 (Nocard and Roux, 1898) from a case of contagious bovine pleuropneumonia. Similar organisms, isolated from numerous animal diseases, were called pleuropneumonia-like organisms, because of their great resemblance to the agent causing bovine pleuropneumonia. In 1929 the term *Mycoplasma* was suggested by Nowak (Nowak, 1929). In 1937 this organism was isolated for the first time from humans, after drainage of a Bartholin gland abscess (Dienes and Edsall, 1937). Since that time, mycoplasmas have been implicated as etiologic agents in a variety of human infections, including pelvic abscesses (Dienes *et al.*, 1948), ovarian abscesses (Gotthardson and Melen, 1953) and blood cultures (Carlson *et al.*, 1951; Slingerland and Morgan, 1952). *Mycoplasma hominis* has also been found to cause puerperal sepsis and febrile episodes following gynecological surgery (Stokes, 1955, 1959).

In 1954 a mycoplasma was isolated from a man with non-gonoccocal urethritis. This organism differed from ordinary mycoplasmas by producing colonies of minute size on mycoplasma agar (Shepard, 1954); for this reason it was called 'T. mycoplasma' (T = tiny colonies). Later these mycoplasmas were found to possess an urease system that breaks down urea to ammonia (Shepard and Lunceford, 1967).

As a result, T. mycoplasma was removed from the genus *Mycoplasma* and a new genus was formed, i.e. *Ureaplasma*. To date only one species in the genus is described: *U. urealyticum*.

U. urealyticum and *M. hominis* presently are called 'genital mycoplasmas', because they are frequently isolated from the genital tract where they can play a role in genitourinary tract infections.

GENITAL MYCOPLASMAS IN NORMAL PREGNANT WOMEN

Genital mycoplasmas are found in men and in women. Acquisition occurs during sexual contact. Mycoplasmas are rarely isolated from individuals who deny having had sexual contact, but are frequently isolated from those who have regular intercourse. The percentage of women who are positive for mycoplasmas increases with the number of their partners (McCormack *et al.*, 1972).

M. hominis is recovered from 14–29% of cervical cultures in pregnant women (Foy *et al.*, 1970; Ross *et al.*, 1981). *U. urealyticum* is found in even larger numbers than *M. hominis*, ranging from 23% (Gnarpe and Friberg, 1972) to 71% (Braun *et al.*, 1970) depending on the community. In our population the prevalence of this organism is 40%.

Mycoplasmas were recovered from placentas and from amniotic fluid. *M. hominis* was isolated in four out of 50 diagnostic or therapeutic amniotic punctures (Harwick *et al.*, 1969). *U. urealyticum* was found in 61 out of 253 placentas (24%) (Naessens *et al.*, 1982). All pregnancies were normal; however, ureaplasmas were more frequently isolated from placentas when the membranes were ruptured for a long time before expulsion. In the majority of positive placental cultures, *U. urealyticum* represents an ascending infection after rupture of the membranes.

This statement notwithstanding, *M. hominis* and *U. urealyticum* also have been isolated from placentas (Caspi *et al.*, 1976) and from decidua (Lamey *et al.*, 1974) at the time of cesarean section performed prior to rupture of the membranes. This latter finding suggests that genital mycoplasmas produce endocervical and endometrial infections that remain strictly asymptomatic.

GENITAL MYCOPLASMAS AS POSSIBLE AGENTS IN SPONTANEOUS ABORTION

Spontaneous abortion affects at least 10% of all human conceptions; in most instances the etiology is not clearly understood. In the light of numerous case reports in which genital mycoplasmas were implicated, studies were conducted to investigate the role of these agents in the causation of fetal wastage. At first, attention was focused on *M. hominis.* Jones (1967), Harwick and colleagues (1970) and Di Musto and colleagues (1973) compared cervical isolation rate of *M. hominis* in patients having spontaneous abortions to a control group of normal pregnant women (Table 15.2). All these workers found the cervical isolation rate of M. hominis to be similar in both groups. When the spontaneous abortion was accompanied by febrile complications, however, a significantly higher isolation rate for *M. hominis* was found (Harwick *et al.*, 1970). The prevalence of antibodies against *M. hominis* was twice as high in the group with spontaneous abortion (Jones, 1967).

Mycoplasmas have also been isolated from lungs of aborted fetuses (Jones, 1967). An ascending infection originating from the cervix was the most likely explanation in all but two cases: in one case histologic examination of the fetal lungs revealed signs of early pneumonia, suggestive of a *M. hominis* infection involving the fetus prior to the abortion. In the second case *M. hominis* was isolated from all the internal organs of the fetus, thus indicating a hematogenous spread of the infection.

These studies indicate that *M. hominis* is probably rarely implicated as an etiologic agent in spontaneous abortion. The ability of the microorganism to invade dead tissue is well established; however, postabortal infection with *M. hominis* is generally mild, suggesting that the organism has a low grade of virulence.

It is more likely that *U. urealyticum* is implicated in spontaneous abortion. Considerable interest in the past decade has centered around this organism (Table 15.3). The first report of a probably deleterious effect of *U. urealyticum* in pregnancy was published in 1967 (Kundsin *et al.*, 1967).

Ureaplasmas were isolated from the chorion, decidua and amnion of an

Table 15.2 Incidence of *M. hominis* in patients with spontaneous abortion

Authors	*Study group*	*Samples*	*Results*
Jones, 1967	70 patients with spontaneous abortion	cervical cultures serum	17% cervical isolation rate* antibodies found in 29% of the samples†
Harwick *et al.*, 1970	53 patients with afebrile abortion 51 patients with febrile spontaneous abortion	cervical cultures cervical cultures	11% cervical isolation rate* 39% cervical isolation rate‡
Di Musto *et al.*, 1973	100 pregnant women with positive cervical cultures	cervical cultures	No more pregenancy wastage than in patients with negative cervical culture

* No difference in isolation rate as compared to normal pregnant women
† Antibodies twice as common as compared to normal pregnant women
‡ $p < 0.01$ as compared to normal pregnant women

Table 15.3 *U. urealyticum* in patients with spontaneous abortion

Authors	*No. of spont. abortions studied*	*Control group*	*Samples*	*Results*
Kundsin *et al.*, 1967	1	none	chroion, decidua, amnion	Positive tissue cultures
Romano *et al.*, 1971	1	none	heart, lungs, placenta	positive organ cultures
Caspi *et al.*, 1972	183	99 induced abortions	cervix	36% vs 25% in the control group
			trophoblast	31% vs 5% in the control group
Sompolinsky *et al.*, 1975	106 2nd trimester	28 2nd trimester induced abortions	placental	37% vs 4% in the control group ($p < 0.001$)
			fetal organs	22% vs 0% in the control group ($p < 0.001$)

abortus of 17 weeks. On histologic examination, necrosis and a subacute inflammatory reaction of the decidua were found, and the membranes and umbilical cord showed an inflammatory reaction as well. Although signs of placentitis different from those found in viral infections were seen, spontaneous rupture of the membranes had taken place 5 days before expulsion and facilitated an intra-amniotic infection.

U. urealyticum was recovered from the placenta, heart and lungs of a fetus aborted in the 19th week of pregnancy (Romano *et al.*, 1971). Histologic exmination showed an inflammatory process involving some respiratory bronchioles and alveoli strongly suggesting that the infection took place prior to the fetal death. Cultures for viruses, bacteria and other mycoplasmas remained negative. An increase in serum antibodies against *U. urealyticum* was suggestive of recent infection in the mother, however. Intrauterine spread of *U. urealyticum* with fetal lung involvement originating from the cervix was an acceptable explanation for the fetal demise.

In a comparative study of spontaneous and induced abortion the incidence of mycoplasma in cervical secretions was found to be 37% and 28% respectively for each type of pregnancy loss (Caspi *et al.*, 1972). The difference of positive fetal tissue was even more significant: mycoplasmas were isolated in 31% of the study group and in only 5% of the control group. These differences were most significant for *U. urealyticum*, suggesting an association between *U. urealyticum* infection and spontaneous abortion.

A cervical isolation rate of 55% found in patients with spontaneous abortion was significantly different from the 40% cervical isolation rate in normal pregnant women (Foulon *et al.*, 1982). Patients having positive cervical cultures for *U. urealyticum* more often appear to have positive fetal tissue cultures if the abortion is spontaneous rather than induced (Table 15.4).

A positive relationship between fetal loss and mycoplasma was found in advanced as well as early pregnancy (Sompolinsky *et al.*, 1975).

In spite of reports showing a positive correlation between isolation rates of *U. urealyticum* and spontaneous abortion, we are unable to conclude that *U. urealyticum* is a major etiologic agent of this condition. Sometimes it may indeed cause a primary infection, but it is quite likely that in most cases of positive cultures the organism has acted as a secondary infective agent in a fetus that has already died.

Table 15.4 Incidence of *U. urealyticum* colonization in cervical smears and in trophoblast cultures in normal pregnant women and in patients with spontaneous abortion

Group	*Cervical colonization*	*Trophoblast colon. in patients with posit. cerv. smears*
Normal pregnant women	40%	–
Induced abortion	49%	22%
One spontaneous abortion	55% ($p < 0.05$)*	58% ($p < 0.001$)†
Two or more spontaneous abortions	67% ($p < 0.025$)*	71% ($p < 0.001$)†

* *p* value in comparison with normal pregnant women
† *p* value in comparison with induced abortion

It is not yet clear how *U. urealyticum* acts. It is known that chromosomal aberrations are responsible for at least 40% of all spontaneous abortions; it is not always appreciated that mycoplasmas may induce chromosome changes in human diploid cells (Allison and Paton, 1966). Ureaplasmas isolated from a mid-trimester abortion were able to induce chromosomal abnormalities (isochromatid gaps, breaks and tetraploidy) (Kundsin *et al.*, 1971). Such *in vitro* findings suggest that *U. urealyticum* can induce chromosomal aberrations in the zygote with a subsequent miscarriage.

A subclinical inflammation of the endometrium is another possible explanation for the mechanism of action of ureaplasma. Such an inflammation was found more often in patients with positive ureaplasma cultures of cervix and urine (Horne *et al.*, 1973). A third possibility is a direct fetal infection across intact membranes. Such an infection has been thought to be responsible for perinatal deaths (Tafari *et al.*, 1976): of 21 stillborn infants, all had signs of congenital pneumonia on autopsy. *U. urealyticum* was the sole organism cultured from the lungs. It is possible that a direct fetal infection can take place early in pregnancy resulting in fetal death and spontaneous abortion.

GENITAL MYCOPLASMAS IN RECURRENT ABORTION

Recurrent abortion is an important and as yet unsolved problem in obstetrics. The role of *U. urealyticum* in this condition is unclear. In 1969 a preliminary report was published on six women with a history of recurrent abortion. In five of them, cervical swabs were cultured for *Mycoplasma* species: four yielded positive cultures; all six women were treated with demethylchlortetracycline (Declomycin) before and during their subsequent pregnancy. Only one of these pregnancies resulted in a spontaneous abortion (Driscoll *et al.*, 1969).

Forty-six patients suffering from habitual abortion were investigated for the presence of *U. urealyticum* in the cervix and endometrium (Stray-Pedersen, 1979). Cervical colonization was higher in the recurrent abortion group (61%) than in the control group (49%). Moreover, endometrial colonization was significantly different in the study group (28%) as compared with normal fertile patients (7%). Doxycycline therapy given to patients positive for *U. urealyticum* resulted in a better outcome in the subsequent pregnancy as compared with patients who did not harbor the organism. The improved pregnancy outcome was noted in the group with positive endometrial colonization and in whom a relation between *U. urealyticum* and recurrent abortion was established. Such an association was also found in an epidemiologic survey which compared normal pregnant women with patients who had two or more spontaneous abortions (Foulon *et al.*, 1982). Cervical colonization was higher in patients with recurrent abortion (Table 15.4), and positive cervical smears more often resulted in positive trophoblast cultures in the study group than in patients with induced abortions.

The pathogenesis of *U. urealyticum* in recurrent abortion is still debated. A chronic inflammation of the endometrium resulting in recurrent miscarriage is one of the possible explanations for the action of ureaplasmas. The low pathogenicity of this microorganism most likely is the reason for the absence of clinical signs of endometrial infection. A question arises how *U. urealyticum* can colonize the endometrium, which is normally free of microorganisms, and how they can pass through the cervical canal which supposedly prevents microorganisms from penetrating the uterine cavity. It is clear that ureaplasmas can gain access to the endometrium when certain pathological conditions are present, such as a dead fetus, an open cervical canal or abnormal bleeding during pregnancy. These circumstances facilitate the spread of *U. urealyticum*. However, endometrium colonization can also be present in patients without any history of pregnancy or abortion (Stray-Pedersen *et al*., 1978); thus other factors facilitating infection of the endometrium must also be considered.

Perhaps spermatozoa play a carrier role in such cases. Scanning electron microscopy of semen samples positive for *U. urealyticum* reveals structures on the midpiece of the sperm cells not observed in samples which are culture negative (Gnarpe and Friberg, 1973b). On the other hand, when semen was cultured on agar, the great majority of colonies of *U. urealyticum* grew out of the spermatozoa. The structures observed in 1973 subsequently were confirmed to be ureaplasmas (Fowlkes *et al*., 1975) and were localized at the junction between the sperm head and the midpiece (Hofstetter, 1978). These findings could explain the endometrial colonization in some patients.

Numerous problems remain to be solved. Many patients colonized by *U. urealyticum* do not suffer from spontaneous abortion. Some women who have had a spontaneous abortion quickly eliminate the microorganism from the endometrium while others remain colonized. Perhaps differences in the immune status of the patient or a variation in the pathogenicity of the strains may be responsible for these discrepancies. More studies have to be done to elucidate these problems.

MANAGEMENT AND THERAPY

Because no etiologic role in spontaneous abortion has been attributed to *M. hominis*, cultures for this microorganism should not be routinely performed.

The association between *M. hominis* and febrile abortion is well established, however. Since most complications are mild and self-limited, it is not necessary to cover *M. hominis* when treating febrile complications of spontaneous abortion. The antibiotics of choice in postabortal sepsis are those active against potentially lethal pathogens such as the coliforms, streptococci and clostridia.

In view of the high frequency of *U. urealyticum* in the cervix of normal pregnant women, it is neither advisable nor necessary to perform routine prenatal cultures for *U. urealyticum*. Similarly it is not necessary to treat all women with a history of spontaneous abortion. In those patients who had two or more successive abortions, however, it is advisable to investigate the etiology of the abortions. In addition to routine investigations of the causes of recurrent miscarriage, we suggest culture of the endocervix, endometrium and sperm for *U. urealyticum*.

If cultures are positive in one of the three samples, doxycycline should be given for 10 days to both partners. Contraception must be provided because of the known harmful effect of the antibiotic on the fetus. One month after therapy a follow-up culture should be done. This is necessary because eradication of ureaplasma is not always easy (Gnarpe and Friberg, 1973; Rehewy *et al.*, 1978). If cultures remain positive after 10 days of therapy a sensitivity testing should be done, as approximately 10% of *U. urealyticum* strains show *in vitro* resistance to tetracycline (Evans and Taylor-Robinson, 1978).

If the isolated strain is resistant to tetracycline, another antibiotic should be chosen in accordance with the sensitivity studies. Treatment must be continued until the cultures of both partners become negative.

References

Allison, A. C. and Paton, G. R. (1966). Chromosomal abnormalities in human diploid cells infected with mycoplasma and their possible relevance to the aetiology of Down's syndrome. *Lancet,* **2,** 1229

Braun, P., Klein, J. O., Lee, Y. H. and Kass, E. H. (1970). Methodologic investigations and prevalence of genital mycoplasmas in pregnancy. *J. Infect. Dis.,* **121,** 391

Carlson, H. J., Spector, S. and Douglas, H. G. (1951). Possible role of pleuropneumonia-like organisms in etiology of disease in childhood. *Am. J. Dis. Child.,* **81,** 193

Caspi, E., Solomon, F. and Sompolinsky, D. (1972). Early abortion and mycoplasma infection. *Isr. J. Med. Sci.,* **8,** 122

Caspi, E., Solomon, F., Langer, R. and Sompolinsky, D. (1976). Isolation of Mycoplasmas from the placentas after cesarean section. *Obstet. Gynecol.,* **48,** 682

Dienes, L. and Edsall, G. (1937). Observations on the L. organism of Klieneberger. *Proc. Soc. Exp. Biol. Med.,* **36,** 740

Dienes, L., Ropes, M. W., Smith, W. E., Madoff, S. and Brauer, W. (1948). The role of pleuropneumonia-like organisms in genito-urinary and joint diseases. *N. Engl. J. Med.,* **238,** 563

Di Musto, J. C., Bohjalian, O. and Millar, M. (1973). Mycoplasma hominis type I infection and pregnancy. *Obstet. Gynecol.,* **41,** 33

Driscoll, S. G., Kundsin, R. B., Horne, H. W. and Scott, J. M. (1969). Infections and first trimester losses: Possible role of mycoplasmas. *Fertil. Steril.,* **20,** 1017

Evans, R. T. and Taylor-Robinson, D. (1978). The incidence of tetracycline resistant strains of Ureaplasma urealyticum. *J. Antimicrob. Chemother.,* **4,** 57

Foulon, W., Naessens, A. and Lauwers, S. (1982). Role of U. urealyticum in spontaneous abortion. Presented at the *International Symposium on 'Abortion Spontaneous and Induced',* 1982, Maui, Hawaii

Fowlkes, D. M., Dooher, G. B. and O'Leary, W. M. (1975). Evidence by scanning electron microscopy for an association between spermatozoa and T-mycoplasmas in men of infertile marriages. *Fertil. Steril.,* **26,** 1203

Foy, H. M., Kenny, G. E., Wenthworth, B. B., Johnson, W. L. and Grayston, J. T. (1970). Isolation of Mycoplasmas hominis, T. strains, and cytomegalovirus from the cervix of pregnant women. *Am. J. Obstet. Gynecol.,* **106,** 635

Freundt, E. A. (1967). The mycoplasmas. In Buchanan, R. E. and Gibbons, N. E. (eds.) *Bergey's Manual of Determinative Bacteriology.* 8th Edn., pp. 929–949. (Baltimore: Williams & Wilkins)

Gnarpe, H. and Friberg, S. (1972). Mycoplasma and human reproductive failure: I. The occurrence of different mycoplasmas in couples with reproductive failure. *Am. J. Obstet. Gynecol.,* **114,** 727

Gnarpe, H. and Friberg, S. (1973*a*). T-mycoplasmas as a possible cause for reproductive failure. *Nature (Lond.),* **242,** 120

Gnarpe, H. and Friberg, S. (1973*b*). T-mycoplasmas on spermatozoa and infertility. *Nature (Lond.),* **245,** 97

Gotthardson, A. and Melen, B. (1953). Isolation of pleuropneumonia-like organisms from ovarian abscesses. *Acta Pathol. Microbiol. Scand.*, **33,** 291

Harwick, H. J., Iuppa, J. B. and Fekety, F. R. (1969). Microorganisms and amniotic fluid. *Obstet. Gynecol.*, **33,** 256

Harwick, H. J., Purcell, R. H., Iuppa, J. B. and Fekety, F. R. (1970). Mycoplasma hominis and abortion. *J. Infect. Dis.*, **121,** 260

Hofstetter, A., Schmeidt, E., Schill, W. B. and Wolff, H. H. (1978). Genital Mykoplasmenstämme als Ursache der männlichen Infertilität. *Helv. Chir. Acta*, **45,** 329

Horne, H. W., Hertig, H. T., Kundsin, R. B. and Kosasa, T. S. (1973). Subclinical endometrial inflammation and T-mycoplasma: A possible cause of human reproductive failure. *Int. J. Fertil.*, **18,** 226

Jones, D. M. (1967). Mycoplasm hominis in abortion. *Br. Med. J.*, **1,** 338

Kundsin, R. B., Driscoll, S. G. and Ming, P. L. (1967). Strain of mycoplasma associated with human reproductive failure. *Science*, **157,** 1573

Kundsin, R. B., Ampola, M., Streeter, S. and Neurath, P. (1971). Chromosomal aberrations induced by T-strains mycoplasmas. *J. Med. Genet.*, **8,** 181

Lamey, J. R., Foy, H. M. and Kenny, G. E. (1974). Infection with Mycoplasma hominis and T-strains in the femal genital tract. *Obstet. Gynecol.*, **44,** 703

McCormack, W. M., Almeida, P. C., Bailey, P. E., Grady, E. M. and Lee, Y. H. (1972). Sexual activity and vaginal colonization with genital mycoplasmas. *J. Am. Med. Assoc.*, **221,** 1375

Naessens, A., Foulon, W., Amy, J. J. and Lauwers, S. (1982). Ureaplasma urealyticum in pregnancy and the relation to birth weight and gestational length. Presented at the *82nd ASM Meeting*, Atlanta

Nocard, E. and Roux, E. (1889). Le microbe de la peripneumonie. *Ann. Inst. Pasteur (Paris)*, **12,** 240

Nowak, J. (1929). Morphologie, nature et cycle evolutif du microbe de la peripneumonie des bovides. *Ann. Inst. Pasteur (Paris)*, **43,** 1330

Rehewy, M. S. E., Jaszczak, C., Hafez, E. S. E., Thomas, A. and Brown, W. J. (1978). Ureaplasma urealyticum (T-mycoplasma) in vaginal fluid and cervical mucus from fertile and infertile women. *Fertil. Steril.*, **30,** 297

Romano, N., Romano, F. and Carollo, F. (1971). T-strains of mycoplasma in bronchopneumonic lungs of an aborted fetus. *N. Engl. J. Med.*, **285,** 950

Ross, J. M., Furr, P. M., Taylor-Robinson, D., Altman, D. G. and Coid, C. R. (1981). The effect of genital mycoplasmas on human fetal growth. *Br. J. Obstet. Gynecol.*, **88,** 749

Shepard, M. C. (1954). The recovery of pleuropneumonia-like organisms from Negro men with and without non-gonococcal urethritis. *Am. J. Syph. Gonorr. Vener. Dis.*, **38,** 113

Shepard, M. C. and Lunceford, C. D. (1967). Occurrence of urease in T strains of Mycoplasma. *J. Bacteriol.*, **93,** 1513

Slingerland, D. W. and Morgan, H. R. (1952). Sustained bacteremia with pleuropneumonia-like organisms in a post partum patient. *J. Am. Med. Assoc.*, **150,** 1309

Sompolinsky, D., Solomon, F., Elkina, L., Weinraub, Z., Bukovsky, I. and Caspi, E. (1975). Infections with mycoplasmas and bacteria in induced midtrimester abortion and fetal loss. *Am. J. Obstet. Gynecol.*, **121,** 610

Stokes, E. J. (1955). Human infection with pleuropneumonia-like organisms. *Lancet*, **1,** 276

Stokes, E. J. (1959). P.P.L.O. in genital infections. *Br. Med. J.*, **1,** 510

Stray-Pedersen, B. (1979). Female genital colonization with Ureaplasma urealyticum and reproductive failure. *Curr. Ther. Res.*, **26,** 771

Stray-Pedersen, B., Eng, J. and Reikvam, T. M. (1978). Uterine T Mycoplasma colonization in reproductive failure. *Gynecology*, **130,** 307

Tafari, N., Ross, S., Naeye, R. L., Judge, D. M. and Marboe, C. (1976). Mycoplasma T-strain and perinatal death. *Lancet*, **1,** 108

16
Endometriosis and spontaneous abortion

J. D. NAPLES and R. E. BATT

Endometriosis is a major cause of infertility and currently is identified in 21% of infertile women (Strathy *et al.*, 1982). Recently endometriosis has been recognized as a cause of spontaneous abortion (Petersohn, 1970; Jones and Jones, 1971; Rock *et al.*, 1981; Naples *et al.*, 1981; Olive *et al.*, 1982). This has important therapeutic implications; treatment of endometriosis in the infertile couple should correct both problems – the inability to conceive and the fetal wastage. The objective of treatment is a healthy newborn.

DETERIORATION OF FERTILITY

Endometriosis does not cause absolute infertility, for some women with untreated endometriosis do conceive. The study of secondary infertility caused by endometriosis provides valuable insight into the natural history of the disease. Examination of the reproductive performance of 100 women with secondary infertility and endometriosis (i.e. the reproductive performance prior to the diagnosis of endometriosis), reveals a deterioration of fertility. This deterioration is characterized by a decreasing conception rate, an increasing spontaneous abortion rate and finally – during the 2 years prior to the diagnosis of endometriosis – a fetal wastage rate of 81% (Naples *et al.*, 1981).

INCREASING SPONTANEOUS ABORTION RATE

Women who conceive more than 10 years before the diagnosis and treatment of endometriosis experience a term livebirth rate of 92% and a spontaneous abortion rate of 7%. As the endometriotic process progresses the conception rate decreases. The term livebirth rate also decreases while the spontaneous abortion rate rises sharply (Figure 16.1). The few women who conceive within the 2 years immediately preceding the diagnosis and treatment of endometriosis suffer a 63% spontaneous abortion rate, 12% ectopic pregnancy rate, 6% stillbirth rate with only a 19% term livebirth rate.

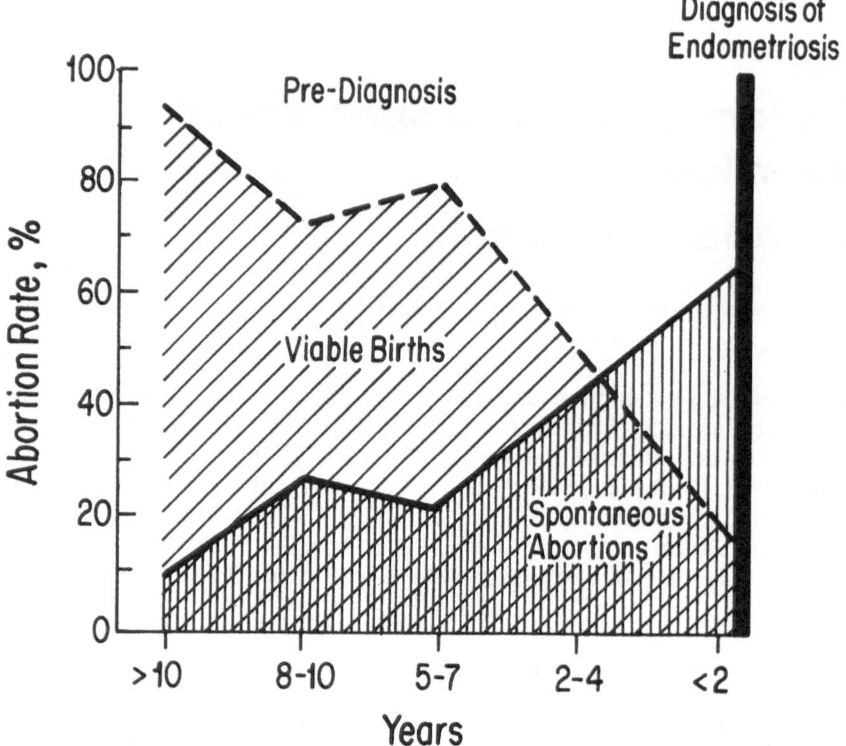

Figure 16.1 Decreasing viable births and increasing spontaneous abortions prior to diagnosis of endometriosis.

Most women with endometriosis present with primary infertility. Presumably their fertility potential has deteriorated to the point that conception will not occur without treatment. Like the women with secondary infertility, they are at risk for spontaneous abortion unless the endometriotic process is completely treated.

RESTORATION OF FERTILITY

Spontaneous abortion rate is a good monitor of the effectiveness of treatment of endometriosis. This is clearly demonstrated by comparing the results of expectant treatment of mild endometriosis to conservative surgical treatment of moderate and severe endometriosis. Effective treatment should restore fertility in a high percentage of patients – resulting in a high conception rate, a high term livebirth rate and a low spontaneous abortion rate.

EXPECTANT MANAGEMENT OF ENDOMETRIOSIS

After the diagnosis of endometriosis was made at laparoscopy or laparotomy in the study group of 100 women, 40 of the patients with mild endometriosis (AFS Stage I, Acosta Stage I) who desired to conceive were treated expectantly (Table 16.1). Expectant treatment means a complete infertility evaluation with diagnosis and treatment of all factors in both husband and wife – except direct treatment of the endometriosis and associated surgical lesions like leiomyomas (Batt and Naples, 1982). Expectant treatment includes correction of anovulation and ovulatory dysfunction (Schenken and Malinak, 1982). Seventy percent of the women conceived with expectant treatment but 25 % of the conceptions terminated in spontaneous abortion. The spontaneous abortion rate prior to treatment was 36 %.

Table 16.1 Pregnancy outcome before and after expectant treatment for mild endometriosis – 40 patients (30 without clomiphene citrate (Clomid), 10 with clomiphene citrate (Clomid)

	Before treatment		*After treatment*	
Outcome	*No.*	*Percent*	*No.*	*Percent*
Term	25	53	27	68
Premature	0	0	2	5
Ectopic	2	4	0	0
Legal abortion	3	6	1	2
Abortion	17	36	10	25
Totals	47		40	

CONSERVATIVE SURGERY FOR ENDOMETRIOSIS

A second group of patients with moderate (AFS Stage II, Acosta Stage II) and severe endometriosis (AFS Stage III, Acosta Stage III) was treated with conservative surgery (Sadigh *et al.*, 1977). Fifty-seven percent of the patients conceived and only 8 % of the conceptions were lost by spontaneous abortion (Table 16.2). The spontaneous abortion rate before surgery was 46 %. The conservative surgery study group demonstrates that the high fetal wastage in

Table 16.2 Pregnancy outcome before and after conservative surgery – 65 patients (23 moderate, 42 severe endometriosis)

	Before surgery		*After surgery*	
Outcome	*No.*	*Percent*	*No.*	*Percent*
Term	19	51	43	86
Premature	0	0	3	6
Stillborn	1	3	0	0
Ectopic	0	0	0	0
Abortion	17	46	4	8
Total	37		50	

patients with endometriosis is corrected by surgery. Conservative surgery for endometriosis means a complete infertility evaluation with diagnosis and treatment of all factors in both husband and wife prior to the sharp excision of all endometriosis and correction of associated surgical lesions (Batt and Naples, 1982).

Conservative surgery is effective because, by the removal of visible endometriotic lesions, the disease process is forced to retreat to stage zero. Following conservative surgery with sharp excision of endometriosis, the spontaneous abortion rates consistently run between 7.7% and 14%, with term livebirth rates between 83 and 91% (Green, 1966; Rogers and Jacobs, 1968; Petersohn, 1970; Acosta *et al.*, 1973; Sadigh *et al.*, 1977; Buttram, 1979; Rock *et al.*, 1981).

PREVENTION OF SPONTANEOUS ABORTION

The term livebirth rate of 86% with conservative surgery is decidedly better than the term livebirth rate of 68% with expectant treatment of endometriosis. The difference is striking because expectant treatment was used for mild endometriosis while conservative surgical treatment was used for moderate and severe endometriosis. The difference is even more striking when it is realized that expectant treatment lowered the spontaneous abortion rate from 36% to 25% whereas the conservative surgical treatment reduced the spontaneous abortion rate from 46% to 8%.

The significant difference between expectant treatment and conservative surgery for endometriosis is that with surgery the endometriotic lesions are removed while with expectant treatment the endometriotic lesions are allowed to remain intact.

Endometriotic tissue of humans has been shown to contain significantly higher levels of prostaglandins than the non-endometriotic tissue of the same organ (Moon *et al.*, 1981). Removal of endometriosis by conservative surgery eradicates this source of prostaglandins. Since prostaglandins are known abortifacients, their removal along with the endometriosis may be the mechanism by which conservative surgery prevents spontaneous abortion. Conversely, continued production and release of prostaglandins by endometriotic tissue may explain the persistently high spontaneous abortion rate in patients treated expectantly.

CONCLUSIONS

Endometriosis is a cause of spontaneous abortion as well as a cause of failure to conceive. Treatment should correct both problems. Each couple should be offered the treatment which affords the best chance for a healthy baby and the lowest risk for spontaneous abortion.

Acknowledgement

Information, tables and figure previously published in Naples *et al.*, (1981) are reproduced by permission of *Obstetrics and Gynaecology* and Elsevier Science Publication Company, New York.

References

Acosta, A. A., Buttram, V. C., Besch, P. K., Malinak, R. L., Franklin, R. R. and Vanderhayden, J. D. (1973). A proposed classification of pelvic endometriosis. *Obstet. Gynecol.*, **42,** 19

Batt, R. E. and Naples, J. D. (1982). Conservative surgery for endometriosis in the infertile couple. *Curr. Probl. Obstet. Gynecol.*, **VI,** 1

Buttram, V. C. Jr (1979). Conservative surgery for endometriosis in the infertile female: A study of 206 patients with implications for both medical and surgical therapy. *Fertil. Steril.*, **31,** 117

Green, T. H. (1966). Conservative surgical treatment of endometriosis. *Clin. Obstet. Gynecol.*, **9,** 293

Halme, J., Becker, S., Hammond, M. G., Raj, M. H. G. and Raj, S. (1983). Increased activation of pelvic macrophages in infertile women with mild endometriosis. *Am. J. Obstet. Gynecol.*, **145,** 333

Jones, G. S. and Jones, H. W. Jr. (1971). Editorial. *Obstet. Gynecol. Survey*, **26,** 539

Moon, Y. S., Leung, P. C. S., Yuen, B. H. and Gomel, V. (1981). Prostaglandin F in human endometriosis tissue. *Am. J. Obstet. Gynecol.*, **141,** 344

Naples, J. D., Batt, R. E. and Sadigh, H. (1981). Spontaneous abortion rate in patients with endometriosis. *Obstet. Gynecol.*, **57,** 509

Olive, D. L., Franklin, R. R. and Gratkins, L. V. (1982). The association between endometriosis and spontaneous abortion. *J. Reprod. Med.*, **27,** 333

Petersohn, L. (1970). Fertility in patients with ovarian endometriosis before and after treatment. *Acta Obstet. Gynecol. Scand.*, **49,** 331

Rock, J. A., Guzick, D. S., Sengos, C., Schweditsch, M., Sapp, K. C. and Jones, H. W. Jr. (1981). The conservative surgical treatment of endometriosis: evaluation of pregnancy success with respect to the extent of disease as categorized using contemporary classification systems. *Fertil. Steril.*, **35,** 131

Rogers, S. F. and Jacobs, W. M. (1968). Infertility and endometriosis: Conservative surgical approach. *Fertil. Steril.*, **19,** 529

Sadigh, H., Naples, J. D. and Batt, R. E. (1977). Conservative surgery for endometriosis in the infertile couple. *Obstet. Gynecol.*, **49,** 562

Schenken, R. S. and Asch, R. H. (1980). Surgical induction of endometriosis in the rabbit: Effects on fertility and concentrations of peritoneal fluid prostaglandins. *Fertil. Steril.*, **34,** 581

Schenken, R. S. and Malinak, L. R. (1982). Conservative surgery versus expectant management for the infertile patient with mild endometriosis. *Fertil. Steril.*, **37,** 183

Strathy, J. H., Molgaard, C. A., Coulam, C. B. and Melton, L. J. III (1982). Endometriosis and infertility: A laparoscopic study of endometriosis among fertile and infertile women. *Fertil. Steril.*, **38,** 667

17
Asymptomatic bacteriospermia in spontaneous abortion

B. DAHLBERG

ABORTION IN EARLY PREGNANCY

The true rate of spontaneous abortion in early pregnancy is not well known. A prospective study (Miller *et al.*, 1980) in 197 women based on the presence of elevated urinary human chorionic gonadotropin (hCG) during the luteal phase of the menstrual cycle shows evidence of conception in 24% (152) of 623 menstrual cycles. Of these, only 57% (87) advanced beyond 20 weeks' gestation. Spontaneous abortion was apparent in 14% of 102 recognized pregnancies. Of the lost conceptions only one-fourth are clinically recognized abortions. The conceptions identified by raised β-hCG levels are considered to be postimplantation conceptions. The causes of the early preamenorrhoic abortions are yet to be interpreted. Clinically registered abortions are reported at lower levels, between 10 and 15%.

The risk of a new abortion is 24% after one abortion (Glass and Golbus, 1978). About 25–30% remain infertile after the first abortion (Dahlberg, 1982). The prognosis for a subsequent normal pregnancy may thus be around 50%. Spontaneous abortion, although a sign of apparent fecundity, could be the sign of infertility in a marital unit.

Pathogenesis

The pathogenesis of abortion may be found in the mother, in the embryo and in the spermatozoa.

Etiologies

The difficulty in establishing whether an apparent factor is a primary or a secondary cause of abortion is reflected in the reports with multifactorial etiologies.

Anomalies

Anomalies found in the mother may have been the cause of abortion if subsequent pregnancies are normal after treatment. Most women with anomalies have normal pregnancies brought to term.

Chromosomal aberrations

Chromosomal aberrations are found in 47–60% of early pregnancies (Poland, 1971; Boué *et al.*, 1975; Tolksdorf, 1979) and are believed to be the cause of abortions. Investigations of parents usually give negative chromosomal findings (Poland, 1971; Lauritsen, 1976; Leodolter *et al.*, 1979). The frequency of chromosome aberration in the parents is 0.76% (Lauritsen, 1976). Chromosomal aberrations may thus not be a primary cause but are definitely secondary with disturbances of implantation and evolution.

Hormonal dysfunction

Hyperthyroidism has been suggested as a cause of abortion but no certain evidence has been found.

Dysfunction in the ovarian hormone system is considered to give pathologic changes in:

(1) Growth of embryoblast
(2) Nutrition of blastocyte (trophoblast cell)
(3) Contact between trophoblast and endometrium
(4) Cytology of endometrium

Even with endocrine tests, the therapeutic possibilities of a hormonal treatment are not promising (Beier, 1979).

Infection

See the following section on Habitual Abortion.

HABITUAL ABORTION

Abortions after the first trimester often mean the loss of a normal fetus, whereas spontaneous abortion in the first trimester seems to be the result of disturbed or blighted ova. Efforts to conserve an early threatened pregnancy may not only be in vain, but unnecessary.

Incidence

The frequency of habitual abortion varies from one in 122 deliveries (Harger, 1980) to one in 777 (Peters *et al.*, 1979) judged by the incidence of cervical incompetence.

Etiology

Anomalies, chromosomal aberrations and hormonal dysfunction considered as possible causes in single abortion are also found in cases of habitual abortion.

The risk of having another abortion after a previous one is 33 %, influenced by the karyotype of the index aberration. The frequency of a subsequent abortion where the index abortus has a normal karyotype is as high as 45 % (Lauritsen, 1976). Glass and Golbus (1978) calculate the risk of a new abortion to be 24 % after one abortion, 26 % after two abortions, and 32 % after three abortions. The frequency of remaining infertility, be it voluntary or involuntary, is not well known.

Cervical incompetence

The loss of a normal fetus is infrequently considered to be due to cervical incompetence. This is a diagnosis that is not well defined. It is based solely on past obstetric history and follow-up of cases with habitual abortion. Cervical incompetence may be the direct cause in a few cases where there is visual evidence of previous surgical or obstetric trauma to the cervix. In most cases cervical incompetence is not a primary, but a secondary cause.

An asymptomatic chorioamnionitis can start the progressive dilatation of the cervix (Curbelo *et al.*, 1981).

Treatment

Surgical treatment with cerclage of the cervix after the 14th week of gestation by procedure of Shirodkar or McDonald has resulted in a prevention of premature delivery in about 70 % of cases. Complications to mother and child are noted in about 30 % (Aarnoudse and Huisjes, 1979; Peters *et al.*, 1979; Harger, 1980), such as premature membrane rupture, uterine rupture or infection, untreatable premature labor of fetal death. Indications for operation are suggested by Block and Rahhal (1976). Surgical treatment must be followed by constant obstetric observation.

Coital activity

The effects of intercourse and orgasm on premature delivery have been controversially interpreted. Rayburn and Wilson (1980) compared coital activity of 111 patients, who were delivered after spontaneous premature labor, with that of a control group, who were delivered at term. They concluded that normal coitus was not an etiologic factor in premature delivery.

Infection

Toxoplasma gondii can invade the placenta and fetus but is not a significant factor in habitual abortion. *Listeria monocytogenes* has not been found to cause abortion in women.

The role of *Chlamydia trachomatis* and *Mycoplasma* commonly found in the vagina and the cervix is not established and is doubtful. The role of herpesvirus and cytomegalovirus infections, if any, is not known.

There is an association of premature labor with intrauterine infection or contamination, urinary tract infection and early neonatal sepsis, which suggests that microorganisms might influence labor. Microorganisms have phospholipase A_2 activity (Bejar *et al.*, 1981). Phospholipase A_2 is activated at the onset of labor and hydrolyses phospholipids, producing free arachidonic acid, which is the precursor of prostaglandins E_2 and $F_2\alpha$. Activity is found in *Bacteriodes fragilis*, *Peptostreptococcus*, *Fusobacterium necrophorum*, *Streptococcus viridans*, *Streptococcus faecalis*, *Streptococcus A* and *B*, *Escherichia coli*, *Klebsiella*, *Staph. epidermidis*, *Pneumococcus*, *Lactobacillus* and *Mycoplasma hominis*. Activities are highest in *B. fragilis*, *Peptostreptococcus*, *Fusobacterium* and *S. viridans*. The specific activities of phospholipase A_2 from these organisms are several times higher than that of the membrane phospholiphase A_2 of the amnion and chorion.

Labor may be triggered by this microbially induced increase of prostaglandin synthesis (Block and Rahhal, 1976). Asymptomatic amnionitis may occur in the presence of intact membranes. Diagnostic amniocentesis was tried by Wallace and Herrick (1981), but amnionitis was not demonstrated in a significant number of asymptomatic patients in premature labor. In view of the higher risk associated with amniocentesis in these women it would seem clinically unwarranted.

Asymptomatic bacteriospermia (ABS)

The role of the male in abortion has rarely been questioned or investigated. Recent studies show correlation between male asymptomatic bcteriospermia and spontaneous abortion. Asymptomatic bacteriospermia is a silent infection found in the genital tract of 10–15% of males. It is not to be misinterpreted as ailments such as prostatitis or prostatos, which usually have symptoms. The silent infection found in 90% of the young men in infertile units (Dahlberg, 1973) has been termed asymptomatic bacteriospermia. This condition can affect the female with infections and abortions (Dahlberg, 1976).

Asymptomatic bacteriospermia causes infertility in the male (DelPorto *et al.*, 1975; Dahlberg, 1976; Derrick and Dahlberg, 1976), by inhibition of motility, reduction of survival time or longevity and changes in morphology with increased abnormal spermatozoa. This is caused by aerobic or anaerobic microorganisms. A decrease in longevity will impede the impregnation of the ovum. Antibiotic treatment reverses the infertile sperm to normal.

Motile spermatozoa are able to transport microorganisms (Toth, 1982). Although the female genital tract hinders most deficient spermatozoa, a normal spermatozoon, transporting microorganisms, may reach the fallopian tubes and disturb the impregnation and implantation of the ovum. This may explain the degree of abortions and chromosomal aberrations in the *in vitro* fertilisation experiments.

A new etiology of spontaneous abortion is found in the male partner of women with spontaneous abortions (Dahlberg, 1982). Ninety-one patients with a history of 156 abortions had one abortion in 56 %. Forty-four percent had two or more abortions (Table 17.1). Nine percent had ectopic pregnancies. Male partners examined for asymptomatic bacteriospermia (Dahlberg, 1976) show a variety of positive cultures in 97 %, with *S. fecalis*, 32 %, *Staphylococcus albus*, 26 %, *E. coli* 13 %, *Streptococcus alpha*, 11 %, as the most frequent strains. Twenty-four percent of men have more than one strain of bacteria (Table 17.2). Negative cultures are found in 3 %. Although anaerobic bacteria have previously been found in bacteriospermia, in this study no such cultures were found. This may be due to the pretreatment of *Trichomonas* (6 %) and *Candida albicans* (8 %) with metronidazole, which is an antianaerobic substance, before cultures were taken.

Equivalent positive cultures from 19 out of 20 female cervixes show correlation to the findings of the male (Table 17.3).

This etiology offers a new way of treatment.

Table 17.1

In the 91 cases there were 156 abortions

Number of abortions	1	2	3	4	5–8
Number of cases	51	27	7	3	2–1

Table 17.2

Semen analysis included bacteriologic cultures of semen. Positive cultures were found in 97 % of male semen. Fourteen strains were found. Twenty-four percent had more than one strain of bacteria. Most frequent strains were:

Streptococcus fecalis	32 %
Staphylococcus albus	26 %
Escherichia coli	13 %
Streptococcus alpha	1 %

Although anaerobic bacteria have previously been found in bacteriospermia, in this study no such cultures were found. This may be due to the pretreatment of *Trichomonas* (6 %) and *Candida albicans* (8 %) with metronidazole, which is an antianaerobic substance, before cultures were taken

Table 17.3

Bacteriologic cultures taken from female partners' cervixes (20). The 19 positive cultures were equivalent to their male partners':

Positive cultures	19
Negative cultures	1

Treatment

Female treatment

Antibiotic administration is dependent on the sensitivity of the bacteria. The female is treated for 10–14 days after which period most cervical cultures become negative. To prevent reinfection by the male partner's sperm, the use of the condom is essential.

Male treatment

Antibiotics specifically relevant to cultures are administered. The time of treatment of the male varies between 1 and 6 months, until sperm culture is negative. The couple is then free to try a new conception under the cover of antibiotics for the male. When a conception is achieved, antibiotics are discontinued. This guarantees germ free sperm, at the time of conception. To shield the pregnancy from recurring silent infections in the male that may disturb the female with infections, the use of the condom during the rest of the pregnancy is necessary. This regime shows no complications. Control groups where antibiotics are discontinued too early before conception occurs show a significant difference in recurrent infection in the male.

In the majority of men, with asymptomatic bacteriospermia, there will be a recurrence, after discontinuation of the antibiotic treatment. It is therefore important to suppress ABS until a successful pregnancy is achieved.

Of 56 couples treated 37 (66 %) had full term births without complications. One case was a malformation and died. In this case the male admitted being rather casual about taking antibiotics and did not return for a final sperm examination and culture. This couple have since followed the regime advised, and have a normal child.

Thirty-five couples not receiving treatment acted as controls. No pregnancy was noted in the 2-year time of observation for both groups. The difference in treated and untreated is highly significant.

Remaining infertility in 30 % of cases is due to female immunologic response. This may occur after the first abortion. An early recognition of the possible association with ABS in the male and subsequent treatment may restore the female sensitivity and reverse the hostile effects to sperm (Dahlberg, 1973).

CONCLUDING REMARKS

There are multifactorial apparent causes of abortion. Abortion, single or habitual, should be understood as a sign of disturbed fertility. In a threatened abortion during the first trimester the use of ultrasonography, if available, is an asset for the prognosis. Efforts to treat this condition will be symptomatic as the cause has been asymptomatic until the onset of the abortion. The cause is often an earlier disturbance of the ovum or the implantation. In late abortion, symptomatic treatment is of aid in cases where cervical incompetence is found.

Early antibiotic treatment in suspected cases of habitual abortion may be a future solution. It is important to find a common denominator for the majority of cases of abortions, so that treatment may be directed to the primary cause, and not only to the symptoms.

An etiology found in both early and late abortions is asymptomatic bacteriospermia.

If asymptomatic bacteriospermia is missed, the patient may have one single pregnancy and abortion only, and subsequently suffer from sterility due to infections or immunization caused by the male silent infection. There is a connection between spontaneous abortion and early infection at the time of conception disturbing the normal development of the impregnated ovum. An infection within the ovum will result in an early abortion. An infection resulting in chorioamnionitis will lead to abortion in the later trimesters with the loss of a normal fetus. The treatment suggested offers the patient a normal pregnancy and a normal child.

References

Aarnoudse, J. G. and Huisjes, H. J. (1979). Complications of cerclage. *Acta Obstet. Gynecol. Scand.*, **58**, 255

Block, M. F. and Rahhal, D. K. (1976). Cervical incompetence. *Obstet. Gynecol.*, **47**, 279

Bejar, R., Curbelo, V., Davis, C. and Gluck, L. (1981). Premature II. Bacterial sources of phospholipase. *Obstet. Gynecol.*, **57**, 479

Beier, H. M. (1979). Endocrinolog. und Histolog. Grundlagen des Früaborts. *Fortschr. Fertilitätsforsch.*, **8**, 79

Boué, J., Boué, A. and Lazar, P. (1975). Retrospective and prospective epidemiological studies of 1500 karyotyped spontaneous abortions. *Teratology*, **12**, 11

Curbelo, V., Bejar, R., Benirschke, V. and Gluck, L. (1981). Premature labour I. Prostaglandin precursors in human placenta membrane. *Obstet. Gynecol.*, **57**, 473

Dahlberg, B. (1973). The lethal factor in infertility. An immunologic reaction in the vaginal environment. In *Immunology in Obstetrics and Gynecology. Proceedings of 1st International Congress, Padua*, p. 103. (Amsterdam: Excerpta Medica)

Dahlberg, B. (1976). Asymptomatic bacteriospermia as a cause of infertility in men. *Urology*, **3**, 563

Dahlberg, B. (1982). Asymptomatic bacteriospermia in the male and spontaneous abortion. *Contracept. Deliv. Syst.*, **3**, 394

DelPorto, G., Derrick, F. C. Jr. and Bannister, E. R. (1975). Bacterial effect on sperm motility. *Urology*, **5**, 638

Derrick, F. C. Jr. and Dahlberg, B. (1976). In Hafez, E. S. E. (ed.) *The Human Semen and Fertility Regulation in Men*, pp. 389–397. (St Louis: Mosby)

Glass, R. H. and Golbus, M. S. (1978). Habitual abortion. *Fertil. Steril.*, **29**, 257

Harger, J. H. (1980). Comparison of success and morbidity in cervical cerclage procedures. *Obstet. Gynecol.*, **56**, 543

Lauritsen, J. G. (1976). Aetiology of spontaneous abortion. *Acta Obstet. Gynecol. Scand.*, Suppl. 52

Leodoltér, S., Philipp, K., Schmid, R. and Schneider, W. H. F. (1979). Ergebnisse einer Intensivbetreuung bei Fällen mit Abortus Habitualis. *Fortschr. Fertilitätsforsch.*, **8**, 71

Miller, J. F., Williamson, E., Glue, J., Gordon, Y. B., Grudzinskas, J. G. and Sykes, A. (1980). Fetal loss after implantation. A prospective study. *Lancet*, **2**, 554

Peters, W. A. III, Thiagara, S. and Harbert, C. H. Jr. (1979). Cervical cerclage 20 years experience. *South Med. J.* **72**, 933

Poland, B. J. (1971). Embryonic development in patients with recurrent abortions. *Fertil. Steril.*, **22**, 325

Rayburn, W. F. and Wilson, E. A. (1980). Coital activity and premature delivery. *Am. J. Obstet. Gynecol.*, **137**, 8, 972

Tolksdorf, M. (1979). Chromosomale Ursachen des Spontanabortes. *Fortschr. Festilitätsforsch.*, **8**, 41

Toth, A. (1982). Asymptomatic bacteriospermia and developing female pelvic problems. *Contracept. Deliv. Syst.*, **3**, 524

Wallace, R. L. and Herrick, C. N. (1981). Amniocentesis in the evaluation of premature labor. *Obstet. Gynecol.*, **57**, 483

18
Psychological aspects of spontaneous and adolescent abortions

M. PAJNTAR and J. ROJŠEK

PSYCHOSOMATIC ASPECTS OF SPONTANEOUS ABORTION

Pregnancy and stress

Psychological stress may cause habitual abortion as a result of unresolved unconscious conflicts. Patients frequently have problems accepting a feminine and maternal role (Deutsch, 1945; Squier and Dunbar, 1946; Kroger and Freed, 1951; Javert, 1962; Grimm, 1962; Carlson and Labarba, 1979). In some mammals, psychic stress results in constriction of uterine arteries, reduction of uteroplacentary circulation, reduction of progesterone and MAO (monoaminoxidase), thus provoking abortion (Naaktgeboren and Bontekoe, 1976).

Psychogenic abortion

Psychosomatic studies of spontaneous abortion are rare since most examiners investigate spontaneous abortion only in case of habitual abortion. Habitual abortion is frequently treated by cerclage (suturing of the cervical canal). Cerclage is indicated also in cases of psychogenic abortion (Lancet *et al.*, 1972). In such cases severe underlying emotional conflicts may be manifested and exacerbated after delivery (Van den Bergh *et al.*, 1966).

Personality traits and spontaneous abortion

The reaction to the pregnancy stress depends on the personality structure, dynamics and the intensity of stress. A group of fifty women with threatened abortion were analysed. Personality traits were assessed by E.P.Q. (the Eysenck Personality Questionnaire) and by the P.I.E. (Plutchik Index of Emotions) and by the projective test of incomplete sentences (Bras, 1974). The sample was divided into four groups.

Group A. Women who did not abort in the examined pregnancy with no history of spontaneous abortion and/or preterm delivery.

Group B. Women who did not abort in the examined pregnancy with a history of spontaneous abortion.

Group C. Women whose examined pregnancy terminated in spontaneous abortion, but who had-no history of spontaneous abortion and/or preterm delivery.

Group D. Women whose examined pregnancy terminated in spontaneous abortion and who had a history of spontaneous abortion and/or preterm delivery.

Personality disturbances are the strongest in Groups B and D. Women in Groups A and C were emotionally more stable and less violent. Group A was characterized by slightest symptoms of threatening abortion (bleeding, etc).

Dynamic psychological traits

Group D is the most difficult. These women were strongly attached to their fathers and even accepted some of their fathers' ideals and attitudes as their own. They required a great deal of attention and had a strong desire to be independent. However, in general, they had much distrust for men and felt inferior to and rejected by most men. In fact, they showed little trust in any friends or acquaintance and displayed much anxiety and fear.

Personality – motherhood – threatening, spontaneous and habitual abortion

Motherhood is an integration of instinctive wishes and needs at the highest possible level of Ego potential (Cividini-Stanić, 1975). While motherhood offers satisfaction, it also entails many new problems. Motherhood is not only a progressive process, but also regressive process. Maturity and stability determine whether the progressive behavior will win over the regressive behavior. Each of the four groups of patients is characterized by neurotic behavior, motivations, conflicts and psychodynamics. A personality disturbance consisting of depressive and regressive symptoms prevailed in women with threatening abortion who aborted in the examined pregnancy or had spontaneous abortion and/or preterm delivery before (Group D.) These women displayed anxiety of: transience, spontaneous and self-initiating activity, self-assertion, independence, and any kind of loss. They must control everything, to be the first or last and to be unique. They are egocentric and the child in them takes control.

Group C women are characterized by an anancastic personality structure with a typical retentive-aggressive inhibition. They lack the ability to develop independence and self-respect to face everyday life. They fear changes, risk and transience. These women are constantly trying to achieve consistency and stability. They have a strong desire to be important, recognized, and powerful. Pregnancy may destroy this neurotic balance; only abortion can restore it. These women act very rationally.

Group B women have anancastic personalities. They have somewhat neurotic and aggressive tendencies. Their moral anxieties are very much activated. This is caused by thoughts of the dependence and emotional meaning that children and family bring for these women. They decide to risk having a child precisely because of these moral anxieties and the egocentric emotional benefit the child and family will provide for them, thus establishing security, acceptance and attention.

Group A women are slightly neurotic and depressive. Their psychoreactive experience of anxieties and conflicts, aroused by pregnancy, does not trigger off fatal regression that may provoke abortion. A part of the personality finds the necessary energy in the mother's desire to preserve the family unity. This is of great emotional importance for her, and thus saves the pregnancy.

Therapeutic possibilities

The woman's personality traits are part of the genesis of spontaneous abortion. Abortion cannot be successfully treated by chemical substances or surgical interventions only. A psychological assessment of the actual situation is equally important. In cases of patients with several previous abortions, the cerclage may be decided only after thorough psychological treatment and therapy. Favorable conditions for pregnancy should be created by professional consultation, even if minimal difficulties in pregnancy suggesting abortion are noticed. The psychotherapeutic process should include the husband. Consultations with a professional person should be conducted in a warm, friendly relaxing atmosphere, to promote acceptance and understanding. The changes in life style, relationship between partners and added responsibilities of pregnancy and motherhood should be thoroughly discussed. In cases of intense, anxious conditions psychotherapy treatment may be supported by medication.

The therapeutic objective is delivery of a healthy child and its upbringing in a healthy environment. In some cases, a profound, reconstructively oriented psychotherapy is required.

PERSONALITY CHARACTERISTICS AND PSYCHIC SEQUELAE OF ABORTION IN ADOLESCENTS

Personality characteristics of adolescents seeking abortion

Unwelcome pregnancy and abortion, caused by social and psychological factors, are considered a pathological process. Abortion is a linkage in a long chain of sociopsychopathology involving psychic, cultural, environmental, educational and other factors (Galdston and Calderone, 1958). Adolescent pregnancy is the product of social pathology (Harrison, 1969): parental neglect, lack of love, insecurity, poverty, ignorance and violence. It is the result of irresponsibility or of an unconscious desire for pregnancy: the girl refusing to use any contraceptive technique though she may be unaware of her own motives. The pregnancy is the result of, rather than the cause of, emotional disturbance (Harrison, 1969). Molinski (1980) discusses the dilemma of pregnant women in terms of the 'pregnancy conflict'. He claims that the attitude towards the child depends on the extremely varied motivation pattern in which wishes, but also anxieties and fears, play an important role. The wish for a child originates partly from the archaic, more biologically oriented layers of ourselves, partly from others. Today the subject 'fear of child' is closer to our consciousness and less of a taboo. We have to distinguish between fear due to real, external difficulties, fear because of inner-psychic difficulties and fear because of neurotic difficulties. The decision for or against pregnancy can therefore be regarded as the solution of the pregnancy conflict.

Pregnancy is expected by every woman from her childhood days onward. The archaic wish for a child is, in a special way, present also in the adolescent, since it is a confirmation of her sexuality and of her feminine role. This conscious or subconscious wish to find out whether or not she is a complete women plays a significant role, opposite to the conscious contraceptive tendencies.

The woman's choice of a partner, her use of contraception, her decision for pregnancy or abortion are influenced greatly by social values and acquired knowledge and information, intelligence, emotional maturity and personality traits.

A study was conducted to evaluate personality traits of adolescents seeking abortion. A hundred healthy adolescent girls (15–20 years of age) were selected. Sixty-three ranged from 15 to 18 years of age, 37 were 18–20 years of age. These girls were unmarried and wanted to interrupt their first pregnancy. They were psychologically examined (intelligence, emotional maturity and personality characteristics tests) and interviewed during the week before the operation and a year after.

In comparison with the control groups (the normal population, schoolgirls) these adolescents display a lower intelligence level, frequently a lower emotional maturity and personality deviations, especially those with neurotic tendencies. The younger girls are less intelligent, are introverted and have obvious signs of neuroticism, significant depressive and increasingly unstable traits. The older adolescents are less mature emotionally. This trait is not noticed in the younger group.

The commonest reasons for requesting abortions were very poor economics (especially in home conditions) (25), the need to complete school (38) and unstable relationships with the father of the child (39). The least divergence from the controls is displayed by the adolescents who want to abort in order to complete their studies. Their intelligence and personality traits are basically normal, except for a lower emotional maturity displayed by the older girls. The girls seeking abortion because of poor economic living conditions were mainly employed and only bad economic conditions hindered them from normal sexual life and motherhood. These adolescents are, in comparison with the control group, less intelligent, with strongly pronounced signs of neuroticism and significant depressive features in the younger group.

Young girls seeking abortions because of unsteady relationships have the most deviated personalities. They display lower intelligence, with strong signs of neuroticism. They are depressed, with features of paranoia. The older adolescents of this motivation group display significantly pronounced signs of neuroticism only and are emotionally less mature.

The adolescents in our study requested abortion under pressure from parents or partners. Their own attitude towards abortion, however, was not always identical: one group of adolescents (43 % of them) wanted to have a child in spite of pressure and unfavourable circumstances. The other group (57 %) did not want the child. In the adolescents who did not want the child, significantly more pronounced neurotic tendencies were found than in those who wanted it. Their decision for abortion was probably guided by other motives than those quoted in the interview. These motives most probably originated in their structural personality traits, where we might search for disturbances in the identification of their own feminine role.

Psychic sequelae after induced abortion

In spite of the increasing number of studies on psychic sequelae after induced abortion, no absolute conclusion can be given. Petersen (1980) collected, from international literature, the results of 28 analyses of psychiatric and psychological post-examinations after legal abortion, performed from 1948 to 1974. He found severe chronic sequelae, mainly depressive developments, to have been reported in 4–9 % of the cases, and mild, passing reactions in 15–24 % of the cases. The sequelae are greater in women who have been emotionally unstable before pregnancy. Most normal women are found to react to abortion with mild feelings of depression without any serious after-effects (Jansson, 1965; Pasnau, 1972; Petersen, 1980). Women with unstable mental structures and in unstable situations are likely to react with disturbances in any case, whether they carry to term or not (Petersen, 1980).

In adult women, interviewed and tested 1 year after having an abortion, 15 % would not have done it again and 23 % had psychic problems, of the reactive nature, after abortion (Pajntar, 1968). They were more nervous, sensitive, depressed, vulnerable and disappointed. In a year's time, however, those symptoms had disappeared. Even objective psychological tests did not show deterioration in psychoneurotic tendencies which existed at the time of abortion, except in individual cases of psychoneurotically disturbed women who include abortion in their total neurotic behavior.

Studies on psychic sequelae to abortion usually do not distinguish between adolescents and adult women. Adolescents are not yet economically independent. Pregnancy hinders their economic independence. Being pregnant is a new experience to them. Abortion may affect their fertility, because they are young and their personality has not yet been fully developed to its potential.

In a study of psychic sequelae, a year after abortion, 30 % of these girls did not want to experience another abortion, especially the older adolescents. Some of these girls decided they definitely would seek contraceptive methods in the future. They felt the experience of an abortion had somewhat matured their attitudes. They now realized the consequences of their slightly immature previous behavior.

In adult women, guilt and depression are frequently felt after experiencing an abortion (Simon, 1966). Twenty-nine percent of our studied adolescents experienced guilt feelings after abortion. The younger adolescents feel guilty for disposing of the unborn child (a moral point). The older girls feel guilty because they might now be sterile. Thirty-three per cent of the girls believe they have not changed after abortion; 36% think they have psychically changed for the better and have become more sensible and psychically more mature. However, 31% feel that abortion has caused a more adverse effect. They have become more nervous, depressed and irritable after the abortion.

The objective psychological tests, completed a year after abortion, reveal that the entire adolescent population now possesses significantly higher neurotic tendencies. In these neurotic tendencies, manic and schizoid features are significantly more pronounced. A year later only reactive depression is significantly lower. In comparison with adult women, especially those who have children and stable family, the adolescents are more inclined to neurotic reactions of developmental characteristics, e.g. immaturity and undeveloped personality. They cannot adequately overcome the psychological stress resulting from abortion. They cope with the arising fears and feelings of guilt through neurotic symptoms.

Adolescent girls and adult women must not be equated when indications for abortion are being considered. In particular, adolescents must not be equated with adult women who have children and stable family.

The problems of unwelcome pregnancy in adolescents and of interrupting this unwelcome pregnancy were an important aspect of the mental and psychical health of this population. Each adolescent girl seeking abortion should receive careful, individual treatment. Some cases should be disuaded from abortion, since older adolescents believe their abortion to have been a mistake. Better sexual education should be provided, in particular for the population at risk, i.e. emotionally and intellectually immature adolescents and those with neurotic tendencies. This education should not focus on harmfulness of sexual intercourse, but rather on the instinctive behavior in their age group, sexual experiences in superficial relationships, and especially the importance of using contraceptive methods.

References

Bras, S. (1974). Projekcijski preizkus nedokončanih stavkov. *Zavod SR Slovenije za produktivnost dela,* Ljubljana

Carlson, D. C. and Labarba, R. C. (1979). Maternal emotionality during pregnancy and reproductive outcome: A review of the literature. *Int. J. Behav. Devel.*, **2,** 343

Cividini-Stanić, E. (1975). Psihodinamika i klinička slika psihosomatskih reakeija. In Blažević, D. (ed.) *Dinamska psihologija, psihoterapija.* (Zagreb: Yugoslavenska medicinska nablada)

Deutsch, H. (1945). *The psychology of women.* (New York: Grune & Stratton)

Galdston, I. and Calderone, M. (1958). In Steichen-Calderone, M. (ed.) Abortion in the United States (New York: Harper & Row) p. 113

Grimm, E. (1962). Psychological investigation of habitual abortion. *Psychosom. Med.*, **24,** 368

Harrison, C. P. (1969). Teenage pregnancy – Is abortion an answer? *Pediatr. Clin. N. Am.*, **16,** 363

Jansson, B. (1965). Mental disorders after abortion. *Acta Psychiatr. Scand.*, **41,** 87

Javert, C. T. (1962). Further follow-up on habitual abortion patients. *Am. J. Obstet. Gynecol.*, **84,** 1149

Kroger, W. S. and Freed, S. C. (1951). *Psychosomatic Gynecology*, p. 142. (Philadelphia and London: Saunders)

Lancet, M., Borenstein, R. and Katz, Z. (1972). A psychologic indication for cervical cerclage. In Morris, N. (ed.) *Psychosomatic medicine in obstetrics and gynecology*, p. 192. (Basel: Karger)

Molinski, H. (1980). Pregnancy as a conflict – Induced abortion and solution of pregnancy conflict. *Abstracts, 6th International Congress of Psychosomatic Obstetrics and Gynecology*, Berlin, 9

Naaktgeboren, C. and Bontekoe, E. M. H. (1976). Vergleichend-geburtskundliche Betrachtungen experimentelle Untersuchungen über psychosomatische Störungen der Schwangerschaft und das Geburtsablaufes. *Z. Tierzücht. Zühtungsbiol.*, **91**, 287

Pajntar, M. (1968). Some consequences of the legally interrupted pregnancy. *Zdrav. Vestn.*, **37**, 246

Pasnau, R. O. (1972). Psychiatric complications of the therapeutic abortion. *Obstet. Gynecol.*, **40**, 252

Petersen, P. (1980). Psychic consequences after legally induced abortion. *Abstracts, 6th International Congress of psychosomatic obstetrics and gynecology*, Berlin, 9

Simon, N. M. (1966). Psychiatric sequelae of abortion. *Arch. Gen. Psychiatry.*, **15**, 378

Squier, R. and Dunbar, F. (1946). Emotional factors in the course of pregnancy. *Psychosom. Med.*, **8**, 161

Van den Bergh, R. L., Taylor, E. S. and Drose, V. (1966). Emotional illness in habitual aborters following suturing of the incompetent cervical os. *Psychosom. Med.*, **28**, 257

Part III

Diagnostic Endocrinology and Ultrasound

19
Pregnancy evaluation with β-hCG and ultrasound in the first 42 days of gestation

F. R. BATZER, S. WEINER and S. L. CORSON

Diagnosis of early pregnancy and prediction of outcome are now possible even before clinical signs and symptoms of first trimester pregnancy failure are apparent. Combined use of beta human chorionic gonadotropin radioimmunoassay (β-hCG-RIA) measurement and ultrasound gives accurate diagnoses in the first 7 weeks of gestation. This chapter will highlight the recent use of these modalities for early pregnancy evaluation and their synergism when combined or used serially. Within the context of this paper 'weeks gestation' denotes time from ovulation defined by the thermal nadir of the basal body temperature (BBT).

HUMAN CHORIONIC GONADOTROPHIN

Though human chorionic gonadotropin (hCG) is the primary marker for pregnancy detection, little is known about its actual physiologic role. Identified first in 1927 by Ascheim and Zondeck, it was not until 1940 that serial quantitative measurements were recommended by Rakoff for pregnancy prognosis (Rakoff, 1940). Since then techniques with increasing sensitivity have been developed to detect and quantitate hCG in early pregnancy. An understanding of the various differences, advantages and exactly what is being measured is imperative for proper utilization of pregnancy test results.

TECHNIQUES OF hCG MEASUREMENT

Biologic assays were originally utilized for quantitation and detection of hCG. As first developed they were relatively non-specific, insensitive, costly and time-consuming. Several days were required for results. Serial studies were rarely performed.

The modern age of pregnancy testing began with the application of

Table 19.1 Assays for human chorionic gonadotropin

Test	*End-point*	*Time involved* (HR)	*Approx. sensitivity* (i u/ml)
Ascheim–Zondek	Hemorrhagic follicles and corpora lutea in immature mice (urine)	120	3–5
Friedman	Ovulation in rabbits (urine)	24–46	3–5
Kupperman	Hyperemia in rat ovaries (serum)	2	3–5
Latex slide test	Immunologic agglutination of latex particles on a slide (urine)	(2 min)	3–5
Hemagglutination	Inhibition of hemagglutination reaction (urine)	2	0.75
Latex inhibition tube test	Immunologic flocculation of β-subunit specific latex particle in a tube (urine)	1.5	0.250
Radioimmunoassay	Competitive binding of labeled antigen (serum)	24–48	0.010
β-Subunit radio-immunoassay (1972)	Competitive binding of labeled antigen with β-subunit specific antibody	3–6	0.003
Radioreceptorassay (1974)	Binding of hCG-LH to specific sites on bovine corpora lutea	1	0.001
In vitro bioassay (1974)	Adult rat Leydig cell testosterone production	48	0.001

immunoassay techniques to hCG measurement in 1962 (Wide, 1962). Because hCG is a glycoprotein hormone able to evoke a specific antibody response, antisera for immunologic testing could be developed. Immunoassay techniques widely utilized today such as hemagglutination inhibition tube tests, latex flocculation inhibition slide tests and so forth were hampered by the structural similarity between hCG and human luteinizing hormone (LH). Detection levels or sensitivity were necessarily set high to preclude false positive results on this basis. A positive urinary test therefore was not reliably encountered until 2 weeks after the first missed menses, 24–28 days post-ovulation (Figure 19.1). The ease and rapidity of performance, coupled with quick results, lack of major accessory equipment, and reproducibility in different laboratories and offices have made immunoassay pregnancy testing the most widely utilized technique. Further refinement in the antibody utilized has permitted the development of a new generation of increasingly sensitive tube tests (Corson *et al*, 1981*a*). With these, positive testing at the time of missed menses or within the first 5 days thereafter is possible even with urine rather than serum (Corson *et al.*, 1981*b*).

Radioimmunoassay (RIA) techniques permitted increasingly sensitive and specific hCG measurement. In any system, sensitivity is the ability to detect the presence of low levels of a substance when present. Specificity is the ability to discern when a substance is not present. Utilizing first a total hCG molecule antibody (Marshall *et al.*, 1968) and then in 1972 a β-subunit hCG specific antibody (Vaitukaitis *et al.*, 1972), hCG could be measured as early as day 8 following induced or spontaneous ovulation (Braunstein *et al*, 1973; Kosasa *et al.*, 1974). The specificity of the β-hCG-RIA assay system is determined by the unique carboxyl terminal of the β-subunit of the hCG molecule. While

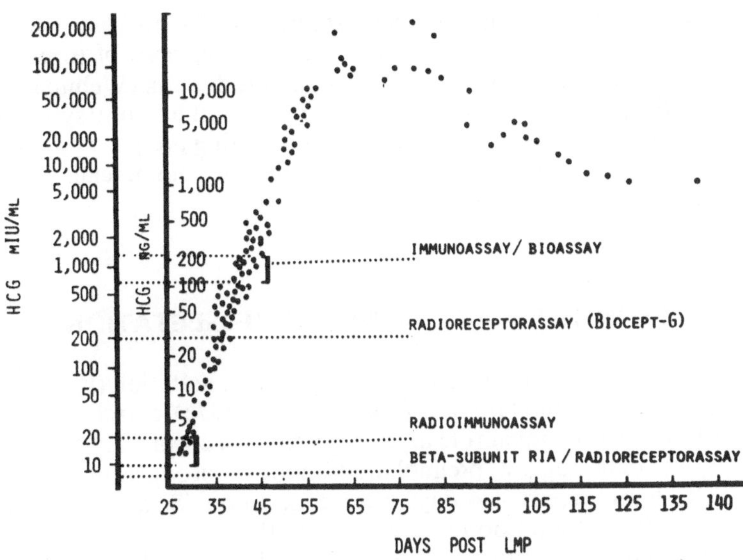

Figure 19.1 Normal β-subunit hCG radioimmunoassay pregnancy curve with comparative sensitivities of various pregnancy tests indicated. (1 ng = 5.7 miu/ml) (Batzer, 1980).

hCG shares a common quaternary structure with pituitary luteinizing hormone (LH), follicule stimulating hormone (FSH), and thyroid stimulating hormone (TSH), only the α-chain of the two-chained structures is common to all. While the β-chain of LH and hCG are very similar, the additional 22 to 30 aminoacid carboxyl terminal of the hCG β-chain is unique and permits antigenic, though not functional, distinction between the two molecules (Ross, 1977). Although values of hCG obtained by β-subunit RIA correlate well with values obtained by other techniques, no real assessment of biologic activity can be made because only the presence of the β-subunit is measured. Discrepancies noted between biologic and immunologic measurement of hCG can be explained on this basis (Vaitukaitis, 1974).

The radioreceptor technique (RRA) applied to hCG measurement (Saxena *et al.*, 1974) is biologically specific. It measures the presence of a whole biologically intact molecule as it binds *in vitro* to receptor sites, usually on bovine corpora lutea. The advantages of the RRA system are short laboratory time and ability to measure biologically active hormone. But the RRA system is unable to distinguish between LH and hCG, since both bind equally well to the receptor. This can be advantageous as the same system can be utilized to monitor ovulation induction as well as early pregnancy (Saxena *et al.*, 1978). It can also be disadvantageous when used diagnostically for pregnancy ascertainment as the magnitude of an LH surge can register as a false positive. Both RIA and RRA assay systems have the major disadvantage of being laboratory tests, not office tests, requiring a gamma counter and special equipment for the handling of radioactive materials. However, the unique sensitivity, especially of the β-hCG-RIA, has specific application in problem pregnancy evaluation and prognosis (Seppälä *et al.*, 1981) and in cases of trophoblastic neoplasm or other ectopic neoplastic hormone production (Wehmann *et al.*, 1981). Knowledge of the sensitivity and specificity of the testing system being utilized and the differences in serum and urine testing are paramount to the interpretation of the results (for complete listing of commercially available tests, see Corson *et al.*, 1981*a*).

HCG LEVELS IN THE FIRST 10 WEEKS OF GESTATION

Peripheral measurement of hCG as early as day 8 of gestation (Kosasa *et al.*, 1973*a*) shortly after implantation (Hertig *et al.*, 1975) correlates with the concept of hCG's functional role in the rescue of the corpus luteum. Though radioreceptor data suggest preimplantation hCG production with measurable hCG levels reported 4 days after conception (Saxena *et al.*, 1974), bioassay and RIA studies do not corroborate this.

Exogenous administration of hCG or LH has long been known to prolong the luteal phase of spontaneously ovulating women and to increase plasma progesterone production (Hanson *et al.*, 1971). The early tropic action of hCG is further supported by the timing precision needed to duplicate these events. In an ovulatory but nonconceptual cycle, levels of estradiol (E_2), progesterone (P), and 17-hydroxyprogesterone (17-OHP) begin to decline about 10 days after the midcycle LH peak (Thorneycroft *et al.*, 1971). HCG injections begun prior to this time delay menses. When begun later, no menstrual timing change could be demonstrated. Except for the notable differences in half-life, 20–36 h for hCG (Ross, 1977) as opposed to approximately 50 min for LH (Kohler *et al.*, 1968), no functional differences could be noted between LH and hCG (Hanson *et al.*, 1971). Addition of antisera to the unique β-subunit tailpiece also failed to neutralize the biological activity of hCG (Louvet *et al.*, 1974). Thus, though luteal phase hCG levels are not much higher than basal LH levels, the markedly prolonged half-life of hCG due to the additional sugar moieties increases its potency manyfold during this crucial period.

Peak values as high as 100 000 miu/ml of hCG may be measured during the first trimester with decreases to 10% of this for the remainder of the pregnancy (Braunstein *et al.*, 1976). Despite the increasing levels of hCG, corpus luteum function as measured by 17-OHP levels begins to decline after the 4th week of gestation (Yoshimi *et al.*, 1969) (Figure 19.2). Luteectomy studies further support this declining role of the corpus luteum of pregnancy in deference to the placenta's increasing dominance as a steroid producer. Removal of the corpus luteum of pregnancy before 6 weeks' gestation results in spontaneous abortion, while after 7 weeks' gestation there is little change (Csapo and Pulkkinen, 1978). Evidence supports placental hCG as crucial to corpus luteum transformation and early pregnancy support; physiologic significance of the other roles suggested for hCG has not been proven (Ross, 1977).

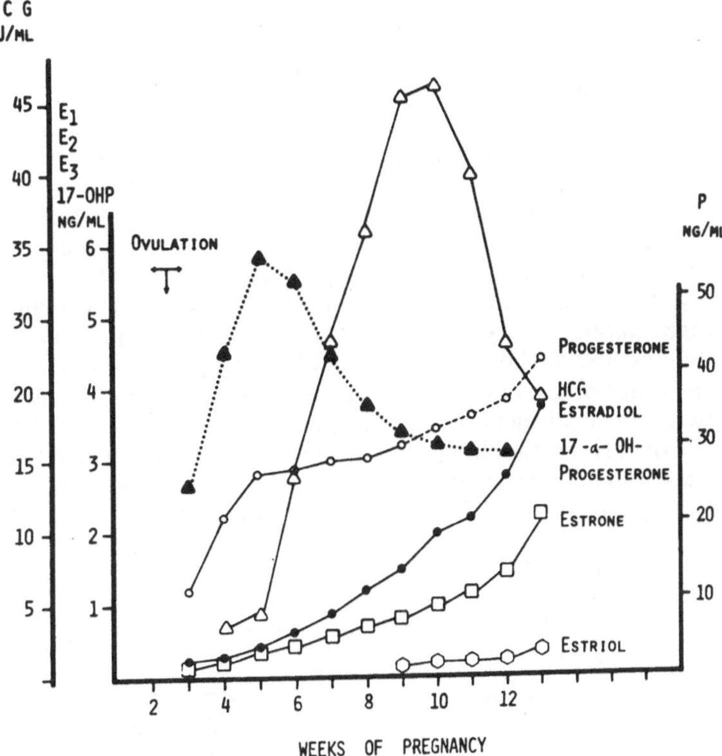

Figure 19.2 Mean plasma values of hCG, P, 17-OHP, and unconjugated E_1, E_2, and E_3 for 10 normal patients followed weekly from 3rd to 13th week of pregnancy. Arrow indicates the presumed time of ovulation. Weeks of pregnancy = weeks from last menstrual period (Tulchinsky and Hobel, 1973).

CLINICAL USES OF hCG

The early presence of hCG and its known exponential increase make monitoring of hCG during early pregnancy particularly useful. Since maternal hCG reflects beginning trophoblastic growth, its value as an indication of disturbed placental function has been recognized (Rakoff, 1940).

Spontaneous abortion rates in women defined as occurring after known missed menses have been reported as 16–19 % (Warburton and Fraser, 1964). On the basis of morphologic studies, Hertig estimated that 28 % of pregnant women who missed one menstrual period abort (Hertig, 1975). The actual incidence of postimplantation pregnancy loss as defined by the presence of a positive β-hCG-RIA in the luteal phase is probably much higher (Block, 1976). In a prospective evaluation of pregnancy outcome in a normal population, a 43 % spontaneous abortion rate was defined on the basis of a positive β-hCG-RIA after day 21 of the luteal phase (Miller *et al.*, 1980). Pertinent is the fact that only 10 % of those were clinically apparent abortions with delayed menses and pregnancy symptoms, while 33 % were evidenced by positive luteal phase testing alone. Other workers have concurred with similarly high abortion rates (Karow and Gentry, 1976; Chartier *et al.*, 1979).

The exponential increase of hCG in the first few weeks of gestation has been correlated with the doubling time of trophoblastic cell number (Braunstein *et al.*, 1973). Normal early gestational growth has been associated with hCG doubling times of 1.4–2.2 days (Marshall *et al.*, 1968; Chartier *et al.*, 1979) (doubling time is calculated by dividing the logarithm of 2 by the slope of the line derived from serial hCG values). On the basis of hCG doubling time in the first 22 days postovulation Chartier *et al.*, (1979) were able to distinguish two early pregnancy populations. In 57 pregnancies that evolved normally to term an average doubling time of 1.4 days was defined, while 14 pregnancies which aborted in the first 60 days averaged a doubling time of 2.1 days. In a similar study, the range of doubling times in the aborter population was too great to generate a statistical mean of useful significance (Batzer *et al.*, 1981). The frequency of various doubling times was obviously not a normal distribution but appeared to be constant over a range of 0.5–10 days, probably indicative of the multiple etiologies of early pregnancy wastage.

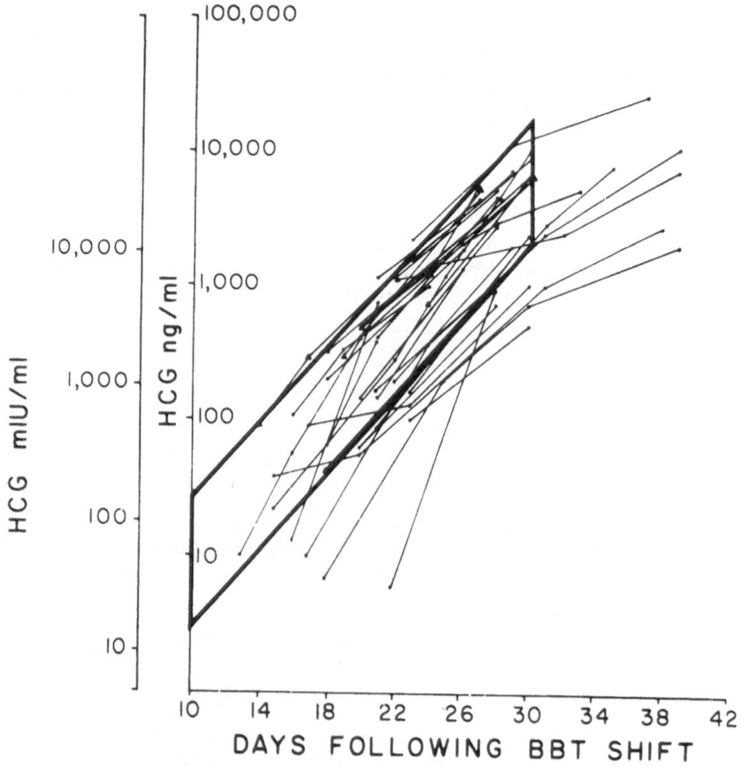

Figure 19.3 Serial β-hCG-RIA values during first 30 days of successful pregnancies in 38 pregnancies. ▲, Twin gestation. The solid line encloses the 95 % confidence limits in successful pregnancies (Batzer *et al.*, 1981).

Using the concept of hCG doubling time for prospective pregnancy prognosis in an infertile population has proved both useful and practical. It obviates the need for ovulation dating in order to avoid false identification of a low-for-dates value; since most patients are not on a BBT this is of great use in interpretation as each patient becomes her own control. It is available as a predictive index long before other reliable pregnancy changes have occurred, either hormonal (Tulchinsky and Hobel, 1973) or anatomical (Jouppila, 1980*b*). It increases predictive accuracy for both successful pregnancies and (especially) pregnancies associated with low-for-date values (Batzer *et al.*, 1981) (Figure 19.3). Application of the same concept of immunologic pregnancy testing using a semiquantitative technique for urine proved similarly useful and predictive (Corson *et al.*, 1981*b*) (Figure 19.4). The immediacy of results, ease and cost of performance and ready availability within the office setting are of importance.

In a prospective monitoring of 29 pregnancies of which nine aborted, hCG values were abnormal at the time of abortion in all but one pregnancy, correlating with abnormal ultrasound scans (Ho Yuen *et al.*, 1981) Human chorionic gonadotropin values were, however, normal in two of seven of the pregnancies at a point when simultaneous ultrasounds demonstrated abnormalities. In our series, β-hCG-RIA and ultrasound diagnoses were usually in agreement (Batzer *et al.*, 1982). Since both are expressive of trophoblastic function this is not surprising.

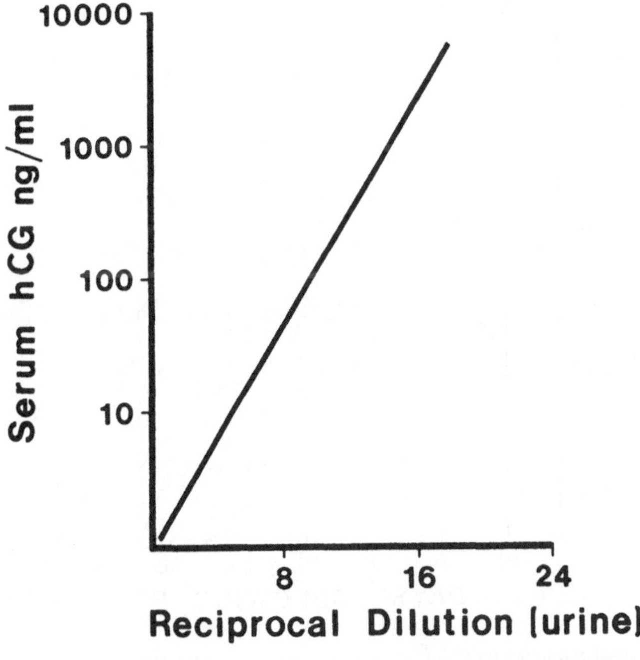

Figure 19.4 Regression analysis of urinary and serum hCG titers ($r = 0.99$) in successful pregnancies during first 30 days following ovulation (Corson *et al.*, 1981*b*).

Within the context of early pregnancy growth, several repetitive patterns of abnormal hormonal values have been identified. Since hCG seems to be easily measurable, reasonably unique to pregnancy, and normally given to exponential increase during this crucial period, it is the prototype. Pregnancy-specific β-glycoprotein and other pregnancy hormones may prove valuable as markers as well (Braunstein *et al.*, 1980). Repetitive patterns of hCG doubling time (Figure 19.5) included the negative slope associated with subclinical abortion or occult pregnancy (Block, 1976; Braunstein *et al.*, 1978). A persistently low doubling time or low slope was noted in cases several weeks before the time of clinical abortion (Batzer *et al.*, 1981). A similar sequence in patients aborting with 'blighted ova' is reported (Schweditsch *et al.*, 1979). A normal slope was identified in patients who aborted after the confirmation of fetal heart tones (FHT) by ultrasound in the second trimester (Batzer *et al.*, 1982). The latter pattern suggests a non-trophoblastic cause for abortion.

Steroid hormone data, though useful perhaps in discerning etiologies of pregnancy failure, are problematic for immediate early pregnancy prognosis. Individual steroid hormones cannot be uniquely identified as corpus luteum

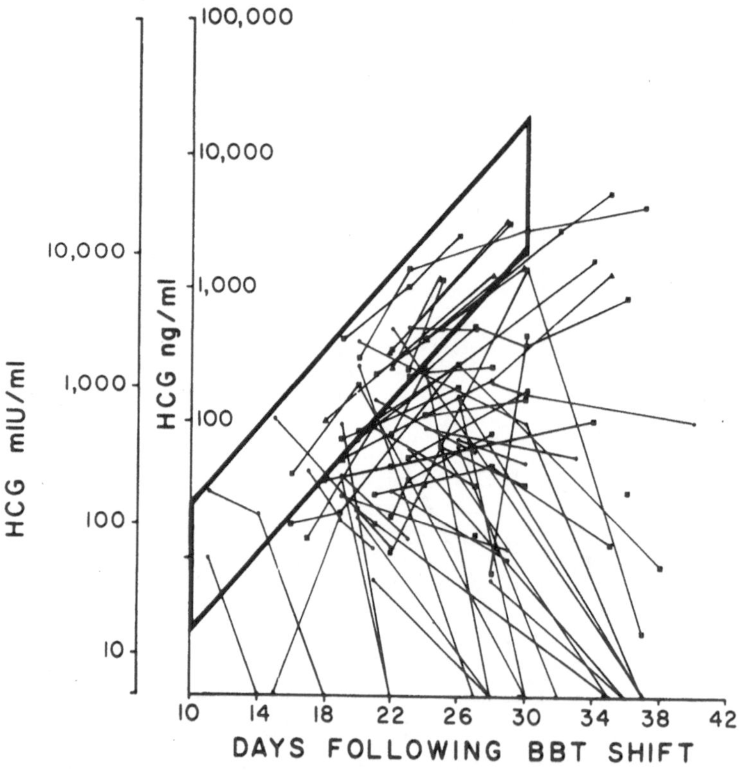

Figure 19.5 Serial β-hCG-RIA values in 53 patients who aborted spontaneously. Twenty-six patients had a negative slope. Five patients with a normal slope aborted in the second trimester. The solid line encloses the 95% confidence limits in successful pregnancies (Batzer *et al.*, 1981)

or fetal. Ranges of normal are very broad. In combination E_2, P and prolactin (PRL) have proved useful though usually applied to later pregnancy or patients already symptomatic for pregnancy loss (Kunz and Keller, 1976; Jovanovic *et al.*, 1978).

hCG AS PROGNOSTIC INDEX

Most data on the use of hCG values for pregnancy prognosis are generated in patients already symptomatic with vaginal bleeding. In a symptomatic population sample, random hCG values have been found to be 79–100% predictive of abortion, and 71–92% predictive of successful pregnancy outcome (Nygren *et al.*, 1973; Kunz and Keller, 1976; Jouppila *et al.*, 1980*b*). Prospective evaluation in an asymptomatic population utilizing single β-hCG-RIA values is 82% accurate for good outcome and 56–58% predictive of spontaneous abortion (Braunstein *et al.*, 1978; Batzer *et al.*, 1981). Serial studies improve the accuracy of prediction in both studies. In particular in the spontaneous abortion group (Figure 19.5) a slow hCG doubling time was 76% predictive in the first 30 days of gestation of a first trimester abortion while a normal hCG doubling time was 88% predictive of a good pregnancy outcome (Figure 19.3) (Batzer *et al.*, 1981). Sampling obtained at 2-week intervals permitted 88% accuracy in diagnosis of spontaneous abortion in Braunstein's studies (Braunstein *et al.*, 1978) and was predictive in all normal and ectopic pregnancies. Reports with serial application of radioreceptor techniques (Jovanovic *et al.*, 1978) and immunologic urinary pregnancy testing (Corson *et al.*, 1981*b*) have varied from 75% to 90% in normal pregnancy outcome prediction.

ECTOPIC PREGNANCY

The availability of a definitive early pregnancy test in the form of β-hCG-RIA was heralded as a useful diagnostic test for ectopic pregnancy prior to the appearance of catastrophic clinical symptoms and signs. Immunologic urinary pregnancy tests are negative or equivocal in over 50% of ectopic pregnancies (Sandvei *et al.*, 1981). The presence of a low hCG-RIA was considered at first to be diagnostic of ectopic pregnancy (Kosasa *et al.*, 1973*b*). A low β-subunit RIA or radioreceptor result is now interpreted with greater caution. It raises the clinical suspicion of an extrauterine gestation or impending or missed abortion (Saxena and Landesman, 1978). A negative β-hCG-RIA test rules out significant trophoblastic activity at any site (Seppälä *et al.*, 1980). A hormonal pregnancy test can detect the presence of trophoblastic cell mass activity but cannot differentiate the site of implantation. The importance of utilizing a specific β-hCG-RIA testing system in these instances is to be emphasized. Serial application of β-hCG-RIA testing to establish a rate of hCG rise in combination with a search for ultrasound landmarks has proved most useful (Batzer *et al.*, 1982; Kadar *et al.*, 1981*a,b*).

COMBINED APPLICATION OF β-HCG AND ULTRASOUND

The sonographic features of normal and abnormal development of the early gestational sac and fetus have been studied extensively. But simultaneous development of β-hCG levels and the morphological changes noted on ultrasound in the first trimester of human pregnancy have not.

Among 188 symptomatic patients admitted with vaginal bleeding who subsequently aborted, Jouppila *et al.*, (1980*b*) found that the presence or absence of fetal life on scan predicted success or failure of the pregnancy with 90 and 100 % certainty, respectively, if studied at or later than 9 weeks from the last menstrual period (LMP). Low levels of hCG or progesterone (P) were noted in 93 %, while low levels of both hormones predicted abortion in 100 %. Of ten patients who aborted within 2 weeks of fetal life being detected on scan, all had normal plasma levels of hCG, E_2 and P, except for one with a low hCG at 7 weeks. Of 50 patients who demonstrated an empty sac on scan, hCG was normal in 34 % and P was normal in 28 %. E_2, however, was low in 92 %, and hCG, E_2, and P all decreased after 11 weeks. Among patients with an incomplete abortion, the levels of all three hormones were low.

In a similar series (Sande *et al.*, 1980), 104 patients with bleeding were studied between 6 and 25 weeks of pregnancy; 48 had ultrasound examinations, mostly to look for evidence of fetal life. Falling or low hCG levels were ominous, although a proposed leakage of hCG to the maternal circulation at the time of bleeding was thought to result in some falsely high levels.

In a prospective series, nine patients who aborted showed low levels of β-hCG and P even when an embryo was present on ultrasound, while E_2 and prolactin levels were normal in three (Ho Yuen *et al.*, 1981). Ultrasound was 88 % accurate in suggesting the absence of an embryo. Subnormal levels of β-hCG (89 %), E_2 (100 %) and P (57 %) occurred in four of these patients, with 80 % of the abortuses having an abnormal karyotype. These data suggest that E_2 may be the key hormonal tag in the endocrine failure of embryopathic pregnancies, and ultrasound may show earlier signs of this abnormality (i.e. absence of an embryo). Jouppila reports similar hormonal findings (Jouppila, 1980*a*).

Criteria for early pregnancy normalcy by ultrasound (Hellman *et al.*, 1973) are approximately 80 % accurate in predicting abortion when a poorly defined sac, small sac for dates, abnormal intrauterine echoes, low implanted sac, growth failure or a double sac are seen. Up to 6 weeks' gestational age, simultaneous assay of hCG is helpful, and a normal doubling time should be maintained.

As pregnancy progresses, Robinson (1975) defines fetal heart motion (FHM) detection on ultrasound when the gestational sac volume is greater than 2 ml, and sac volume doubling each week until it reaches 5 ml. The absence of FHM in a sac greater than 2.5 ml or less than 75 % increase in sac volume over 1 week predicts pregnancy failure with nearly 100 % accuracy. Bennett (Bennett and Kerr-Wilson, 1980) expects FHM by the time the fetus reaches a crown–rump length of 15 mm, and Levine (Levine and Filly, 1977) anticipates FHM in all viable pregnancies by 8 menstrual weeks. The presence of FHM suggests successful continuation of the pregnancy in 90 % of cases in several studies despite uterine bleeding, although the subsequent risk of premature delivery is increased several-fold. Since the levels of β-hCG may be plateaued or declining by this time, its measurement is of less predictive value than earlier in pregnancy, and the 'doubling time' concept no longer applies.

After FHM is noted, the development of normal fetal activity patterns follows (Shawker *et al.*, 1980; Van Dongen and Goudie, 1980). A poor prognosis may be predicted by delayed or abnormal fetal movement patterns, or a disproportion between the size of the fetus and the gestational sac.

When ultrasound examination and β-hCG assay are combined, the status of the trophoblastic cell mass can be more thoroughly defined than with either test used separately. Application of this combined prospective approach in early pregnancy (< 42 days post ovulation or < 8 menstrual weeks) in asymptomatic first trimester women permitted greater than 90 % accuracy in predicting outcome for the patients studied (Batzer *et al.*, 1982).

Serial ultrasound examinations and simultaneous β-hCG assays were performed in 80 pregnancies between 26 and 45 days postovulation (Batzer *et al.*, 1982). The gestational sac mean diameter (GSMD) was determined by averaging the largest transverse sagittal and perpendicular diameters as measured with a linear array real-time scanner, using the full bladder technique. Fetal heart motion was noted as a distinct flicker in the fetal parts' echoes at a rate of 150–200 beats per minute. Measurements of β-hCG-RIA were performed utilizing a double antibody system. Specifics of both techniques have been previously described (Batzer *et al.*, 1982).

The following predictable patterns and landmarks of normal early gestational development are easily recognizable.

Prior to 26 days postovulation, measurement of plasma levels of β-hCG is most useful, as ultrasound demonstrates only the loss of the central uterine cavity echo (Callen *et al.*, 1979) and the increasingly distinct echoes of the decidual reaction are evidence of the hypersecretory state of the endometrium. When the ovulation date is known, a single assay of β-hCG is 82 % predictive of success if it is normal and 56 % predictive of pregnancy failure if it is low (Batzer *et al.*, 1981). If the results are borderline or the date of conception uncertain (as often happens when bleeding complicates early pregnancy), serial β-hCG assays at 4–8 day intervals must be obtained and the results compared to the expected doubling time. By this technique predictive accuracy can be increased: 88 % predictive when normal and 76 % predictive of abortion when abnormal (Batzer *et al.*, 1981). Perhaps quantitation of the ultrasonic 'tissue signature' of the decidual reaction will prove to be a useful complementary study in the future.

Between 26 and 36 days postovulation, both ultrasound and β-hCG assays are useful. Again, if the duration of pregnancy is known, the β-hCG value should be compared to a simultaneous measurement of the GSMD. If both values are normal, the outlook for the pregnancy is good, despite the presence of uterine bleeding. If the β-hCG is low for dates or the GSMD is smaller than expected with no FHM seen, the prognosis is guarded.

When the ovulation is uncertain, the situation is more complex. If FHM is noted on scan, the prognosis is good in 90 % of cases. Figure 19.6 is useful for

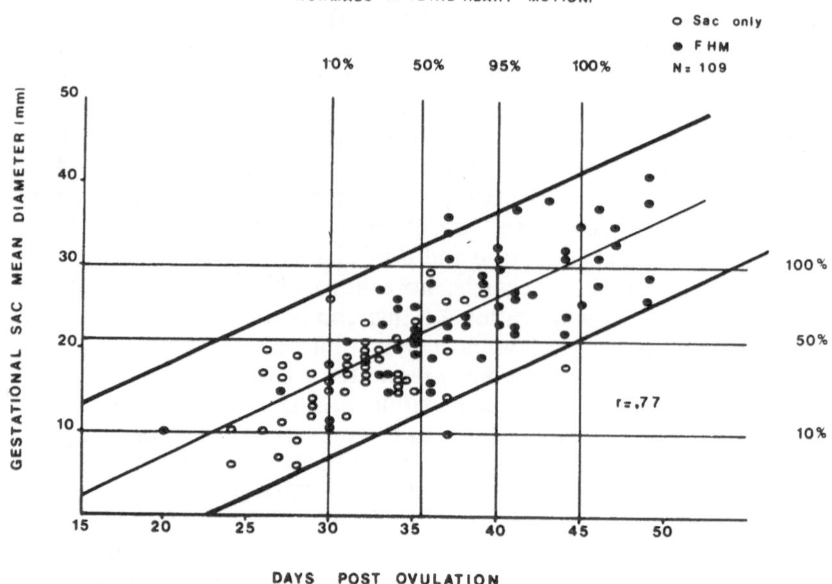

Figure 19.6 Growth of gestational sac mean diameter (GSMD) during first 50 days postovulation in 109 observations (71 pregnancies). Diagonal lines represent the mean ±2 SEM in these successful pregnancies ($r = 0.77$). ○ = presence of a gestational sac only; ● = simultaneous fetal heart motion (FHM). Vertical and horizontal grids indicate the increasing percentage of cases in which FHM was noted; vertical grid by days postovulation, horizontal grid by GSMD) (Batzer *et al.*, 1983).

indicating the probability of finding FHM for any given sac size (GSMD) during this time interval, obviating the need to know the gestational age precisely. If FHM is not seen on scan, serial assays of β-hCG and repeat ultrasound examination (in 1 week) should define the viability and age of the pregnancy.

Finally, comparison of the β-hCG and GSMD may be useful. A close correlation between these two during early pregnancy development is demonstrated (Figure 19.7). When the pregnancy aborts (Figure 19.8), these values were usually both abnormal and proportionate. While a simultaneous finding of low β-hCG and small GSMD in a patient with bleeding usually predicts abortion, an alternate possibility is a viable pregnancy with a delayed ovulation. Serial testing in these cases is necessary. Highly discrepant values between the β-hCG and GSMD may help to differentiate endocrinopathy from embryopathy as the etiology of abortion.

After 36 days postovulation, ultrasound becomes quite definitive in its ability to predict first trimester pregnancy viability, while β-hCG measurement is less useful. When the conception date was known, the GSMD was below normal in all patients studied after 36 days who aborted. Most useful was the presence or absence of FHM, as it was present in over 95% of normal

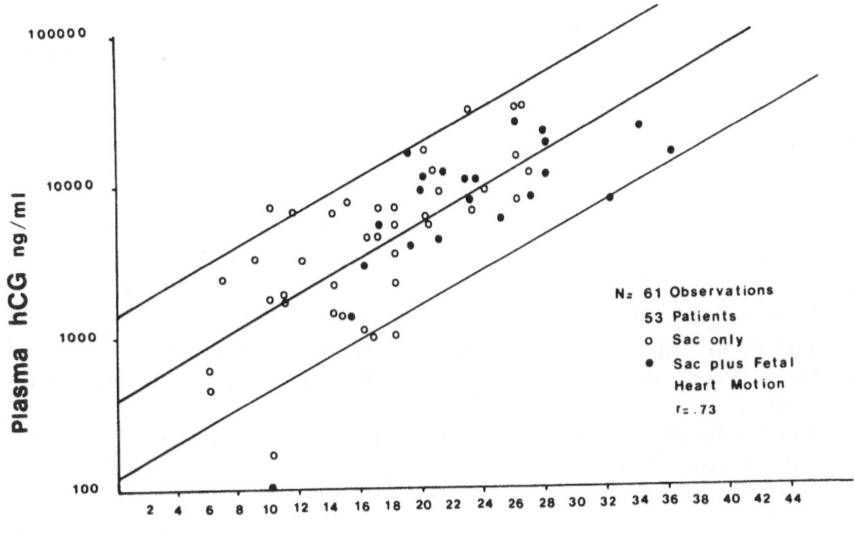

Figure 19.7 Simultaneous measurement of plasma hCG and GSMD in 53 pregnancies (61 observations) during first 42 days postovulation. The lines represent the linear regression ±2 SEM in these successful pregnancies ($r = 0.73$). ○ = presence of a gestational sac only; ● = simultaneous FHM (Batzer *et al.*, 1983).

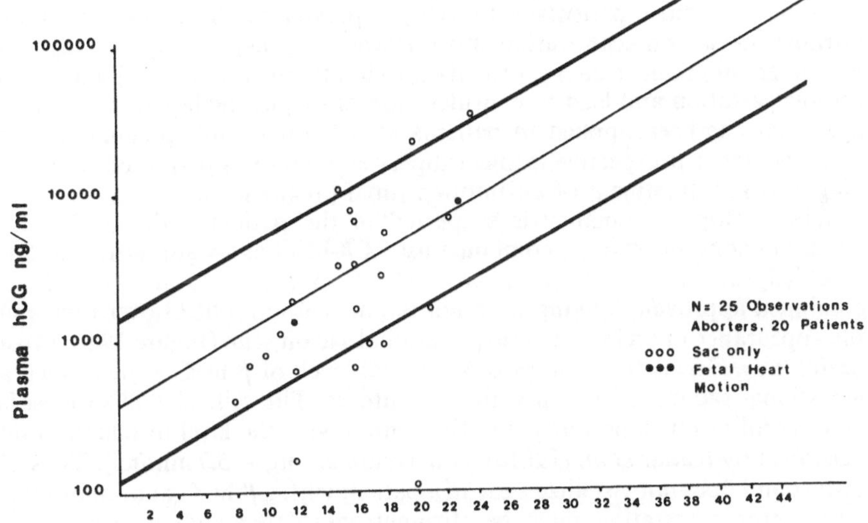

Figure 19.8 Simultaneous measurement of plasma hCG and GSMD in 20 pregnancies (25 observations) which aborted in first trimester. The solid lines indicate the mean ±2 SEM confidence limits in successful pregnancies. ○ = the presence of a gestational sac only; ● = simultaneous FHM. Only two pregnancies in this group demonstrated FHM (Batzer *et al.*, 1983).

pregnancies by 42 days postovulation or 8 menstrual weeks and 100% by 45 days (Figure 19.6). The absence of FHM at greater than 45 days uniformly predicted abortion accurately.

If the gestational length is uncertain, and the patient is bleeding, measurement of GSMD should permit accurate predictions, as FHM was noted in 100% of normal pregnancies with a GSMD greater than 30 mm. If the sac is larger than this, suggesting a pregnancy age >44 days postovulation, and no FHM is seen, the pregnancy is not viable. By comparison Jouppila *et al.*, 1980*a* predicted pregnancy failure by the absence of fetal life on the first scan after the 13th week if the gestational age was uncertain, while Anderson's results on symptomatic patients are similar to ours (Anderson, 1980). If FHM is not noted in a sac smaller than 30 mm in mean diameter, β-hCG and serial ultrasonic studies must be pursued. Any uncertainty can be resolved with repeat studies in 1 week.

Ectopic pregnancy revealed a variable pattern of β-hCG secretion, but the simultaneous application of ultrasound was helpful here too. Ultrasound is most useful in ruling out an ectopic pregnancy by demonstrating the presence of an intrauterine gestational sac (Kelly *et al.*, 1979). Caution must be exercised so that the 'pseudosac' which may be seen when fluid or blood collect in the uterus is not interpreted as a gestational sac (Weiner, 1981). Nevertheless, the absence of a sac in the uterus must be interpreted cautiously unless the exact duration of pregnancy is known. In our series, the smallest sac detected had a GSMD of 6 mm, compatible with 21 days postovulation (5 menstrual weeks). This is earlier by 2–3 weeks than the onset of clinical symptoms in most patients with ectopic pregnancy. The absence of an intrauterine sac on scan during this interval in an asymptomatic pregnant patient greater than 28 days postovulation should suggest the possibility of an ectopic gestation and lead to consideration of diagnostic laparoscopy. This approach has been applied to patients at risk for ectopic pregnancy who conceive under prospective medical supervision and has permitted the early diagnosis and treatment of unruptured tubal pregnancies.

When ectopic pregnancy is suspected in the patient with bleeding or uncertain conception date, combined use of β-hCG assay and ultrasound is most helpful. Others (Jouppila *et al.*, 1980*b*; Kadar *et al.*, 1981*a,b*) describe a combined approach, looking for a normal increase in β-hCG over time and the appearance of an intrauterine gestational sac on scan (Figure 19.9). Most useful, however, is the concept of a 'critical level' of β-hCG above which a gestational sac must be seen within the uterus. The critical β-hCG level is 1000 ng/ml in our laboratory and this agrees with the level of 6000 miu/ml described by Kadar *et al.* (1981*a*) (conversion is 1 ng ~ 5.7 miu/ml). Thus, if ultrasound does not visualize a sac in a patient with a β-hCG at or above this level, ectopic gestation must be strongly considered and laparoscopy is indicated. This concept, too, has led to the efficient management of ectopic pregnancy in several patients, both with and without symptoms.

The simultaneous use of β-hCG assay and ultrasound examination in the prospective evaluation of very early human pregnancy has been described. Unfortunately, little information is revealed by this approach as to the pathogenesis of spontaneous abortion, as both techniques measure the

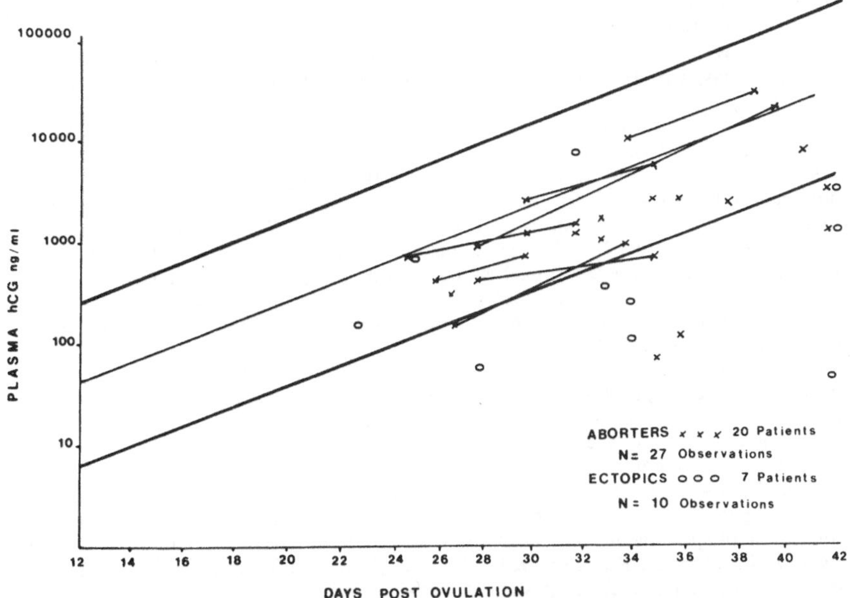

Figure 19.9 β-hCG-RIA values in 20 pregnancies (27 observations) which aborted during first trimester. Serial values are indicated by connecting lines. The solid lines enclose the mean +2 SEM in successful pregnancies. 500 observations in 300 pregnancies ($r = 0.81$) (1 ng/ml = 5.7 miu/ml). Seven ectopic pregnancies are indicated by open circles (10 observations) (Batzer *et al.*, 1982).

viability of the trophoblast. When abortion occurs, it appears that β-hCG and the gestational sac fail nearly simultaneously in most cases. Estradiol may be the first hormone to decline before abortion when no embryo is present according to Yuen (Yuen *et al.*, 1981). When applied to the clinical situation of a patient with bleeding in early pregnancy, β-hCG assay is most useful up to 26 days postovulation, both β-hCG and ultrasound are equally useful between 26 and 36 days, and ultrasound becomes increasingly superior and definitive after that. An approach to the common problem of uncertain gestational length and possible ectopic pregnancy is also offered by this combined application. In the future, further improvements in ultrasonic technologies with histologic hormonal and karyotypic correlations should enable the clinician to better understand and perhaps treat the pathogenesis of early pregnancy failures.

References

Anderson, S. G. (1980). Management of threatened abortion with real-time sonography. *Obstet. Gynecol.*, **55**, 259

Batzer, F. R. (1980). Hormonal evaluation of early pregnancy. *Fertil. Steril.*, **34**, 1

Batzer, F. R., Schlaff, S., Goldfarb, A. F. and Corson, S. L. (1981). Serial β-subunit human chorionic gonadotrophin doubling time as a prognosticator of pregnancy outcome in an infertile population. *Fertil. Steril.*, **35**, 307

Batzer, F. R., Weiner, S., Schlaff, S., Otis, C. and Corson, S. L. (1983). Gestational landmark in the first 42 days with beta-chorionic gonadotropin and ultrasound. *Am. J. Obstet. Gynecol.*, **146**, 973

Bennett, M. J. and Kerr-Wilson, R. H. J. (1980). Evaluation of threatened abortion by ultrasound. *Int. J. Gynaecol. Obstet.*, **17**, 382

Block, S. K. (1976). Occult pregnancy – a pilot study. *Obstet. Gynecol.*, **48**, 365

Braunstein, G. D., Grodin, J. M., Vaitukaitis, J. L. and Ross, F. T. (1973). Secretory rates of human chorionic gonadotropin by normal trophoblast. *Am. J. Obstet. Gynecol.*, **115**, 447

Braunstein, G. D., Rasor, J., Adler, D., Danzer, H. and Wade, M. E. (1976). Serum human chorionic gonadotropin levels throughout normal pregnancy. *Am. J. Obstet. Gynecol.*, **126**, 678

Braunstein, G. D., Karow, W. G., Gentry, W. C., Rasor, J. and Wade, M. E. (1978). First-trimester chorionic gonadotropin measurement as aid in the diagnosis of early pregnancy disorders. *Am. J. Obstet. Gynecol.*, **131**, 25

Braunstein, G. D., Rasor, J. L., Engvall, E. and Wade, M. E. (1980). Interrelationships of human chorionic gonadotropin, human placental lactogen, and pregnancy-specific B1-glycoprotein throughout normal human gestation. *Am. J. Obstet. Gynecol.*, **138**, 1205

Callen, P. W., DeMartini, W. J. and Filly, R. A. (1979). The central uterine cavity echo: A useful anatomic sign in the ultrasonographic evaluation of the female pelvis. *Radiology*, **131**, 187

Chartier, M., Roger, M., Barrat, J. and Michelson, B. (1979). Measurement of plasma human chorionic gonadotropin (hCG) and B-hCG activities in the late luteal phase: Evidence of the occurrence of spontaneous menstrual abortions in infertile women. *Fertil. Steril.*, **31**, 134

Corson, S. L., Derman, R., Horwitz, C. A., Lau, H. L. and Soderstrom, R. (1981*a*). Early diagnosis of pregnancy. A symposium. *J. Reprod. Med.*, **26**, 149

Corson, S. L., Batzer, F. R. and Schlaff, S. (1981*b*). A comparison of serial quantitative serum and urine tests in early pregnancy. *J. Reprod. Med.*, **26**, 611

Csapo, A. I. and Pulkkinen, M. (1978). Indispensability of the human corpus luteum in the maintenance of early pregnancy: Luteectomy evidence. *Obstet. Gynecol. Survey*, **33**, 69

Hanson, F. W., Powell, J. E. and Stevens, V. C. (1971). Effects of hCG and human pituitary LH on steroid secretion and functional life of the human corpus luteum. *J. Clin. Endocrinol. Metab.*, **32**, 211

Hellman, L. M., Kebayashi, M. and Cromb, E. (1973). Ultrasonic diagnosis of embryonic malformations. *Am. J. Obstet. Gynecol.*, **115**, 615

Hertig, A. T. (1975). Implantation of the human ovum. In Behrman, S. J. and Kistner, R. W. (eds.) *Progress in Infertility*. 2nd Edn., pp. 411–438. (Boston: Little, Brown)

Ho Yuen, B. Livingston, J. E., Poland, B. J., Wittmann, B. K., Sy, L. and Cannon, W. (1981). Human chorionic gonadotropin, estradiol, progesterone, prolactin, and B-scan ultrasound monitoring of complications in early pregnancy. *Obstet. Gynecol.*, **57**, 207

Jouppila, P. (1980*a*). The evaluation of prognosis in threatened early pregnancy. *J. Perinat. Med.*, **8**, 3

Jouppila, P. (1980*b*). Clinical and ultrasonic aspects in the diagnosis and follow-up of patients with early pregnancy failure. *Acta Obstet. Gynaecol. Scand.*, **59**, 495

Jouppila, P., Tapanainen, J. and Huhtaniemi, I. (1980*a*). Plasma hCG and ultrasound in suspected ectopic pregnancy. *Eur. J. Obstet. Gynecol. Reprod. Biol.*, **10**, 3

Jouppila, P., Huhtaniemi, I. and Tapanainen, J. (1980*b*). Early pregnancy failure: Study by ultrasonic and hormonal methods. *Obstet. Gynecol.*, **55**, 42

Jovanovic, L., Dawood, M. Y., Landesman, R. and Saxena, B. B. (1978). Hormonal profile as a prognostic index of early threatened abortion. *Am. J. Obstet.*, **130**, 274

Kadar, N., DeBore, G. and Romero, R. (1981*a*). Discriminatory hCG zone: Its use in the sonographic evaluation for ectopic pregnancy. *Obstet. Gynecol.*, **58**, 156

Kadar, N., Caldwell, B. V. and Romero, R. (1981*b*). A method of screening for ectopic pregnancy and its indications. *Obstet. Gynecol.*, **58**, 162

Karow, W. G. and Gentry, W. C. (1976). Corpus luteum function during pregnancies of previously infertile women. *Obstet. Gynecol.*, **48**, 603

Kelly, M. T., Santos-Ramos, R. and Duenhoelter, J. H. (1979). The value of sonography in suspected ectopic pregnancy. *Obstet. Gynecol.*, **53**, 703

Kohler, P. O., Ross, G. T. and Odell, W. D. (1968). Metabolic clearance and production rates of human luteinizing hormone in pre and postmenopausal women. *J. Clin. Invest.*, **47**, 38

Kosasa, T., Levesque, L., Goldstein, D. P. and Taymor, M. L. (1973*a*). Early detection of implantation using a radioimmunoassay specific for human chorionic gonadotropin. *J. Clin. Endocrinol. Metab.*, **36**, 622

Kosasa, T. S., Taymor, M. L., Godstein, D. P. and Levesque, L. A. (1973*b*). Use of a radioimmunoassay specific for human chorionic gonadotropin in the diagnosis of early ectopic pregnancy, *Obstet. Gynecol.*, **42**, 868

Kosasa, T. S., Levesque, L., Taymor, M. L. and Goldstein, D. P. (1974). Measurement of early chorionic activity with a radioimmunoassay specific for human chorionic gonadotropin following spontaneous and induced ovulation. *Fertil. Steril.*, **25**, 211

Kunz, J. and Keller, P. J. (1976). HCG, HPL, oestradiol, progesterone and AFP in serum in patients with threatened abortion. *Br. J. Obstet. Gynaecol.*, **83**, 640

Levine, S. C. and Filly, R. A. (1977). Accuracy of real-time sonography in the determination of fetal viability. *Obstet. Gynecol.*, **49**, 475

Louvet, J.-P., Ross, G. T., Birken, S. and Canfield, R. E. (1974). Absence of neutralizing effect of antisera to the unique structural region of human chorionic gonadotropin. *J. Clin. Endocrinol. Metab.*, **39**, 1155

Marshall, J. R., Hammond, C. B., Ross, G. T., Jacobson, A., Rayford, P. and Odell, W. D. (1968). Plasma and urinary chorionic gonadotropin during early human pregnancy. *Obstet. Gynecol.*, **32**, 760

Miller, J. F., Williamson, E., Glue, J., Gordon, Y. B., Grudzinskas, J. G. and Sykes, A. (1980). Fetal loss after implantation. *Lancet*, **2**, 554

Nygren, K. G., Johansson, E. D. and Wide, L. (1973). Evaluation of the prognosis of threatened abortion from the peripheral plasma levels of progesterone, estradiol, and human chorionic gonadotropin. *Am. J. Obstet. Gynecol.*, **116**, 916

Rakoff, A. E. (1940). The hormonal diagnosis of intrauterine fetal death: the value of quantitative serum prolan determinations as a diagnostic procedure. *Pa. Med. J.*, **43**, 669

Robinson, H. P. (1975). The diagnosis of early pregnancy failure by sonar. *Br. J. Obstet. Gynaecol.*, **82**, 849

Ross, G. T. (1977). Clinical relevance of research on the structure of human chorionic gonadotropin. *Am. J. Obstet. Gynecol.*, **129**, 795

Sande, H. A., Reiertsen, D., Fonstelien, O. and Torjesen, P. (1980). Evaluation of threatened abortion by human chorionic gonadotropin levels and ultrasonography. *Int. J. Gynaecol. Obstet.*, **18**, 123

Sandvei, R., Stoa, K. F. and Ulstein, M. (1981). Radioimmunoassay of human chorionic gonadotropin B-subunit as an early diagnostic test in ectopic pregnancy. *Acta Obstet. Gynaecol. Scand.*, **60**, 389

Saxena, B. B., Hasan, S. H. and Haour, F. (1974). Radioreceptor assay of human chorionic gonadotropin: detection of early pregnancy. *Science*, **184**, 793, 795

Saxena, B. B. and Landesman, R. (1978). Diagnosis and management of pregnancy by the radioreceptorassay of human chorionic gonadotropin. *Am. J. Obstet. Gynecol.*, **131**, 97

Schweditsch, M. O., Dubin, N. H., Jones, G. S. and Wentz, A. C. (1979). Hormonal considerations in early normal pregnancy and blighted ovum syndrome. *Fertil. Steril.*, **31**, 252

Seppälä, M., Ranta, T., Tonitti, K., Stenman, U.-H. and Chard, T. (1980). Use of a rapid hCG-Beta-subunit radioimmunoassay in acute gynaecological emergencies. *Lancet*, **1**, 165

Seppälä, M., Ranta, T., Rutanen, E.-M., Stenman, U.-H. and Chard, T. (1981). Improved diagnosis of pregnancy-related gynaecological emergencies by rapid human chorionic gonadotrophin beta-subunit assay. *Br. J. Obstet. Gynaecol.*, **88**, 138

Shawker, T. H., Schuette, W. H., Whitehouse, W. and Rifka, S. M. (1980). Early fetal movement: A real-time ultrasound study. *Obstet. Gynecol.*, **55**, 194

Thorneycroft, I. H., Mishell, D. R., Stone, S. C., Kharma, K. M. and Nakamura, R. H. (1971). The relation of serum 17-hydroxyprogesterone and estradiol-17B levels during the human menstrual cycle. *Am. J. Obstet. Gynecol.*, **111**, 947

Tulchinsky, D. and Hobel, C. J. (1973). Plasma human chorionic gonadotropin, estrone, estradiol, estriol, progesterone, and 17 a-hydroxyprogesterone in human pregnancy. *Am. J. Obstet. Gynecol.*, **117**, 884

Vaitukaitis, J. L. (1974). Changing placental concentrations of human chorionic gonadotropin and its subunits during gestation. *J. Clin. Endocrinol. Metab.*, **38**, 755

Vaitukaitis, J. L., Braunstein, G. D. and Ross, G. T. (1972). A radioimmunoassay which specifically measures human chorionic gonadotropin in the presence of human luteinizing hormone. *Am. J. Obstet. Gynecol.*, **113,** 751

Van Dongen, L. G. R. and Goudie, E. G. (1980). Fetal movement patterns in the first trimester of pregnancy. *Br. J. Obstet. Gynaecol.*, **87,** 191

Warburton, D. and Fraser, F. S. (1964). Spontaneous abortion risks in man: data from reproductive histories collected in a medical genetic unit. *Am. J. Hum. Genet.*, **16,** 1

Wehmann, R. E., Ayala, A. R., Birken, S., Canfield, R. E. and Nisula, B. C. (1981). Improved monitoring of gestational trophoblastic neoplasia using a highly sensitive assay for urinary human chorionic gonadotropin. *Am. J. Obstet. Gynecol.*, **140,** 753

Weiner, C. (1981). The pseudogestational sac in ectopic pregnancy. *Am. J. Obstet. Gynecol.*, **139,** 959

Wide, L. (1962). An immunological method for the assay of human chorionic gonadotropin. *Acta Endocrinol.(Suppl.)*, **70,** 1

Yoshimi, I., Strott, C. A., Marshall, J. R. and Lipsett, M. B. (1969). Corpus luteum function in early pregnancy. *J. Clin. Endocrinol. Metab.*, **29,** 225

20
Endocrinology of luteal phase defects, habitual abortion and trophoblastic-luteal complex during normal and embryopathic gestation

B. HO YUEN, S. M. PRIDE and B. J. POLAND

Progesterone production by the corpus luteum is essential for the normal maintenance of early pregnancy. After the production of progesterone is transferred to the placenta during the first trimester (the luteo-placental shift), the corpus luteum becomes dispensable (Csapo *et al.*, 1972; Csapo and Pullkinen, 1978). Clinical sequelae of disordered progesterone production by the corpus luteum (the luteal phase defect) include infertility and habitual abortion (three consecutive spontaneous losses). The prevalence of luteal defects in infertility patients was 33% in Sydney, Australia (Grant, 1976); 3.5% in Baltimore (Jones, 1976); 8.1% in Farmington, Connecticut (Rosenberg *et al.*, 1980); and 19% in Memphis, Tennessee (Wentz, 1980). In habitually aborting women, the incidence of luteal defects was 64% in Sydney (Grant, 1976), 35% in Baltimore (Jones, 1976), and 38% in Madrid (Botella Llusia, 1962). To a varying extent, patient selection and differing diagnostic criteria accounted for the range in prevalence noted. Since the statistical distribution of luteal phase defects in the normal fertile population has not been compared to that of habitually aborting women, the clinical relevance of luteal phase defects in the pathogenesis of habitual abortion was considered uncertain (Glass and Golbus, 1978). Furthermore, the efficacy of treatment on the outcome of pregnancy in habitually aborting women has not as yet been assessed in stringently controlled clinical trials. While the validity of these concerns is not in doubt, published research data from several countries, and current knowledge of the important role of the corpus luteum in the maintenance of pregnancy during the first trimester in women (Csapo *et al.*, 1972; Csapo and Pullkinen, 1978; Hammerstein, 1974) and in primates (Bosu and Johansson, 1975) illustrate the clinical importance of the luteal defect.

The luteal defect exists in two forms (Cline, 1979). In 22 cycles exhibiting a lag in the endometrial development (Type I defect), no subclinical pregnancies were observed, while in 18 cycles in which the endometrium was in phase but the luteal span less than 14 days (Type II defect), 12 of 18 (67%) cycles had subclinical pregnancies (Cline, 1979).

Possible defects in the 'rescue phenomenon' of the corpus luteum after implantation but before the luteo-placental shift have not been clearly elucidated to date. Nevertheless, in a prospective study of women at risk for spontaneous abortion, diminished human chorionic gonadotropin (hCG) and progesterone production in early pregnancy were demonstrable in women with embryopathic pregnancy destined to abort (Ho Yuen *et al.*, 1981). It is our purpose (1) to review the current status of the endocrine mechanisms relating to the pathogenesis, diagnosis and treatment of the luteal phase defect and (2) to present data on the hormone production from the trophoblastic-luteal complex of normal and embryopathic pregnancies, including patients with luteal defects.

ENDOCRINOLOGY OF LUTEAL PHASE DEFECTS

The etiologic factors in luteal phase defects are multiple (Jones, 1976) and may be the result of disturbances in the control mechanisms involved in folliculogenesis, ovulation and luteinization of the ovarian follicle. These disturbances will be discussed under the headings: central factors, ovarian factors, endocrinopathies, exogenous factors and local factors.

Central factors

Gonadotropin secretion from the anterior pituitary gland is under the control of neural and hormonal signals. In primates (Belchetz *et al.*, 1978) and women (Yen *et al.*, 1972), the secretion of the gonadotropins is of a pulsatile nature. In mature female rhesus monkeys, lesions induced in the median basal hypothalamus abolished this pulsatile pattern. The subsequent decline in the plasma concentrations of the gonadotropins and the ovarian steroids was associated with amenorrhea. Administration of gonadotropin releasing hormone (GnRH) to these animals (Knobil *et al.*, 1980) and women with hypothalamic amenorrhea (Leyendecker *et al.*, 1980) restored normal pituitary–ovarian relationships and ovulation. Follicle-stimulating hormone (FSH) is an important factor in the hormonal control of follicular maturation (Ross *et al.*, 1970). Subtle abnormalities in GnRH production resulting from environmental (stress?) or other as yet unknown phenomena could conceivably interfere with the output of FSH. In women with luteal defects, FSH and 17β-estradiol concentrations were lower during the follicular phase (Ross *et al.*, 1970; Sherman and Korenman, 1974). There was also no tendency for the FSH levels to rise at the end of the luteal phase (Ross *et al.*, 1970). After ovulation, the inadequately stimulated follicle may give rise to a defective corpus luteum (Sherman and Korenman, 1974). The luteinizing hormone (LH) surge at midcycle initiates luteinization of the granulosa cells in the Graafian follicle. A defective corpus luteum may also be the result of an LH surge of inadequate amplitude and duration. Since LH is luteotropic, decreased LH release in the luteal phase may interfere with corpus luteal maintenance and cause inadequate progesterone output (Vande Wiele *et al.*, 1970).

In the postmenarchal stage, there may be a high incidence of anovulatory cycles. In the first 3 postmenarchal years, between 50 and 80% of cycles may be anovulatory (Apter, 1980; Vollman, 1977). Associated with these anovulatory cycles were increased testosterone, androstenedione and LH levels (Apter, 1980). The prevalence of short luteal phases (2–9 days) in the first 3 postmenarchal years approximated 50% (Vollman, 1977). Since androgens may inhibit progesterone production from the corpus luteum, (Rodriguez-Rigau *et al.*, 1979; Smith *et al.*, 1979) a tendency to excess androgen levels in some of these postmenarchal cycles may contribute to luteal phase defects in this age group.

Ovarian factors

Progressive maturation of the ovarian follicle requires stimulation by FSH. FSH also stimulates estrogen production within the maturing follicle. According to the two-gonadotropin–two-cell theory (Moon *et al.*, 1978; Armstrong, 1980), LH stimulates the production of androgens (androstenedione and testosterone) in the vascularized thecal cell layer. These androgens diffuse to the adjacent granulosa cells and into the follicular fluid. Aromatase enzymes induced by FSH in the granulosa cells convert these androgenic precursors to 17β-estradiol (Moon *et al.*, 1978). FSH and 17β-estradiol also stimulate both the mitogenesis of granulosa cells and the induction of LH receptors on them (Fritz and Speroff, 1982). Consequently, exposure to both FSH and 17β-estradiol determines both the number of granulosa cells and the content of LH receptors on each cell contained in the maturing follicle (Fritz and Speroff, 1982). Thus, proper exposure of the developing follicle in terms of the amount and duration of FSH and 17β-estradiol is necessary for normal corpus luteal function. Adequate progesterone secretion in the luteal phase and the maintenance of pregnancy by the corpus luteum depends on an adequate number of granulosa cells with sufficient LH receptors on them. Abnormalities in the FSH and 17β-estradiol mechanism may result in a decreased number of granulosa cells with a diminished LH receptor content. This could be a cause of inadequate progesterone secretion from the corpus luteum in early pregnancy. Although prolactin is required for progesterone secretion by human granulosa cells, high prolactin concentrations *in vitro* inhibited the production of progesterone by these cells (McNatty, 1974). Suppression of prolactin levels by bromocriptine in normally menstruating women also lowers luteal phase plasma progesterone levels (Schulz *et al.*, 1978).

In perimenopausal women, augmentation of follicular phase FSH levels occurs with shortening of the luteal phase (Sherman and Korenman, 1975). The luteal phase deficiency of perimenopausal women may thus be associated with decreased sensitivity of the ovarian follicles to the stimulatory effect of FSH on their maturation.

The luteolytic factor in human beings has not been clearly elucidated.

Intraovarian administration of 17β-estradiol and testosterone induces luteolysis in women (Hammerstein, 1974). Intraovarian prostaglandin $F_2\alpha$ ($PGF_2\alpha$) and 17β-estradiol induces luteolysis in the rhesus monkey (Sotrel *et al.*, 1981), while the physiological luteolytic agent in the ewe is $PGF_2\alpha$ released from the uterus (Hammerstein, 1974). Whatever the physiologic stimulus for luteolysis in the human female may be, it is possible that the premature induction of luteolysis gives rise to short luteal phases or the Type II defect (Cline, 1979).

Endometriotic tissues produce $PGF_2\alpha$ (Moon *et al.*, 1981). Ovarian endometriotic tissues contain higher concentrations of $PGF_2\alpha$ than normal ovarian tissues (Moon *et al.*, 1981). In a group of women with untreated endometriosis, 17 of 37 (46 %) of pregnancies ended in spontaneous abortion. Following resection of the endometriotic implants, only four of 50 (8 %) of pregnancies ended in spontaneous abortion (Naples *et al.*, 1981). These observations are consistent with a role for the prostaglandins produced by endometriotic tissues in the higher abortion rate experienced by women with this disease.

Endocrinopathies

Disordered prolactin secretion

In hyperprolactinemic women with luteal phase defects, normalization of the prolactin levels by bromocriptine restores normal luteal function (Corenblum *et al.*, 1976; Del Pozo *et al.*, 1979). Although marked lowering of prolactin levels may inhibit luteal phase progesterone secretion (Schulz *et al.*, 1978), the role of subnormal prolactin levels in luteal phase defects has not been elucidated.

Hyperandrogenism

Testosterone inhibited the conversion of pregnenolone to progesterone in human corpora lutea *in vitro* (Rodriguez-Rigau *et al.*, 1979). Elevated testosterone concentrations were present in women with hyperandrogenism and short luteal phases (Smith *et al.*, 1979). Women with congenital adrenal hyperplasia in whom 17-ketosteroid levels were elevated had a 90 % rate of spontaneous abortion (Sarris *et al.*, 1978). Treatment with glucocorticoids resulted in a decrease in the rate of spontaneous abortion to 9 %, comparable to that expected in a normal population of women. Taken together, these data are consistent with an etiologic role for testosterone, dehydroepiandrosterone and possibly other androgens in luteal phase deficiency.

Subclinical hypothyroidism

Eleven of 20 patients with subclinical hypothyroidism had inadequate luteal phases (Bohnet *et al.*, 1981). Thyroid replacement therapy improved luteal function with resultant pregnancies in two of these patients. Subclinical hypothyroidism may be an important etiologic factor in infertile women with luteal inadequacy.

Exogenous factors

Exercise

Running exercise in women of reproductive age is associated with amenorrhea and luteal phase deficiency (Shangold *et al.*, 1979; Prior *et al.*, 1982). The mechanisms by which running induces menstrual dysfunction has not been elucidated. A recent study suggested that this may be related to body weight (Feicht Sanborn *et al.*, 1982).

Alcohol consumption and smoking

Alcohol (Kline *et al.*, 1980) and smoking (Kline *et al.*, 1977) increase the risk of spontaneous abortion. It was also suggested that alcohol results in the abortion of karyotypically normal conceptuses (Kline *et al.*, 1980). Whether or not alcohol and smoking could affect luteal function needs further evaluation.

Synthetic progestins

The administration of several progestational drugs including medroxyprogesterone acetate, norethindrone and norgestrel to healthy young women in the luteal phase inhibited the plasma concentrations of progesterone (Johansson, 1971).

Local factors

An apparent progesterone receptor abnormality in the endometrium of a patient with luteal phase deficiency has been identified (Keller *et al.*, 1979). The endometrium from this patient contained cytosol binding sites, one-half in number but of similar affinity to those of two control patients. This receptor abnormality was not corrected with replacement progesterone therapy.

DIAGNOSIS OF LUTEAL PHASE DEFECTS

Luteal phase defects could be suspected on the basal body temperature record (Grant, 1976; Vollman, 1977). The staircase pattern and luteal phases of

Table 20.1 Changes in luteal index while on treatment with clomiphene citrate (Clomid)

Cycle number	*Mean plasma progesterone (P) level* (ng/ml)	*Luteal length* (days) (t)	*Luteal index* $P \times t$ (*normal 137–247*)	*Treatment*
2	5.7	9	51*	None
3	10.9	10	109*	Clomid 50 mg × 5 days
4	20.6	7	144	Clomid 100 mg × 5 days
5	12.8	9	115*	Clomid 150 mg × 5 days
6	13.1	12	157	Clomid 200 mg × 5 days

* Subnormal values. For further details, see text and Figures 20.1 and 20.2

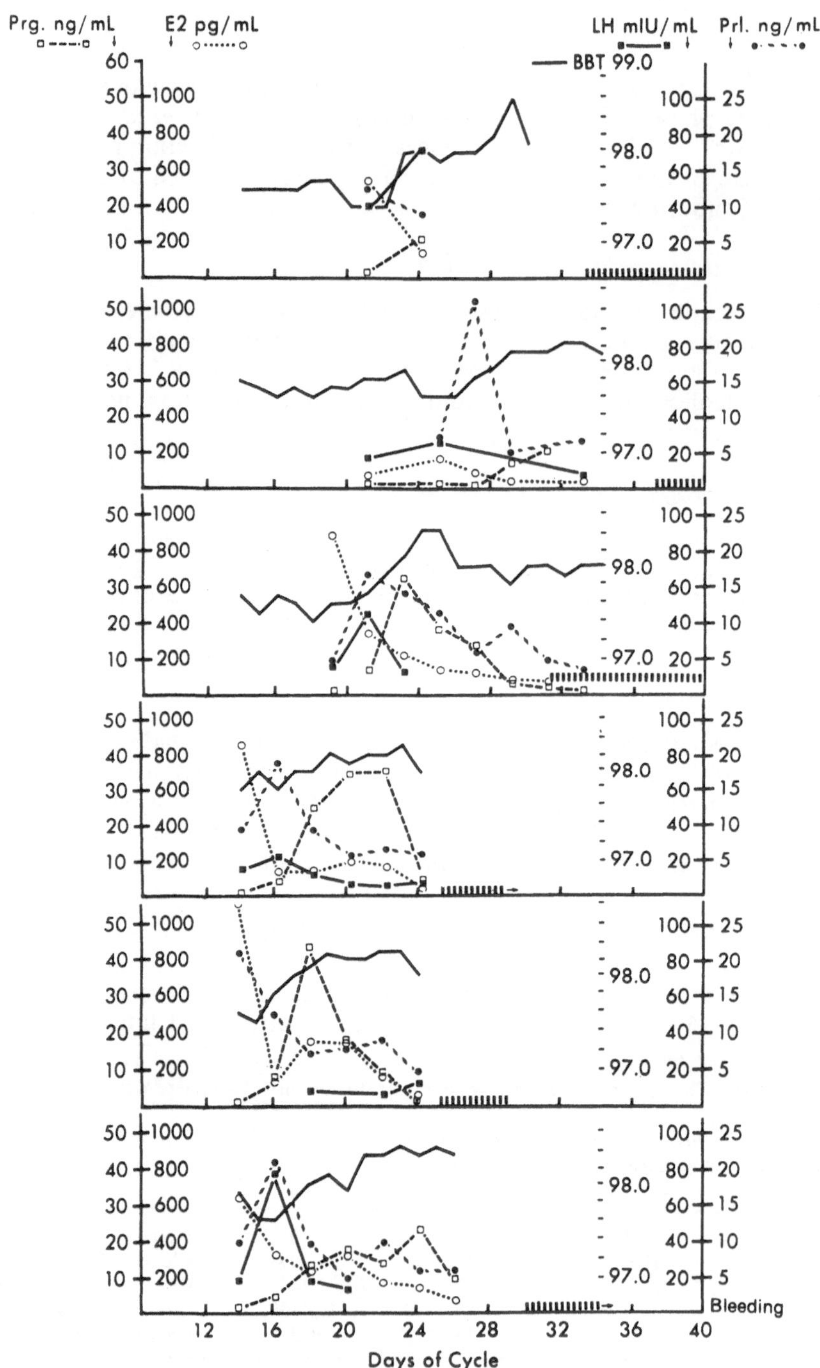
Prg. ng/mL
E2 pg/mL
LH mIU/mL
Prl. ng/mL
BBT 99.0
98.0
97.0
60
50
40
30
20
10
1000
800
600
400
200
100
80
60
40
20
25
20
15
10
5
Bleeding
12
16
20
24
28
32
36
40
Days of Cycle

10 days or less are suspicious. For routine clinical work, the timed endometrial biopsy (Jones, 1976; Wentz, 1980) is practical and useful both for diagnosis and in monitoring treatment, especially in Type 1 defects. Since the Type II defect is not characterized by a lag in endometrial development, it cannot be detected by the biopsy. No single test provides all the desirable information in patients suspected of having luteal phase defects. Apart from the basal temperature record and endometrial morphology, daily or alternate day sampling of progesterone throughout the luteal phase (Del Pozo *et al.*, 1979) may be helpful as confirmation of a Type II defect. We have employed serial sampling during the luteal phase in normal women and women with habitual abortion. The luteal index was calculated (Del Pozo *et al.*, 1979) with minor modifications. A plot of the progesterone levels was made from samples obtained at 1–2 day intervals starting before ovulation through to menstruation in normal women. The values of progesterone before or after the curve intersected the 5 ng/ml line as it rises at the beginning and then falls at the end of the luteal phase are then employed. These values are summed and divided by the number of samples to give the mean progesterone level. The length of the luteal phase is calculated as the number of days between the two points in which the progesterone curve intersects the 5 ng/ml line, as described above, rounded to the nearest day. The luteal index is the product of the mean progesterone concentration and the luteal length (Table 20.1). Occasionally, blood samples were obtained 2–3 days apart and, if bleeding preceded the last sample before the value in the latter has been shown to be below 5 ng/ml, the luteal length is computed up to the day of the onset of bleeding. Data from six cycles studied in one subject are shown in Table 20.1 and Figure 20.1. The first cycle shown on Figure 20.1 was not included in the calculation of luteal index (Table 20.1) because of insufficient data. The maximal luteal index and luteal length was achieved while taking clomiphene 200 mg/day for 5 days. During the evaluation, conception was prevented by barrier methods until the seventh cycle when the same dose of clomiphene was given supplemented with progesterone in the luteal phase (Figure 20.2). A successful conception ensued with a normal outcome at term. Implantation occurred between Days 11 and 12 after the LH surge, as evidenced by initial detection of β-subunit hCG (> 5 mu/ml) on Day 12 following the LH surge. The plasma progesterone levels peaked 2 days after the LH surge, declined to 6 days after the surge despite replacement therapy, then rose slightly around the time of implan-

---

Figure 20.1 Six cycles from a patient (age 32 years, Gravida 3 Para 1) with luteal phase deficiency and two consecutive first trimester abortions within 19 months of the studies. The first and second cycles were without, while cycles 3–6 were with clomiphene citrate in doses shown on Table 20.1. Improvement in the luteal index was shown in cycle 4 (clomiphene 100 mg daily × 5 days) but the luteinizing hormone (LH) surge remained subnormal with a short luteal phase of 7 days. In cycle 6 (clomiphene citrate 200 mg daily × 5 days), the LH surge was restored to normal, as were the luteal index and luteal length (12 days). For further details, see Table 20.1 and Figure 20.2. The normal ovulatory levels of progesterone (Prg.) = 5–40 ng/ml; LH midcycle surge = 40–200 miu/ml (2nd IRP, HMG) and LH follicular and luteal phases = 2–30 miu/ml. During the menstrual cycle, normal levels of estradiol-17β (E_2) = 40–650 pg/ml; prolactin (Prl.) = 5–25 ng/ml. Short luteal length < 10 days (Vollman, 1977) on the basal body temperature record (BBT).

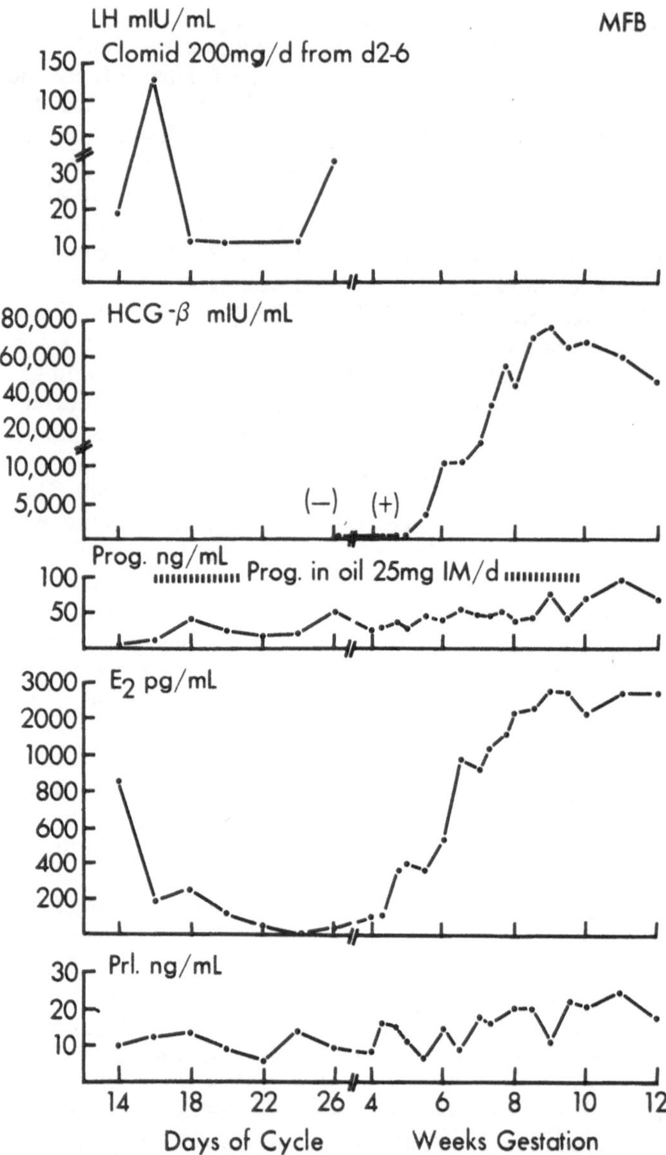

Figure 20.2 The cycle of conception (normal outcome) and the seventh consecutive cycle of observation in the patient shown on Figure 20.1 and Table 20.1. Note treatment with clomiphene citrate (Clomid) 200 mg daily and replacement with progesterone in oil given intramuscularly. The luteinizing hormone (LH) surge is again restored to normal, progesterone (Prog.) and 17β-estradiol (E_2) levels were slightly elevated as compared to the normal, unstimulated cycle (see legend to Figure 20.1). Despite supplemental progesterone therapy, progesterone levels declined between days 22 and 24 with the 17β-estradiol levels subnormal during this interval. Implantation was confirmed at Day 28 by β-subunit human chorionic gonadotropin (hCG-β) levels > 5 miu/ml. Progesterone levels were maintained while on substitution therapy to the 10th week of gestation. The rescue phenomenon by hCG of progesterone secretion is again shown. Prl. = prolactin. See Figure 20.1, for the preceding six cycles of observation in this patient.

tation, with the values being maintained following implantation until the presumed time of the luteo-placental shift, when replacement therapy was discontinued 8 weeks after the LH surge with the endogenous progesterone levels being maintained without further exogenous hormone administration. In contrast, endogenous 17β-estradiol levels declined to subnormal values (< 40 pg/ml) 8 days after the LH surge. Following implantation, the plasma 17β-estradiol levels then rapidly increased concomitantly with β-subunit hCG levels. No abnormalities in prolactin production were observed to the end of the sampling period (Figure 20.2).

ENDOCRINOLOGY OF IMPLANTATION AND PREGNANCY MAINTENANCE

During 3 days traversing the oviduct, the embryo develops to the 12–16 cell stage (Croxatto *et al.*, 1978; Biggers, 1981). Secretion of hCG by the trophoblast is the first recognizable biochemical signal of pregnancy. Employing sensitive competitive protein binding assays specific for hCG, this gonadotropin can be detected in maternal plasma as early as 7–12 days after ovulation (Ross, 1979). The rapid increase in hCG production from the embryo (Figure 20.3) is an important factor in the hormonal regulation of implantation and pregnancy maintenance. The biochemical effect of hCG on the corpus luteum is similar to that of LH. The phenomenon of 'rescue' of the corpus luteum has been attributed to hCG. Its increasing levels in maternal blood after implantation continue to stimulate steroid hormone secretion from the corpus luteum (Figure 20.3). In addition, by preventing the onset of luteolysis, hCG maintains the anatomic and physiologic integrity of the corpus luteum in early pregnancy (Hammerstein, 1974; Bolt, 1979). Following luteectomy during early pregnancy, the corpus luteum was indispensable to the maintenance of human pregnancy, on average in the first 49 days (range 42–57 days of gestation calculated from the last menstrual period) (Csapo and Pulkkinen, 1978; Csapo *et al.*, 1972). In some 10% of patients, careful examination revealed the presence of 'accessory' corpora lutea in the ovaries (Csapo *et al.*, 1972). The secretion of progesterone during the first trimester is therefore not always by a single corpus luteum. This may also explain why some women undergoing ovariectomy bearing the corpus luteum do not abort when the operation is done before the apparent luteo-placental shift has occurred (Csapo *et al.*, 1972).

HORMONE PRODUCTION FROM THE TROPHOBLASTIC-LUTEAL COMPLEX DURING VARIOUS EMBRYOPATHIC PREGNANCIES FROM IMPLANTATION TO ABORTION

During treatment with human menopausal gonadotropin (hMG) and hCG in a patient with hypothalamic amenorrhea, the endocrine events at the time of a normal conception (Figure 20.3) and one which spontaneously aborted are shown (Figure 20.4). Over the initial 5 days of treatment, the estradiol-17β

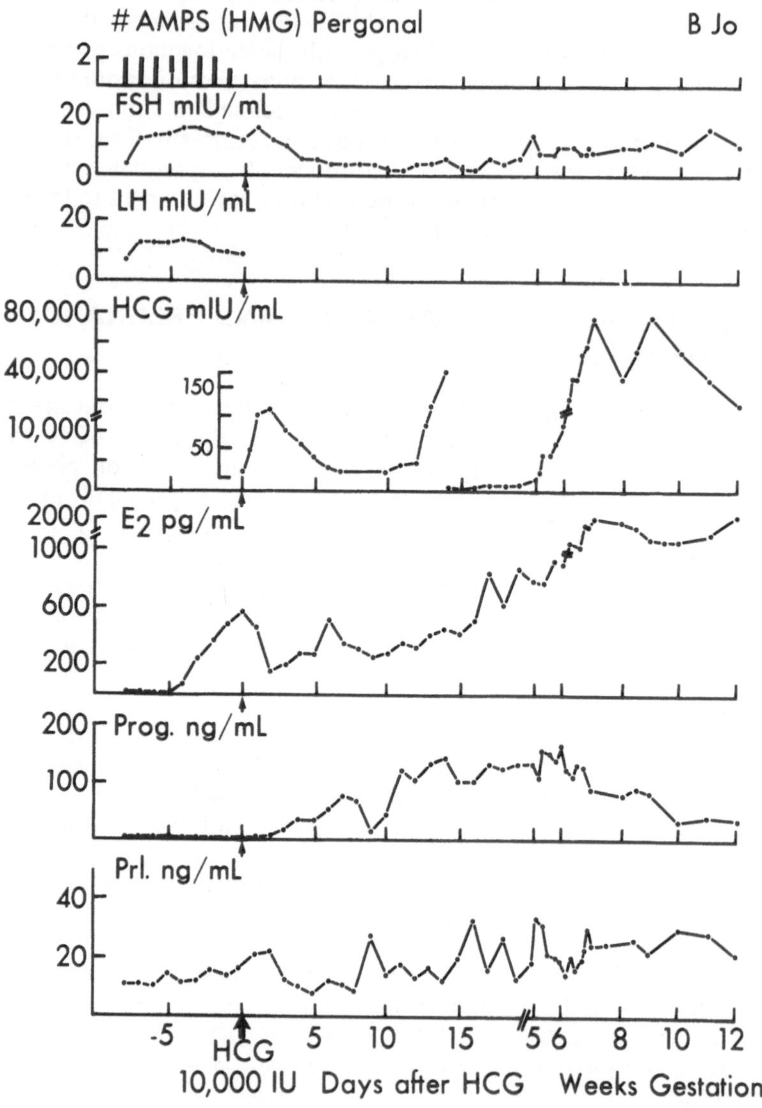

Figure 20.3 Implantation, early corpus luteum function and the rescue phenomenon in a patient conceiving a normal pregnancy on gonadotropin therapy. The initial rise in hCG-β levels is due to the injected exogenous hormone. The increase in hCG levels at levels at Day 10–11 subsequent to hCG administration reflects the production of hCG by the blastocyst at implantation. The declining progesterone levels by 8–9 days after hCG injection is stimulated to increase by Day 10. This is the rescue phenomenon of progesterone production by hCG secreted from the blastocyst. Physiologic patterns of estradiol-17β are shown. The decline of 17β-estradiol after hCG administration is characteristic of the normal profile observed at midcycle in the unstimulated women. FSH = follicle stimulating hormone; Prl. = prolactin. See also Table 20.1 and Figure 20.1.

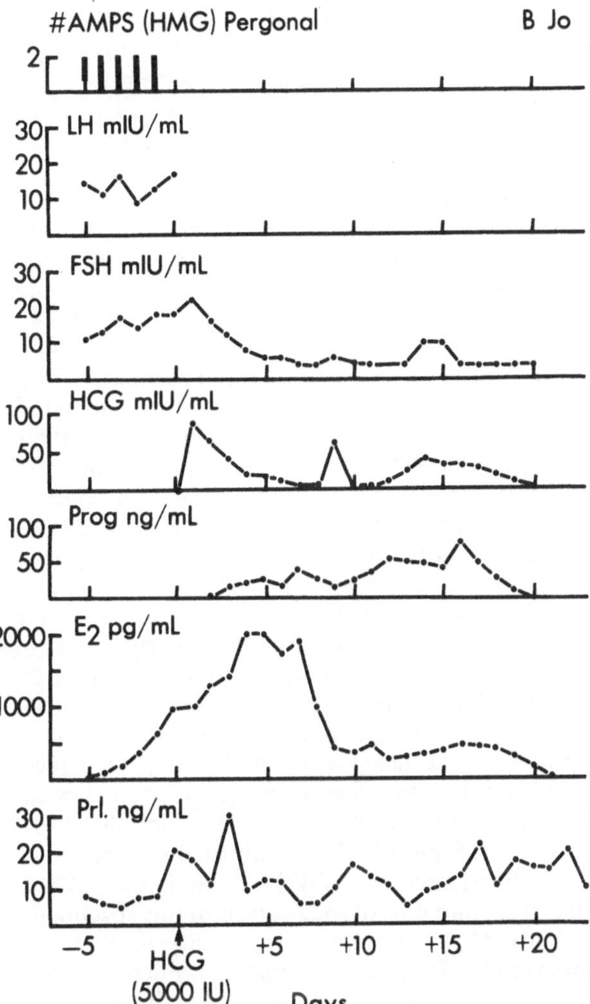

Figure 20.4 Conception and early spontaneous abortion during gonadotropin therapy in the same woman shown on Figure 20.3. The initial rise in β-subunit human chorionic gonadotropin (hCG) is due to the injected exogenous hormone. The rise in hCG on Day 9 after hCG injection was confirmed by repeat assay. The subnormal increase in hCG levels between Days 10–20 after hCG injection reflects a pathological implantation. The 17β-estradiol (E_2) values doubled to 2000 pg/ml over the initial 5 day interval after hCG injection (the early luteal phase). The subnormal hCG levels after implantation reflect the rejection of the blastocyst resulting ultimately in spontaneous abortion. Tissue passed in menstrual blood was never recovered. Prog = progesterone, LH = luteinizing hormone, FSH = follicle stimulating hormone and Prl. = prolactin. See also Figure 20.3.

levels rose consistently; hCG was administered with a further rise in the 17β-estradiol values to 2000 pg/ml over the next five days. Ovulation was reflected by the increased progesterone levels and implantation at Day 8 followed by a spontaneous decline, subsequent consistent rise, then another decline in hCG, progesterone and 17β-estradiol levels with bleeding and passage of tissue *per vaginum* (Figure 20.4). By contrast, the successful pregnancy (Figure 20.3) was associated with a decline in 17β-estradiol levels before hCG administration and then an increase in 17β-estradiol concentrations of a lesser magnitude over the same 5 days after hCG administration. Ovulation was reflected by the increased progesterone levels peaking at Day 7 after hCG administration followed by a sharp decline and a nadir at Day 9. The rescue phenomenon of progesterone secretion by the corpus luteum attributed to hCG is dramatically shown on Figure 20.3, where the rise in hCG associated with implantation was demonstrable by Day 10 after hCG administration.

In the normal menstrual cycle, peak 17β-estradiol levels occur at midcycle corresponding to maximal follicular maturation. Just preceding and concomitant with the LH surge, there is a rapid decline in 17β-estradiol levels. In the luteal phase, the 17β-estradiol levels then rise again but only reach some 50% of the values attained at midcycle (Landgren *et al.*, 1980). Considering that estradiol may be luteolytic in women (Hammerstein, 1974), the increase by twofold to 2000 pg/ml over 5 days during the post-hCG (early luteal) phase of the cycle in which the conceptus was aborted (Figure 20.4) may have been relevant to the unfavorable outcome. The profile of 17β-estradiol levels in Figure 20.3 (the cycle in which a normal pregnancy was conceived) would appear to simulate the normal cycle (Landgren *et al.*, 1980) more closely. It is possible that the rising 17β-estradiol levels in the early luteal phase of the cycle in Figure 20.4 may have had a luteolytic influence and, in this context, the continuously rising 17β-estradiol levels in the early luteal phase (without a preceding decline) may be inappropriate. Further research into the pattern of 17β-estradiol production at midcycle and in the early luteal phase may provide useful information on the endocrine pathology of pregnancy maintenance.

Failure of hCG secretion in a patient with habitual abortion and luteal deficiency is shown in Figure 20.5. The aborted conceptus showed a severe degree of growth disorganization (GD1) (Poland *et al.*, 1981). Although the attempted cell culture and karyotype analysis in this specimen was unsuccessful, the probability of a karyotype abnormality in a growth disorganized specimen approximates 80% (Poland and Ho Yuen, 1978). In this patient, normal progesterone secretion was initially maintained by relatively low levels of hCG. Subsequently, failure of the rescue phenomenon in corpus luteal progesterone secretion appeared to be due to the decreased hCG production by the trophoblast. The low estradiol is of interest since it was dissociated from that of the relatively normal progesterone secretion. Failure of progesterone secretion is demonstrated in Figure 20.6 in another patient spontaneously aborting GD1 twin sacs. The karyotype in one sac was 92,XXXX, while in the other sac, the culture was unsuccessful. The hCG level was normal up to 8 weeks of amenorrhea and then rapidly declined. The progesterone levels were normal at the time of implantation then steadily declined even while hCG was still rising. In contrast to the previous patient (Figure 20.5), the failure of progesterone secretion from the corpus luteum despite adequate tropic stimulation by hCG was consistent with failure of the corpus luteum which preceded failure of trophoblastic hCG secretion. The subnormal 17β-estradiol levels are again shown.

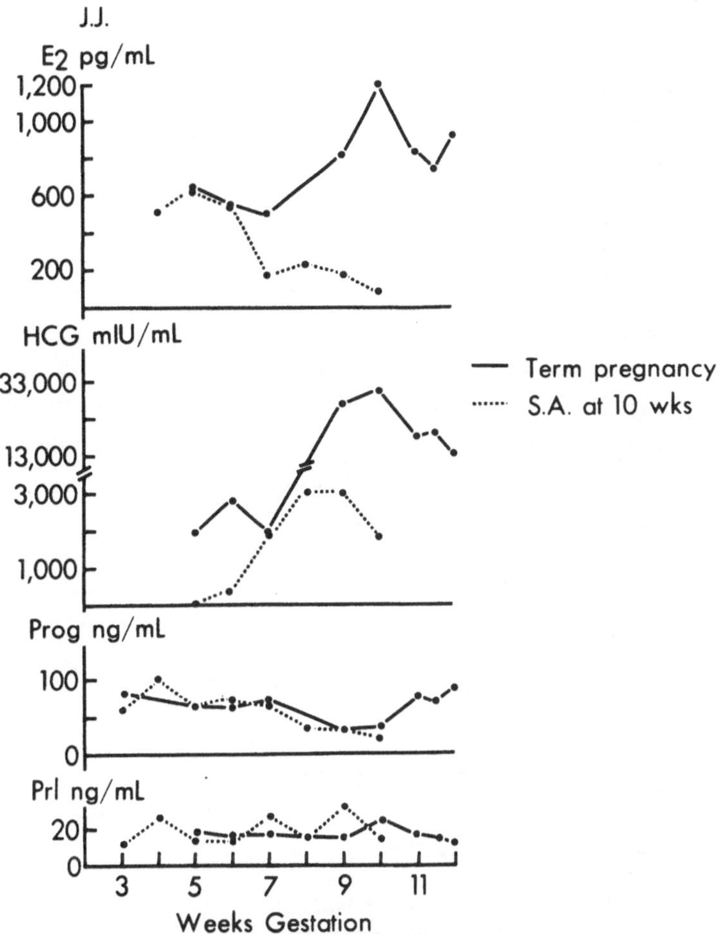

Figure 20.5 Consecutive spontaneously aborted and normal pregnancies in the same patient are shown. The aborted growth disorganized (GD1) pregnancy (see text) is shown with normal progesterone (Prog) and decreased 17β-estradiol (E_2) levels. The failure of human chorionic gonadotropin (hCG) secretion by the trophoblast and 17β-estradiol appeared to be the primary endocrine abnormality in this embryopathic pregnancy. Progesterone levels were initially normal and maintained by relatively low levels of hCG. Failure of the rescue phenomenon of the corpus luteal progesterone production appeared to be secondary to failure of trophoblastic hCG secretion. Prl. = prolactin. See also Figure 20.6.

COMPARISON OF HORMONE PRODUCTION FROM THE TROPHOBLASTIC-LUTEAL COMPLEX BETWEEN NORMAL PREGNANCY, GROWTH DISORGANIZED CONCEPTION AND PREGNANCY ENDING IN ABORTION OF A NORMALLY DEVELOPED EMBRYO

Although women who abort normal fetuses (crown–rump length 30–180 mm) are more likely to have disorders of the maternal environment,

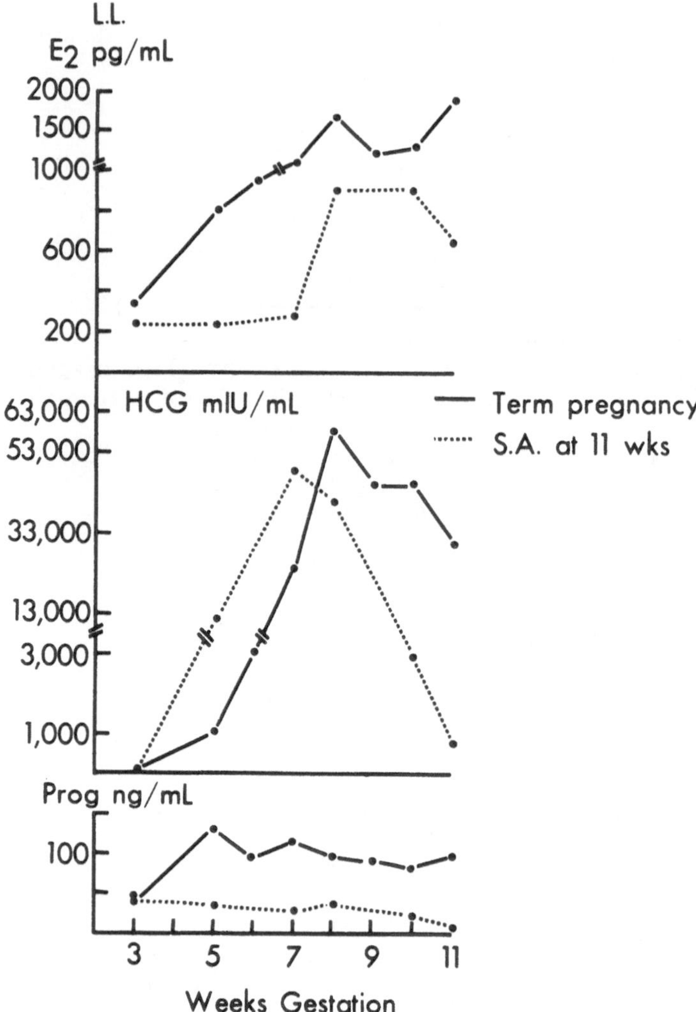

Figure 20.6 Consecutive spontaneously aborted and normal pregnancies in the same patient are shown. The aborted growth disorganized pregnancy (see text) is shown with normal rising β-subunit human chorionic gonadotropin (hCG) up to 8 weeks followed by a rapid decline. Progesterone (Prog) levels, although normal at the time of implantation, showed a low and declining trend even while hCG was rising. This suggests that the corpus luteum was defective in this embryopathic gestation. Low levels of 17β-estradiol are again seen. See also Figure 20.5.

including local intrauterine factors (Poland and Ho Yuen, 1978), data relating specifically to the morphology and karyotype of the abortuses from habitually aborting women with luteal defects are scant. Nevertheless, the mechanisms of the endocrine failure in habitually aborting women who abort recognizable embryos (specimens with crown–rump length < 30 mm) and those who abort severely growth disorganized specimens share similarities and differences

(Figure 20.7). In both types of embryopathic pregnancies, the mean hCG levels are low from implantation and then decline to subnormal values before abortion occurs. The progesterone levels also show a declining trend until abortion has been documented (Figure 20.7). These morphologic types of aborted specimens differed in the pattern of 17β-estradiol production. In contrast to growth disorganization, the presence of an embryo in the aborted specimen was associated with a pattern of rising 17β-estradiol concentrations

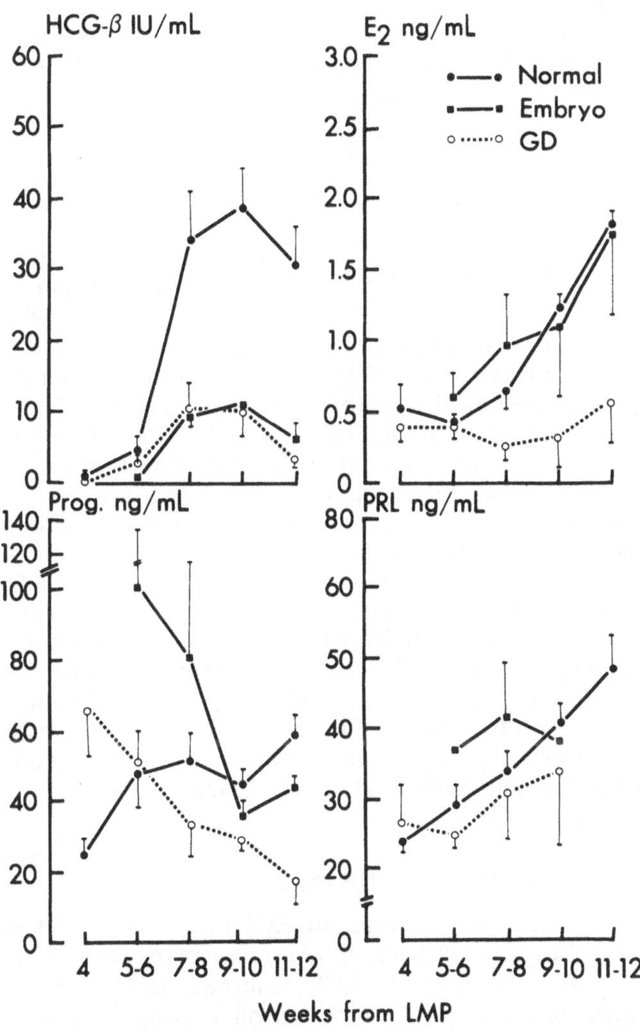

Figure 20.7 Comparison of the mean levels of hCG-β, 17β-estradiol (E_2), progesterone (Prog) and prolactin (PRL) concentrations in pregnancies with normal outcome ($n = 20$), with growth disorganization (GD; $n = 4$) and in pregnancies in which an embryo was aborted ($n = 3$). Bars are standard errors. LMP = last menstrual period. For further details, see text and Ho Yuen *et al.*, 1981 (reprinted with permission of the publisher).

up to the end of the first trimester. The lower mean β-subunit hCG and declining mean progesterone concentrations suggest that endocrine failure of the trophoblast and/or corpus luteum are important factors in both types of embryopathic pregnancy. The normal pattern of 17β-estradiol production in early gestation thus appeared to be dependent on the presence of an embryo, suggesting an embryonic contribution to 17β-estradiol production during early human pregnancy. The role of the embryonic adrenal glands in secreting dehydroepiandrosterone which is then converted to estradiol as early as the first trimester (Seron-Farre *et al.*, 1978) may be the explanation for the lower mean 17β-estradiol concentrations in growth disorganized pregnancies as compared to pregnancies with an embryo present in the aborted specimen.

MANAGEMENT OF LUTEAL PHASE DEFECTS

Removal of known etiologic factors

Where a known etiologic factor is identified, treatment should be directed toward it. Correction of hyperprolactinemia employing bromocriptine corrects the associated luteal defect (Corenblum *et al.*, 1976; Del Pozo *et al.*, 1979). Five of eight hyperprolactinemic women with luteal defects conceived on treatment (Del Pozo *et al.*, 1979). Replacement thyroid hormone therapy in women with subclinical hypothyroidism corrects the luteal defect and allows conception to occur in some (Bohnet *et al.*, 1981). When glucocorticoid therapy was successful in correcting the adrenal androgen excess in women with congenital adrenal hyperplasia, the high abortion rate of untreated women was restored to that expected in a normal population (Sarris *et al.*, 1978). Glucocorticoid therapy may be useful in anovulatory or oligo-ovulatory women with androgen excess. Restoration of ovulation followed suppression of testosterone, androstenedione and urinary excretion of 17-ketosteroids, which was then followed by conception in a few infertile patients (Ho Yuen and Mincey, 1983). Successful treatment of endometriosis has been shown to correct the high abortion rate experienced by women with this disease (Naples *et al.*, 1981), while discontinuation of excessive running exercise was followed by improvement in luteal function and conception in a patient with luteal deficiency (Prior *et al.*, 1982).

Progesterone replacement therapy

In patients with luteal phase defects and regular ovulatory cycles, replacement therapy with natural progesterone alone is effective in correcting these defects (Jones, 1976; Rosenberg, *et al.*, 1980; Andrews, 1979). The use of intramuscular injections with progesterone in oil 12.5 mg daily or intravaginal application of progesterone suppositories 25 mg a.m. and p.m. (Jones, 1976) results in term pregnancies in about 50% of treated women (Jones, 1976; Rosenberg *et al.*, 1980; Andrews, 1979). Treatment is commenced 3 days after the thermal shift in basal temperature and continued until the 9th–10th week of amenorrhea in the cycle of conception (Figure 20.2). This policy is based on the luteectomy data showing that abortion may yet occur in some women when performed as late as Day 57 (8 weeks) from the last menstrual period (Csapo *et al.*, 1972).

We prefer to use natural progesterone in replacement treatment. The physiologic progestins (progesterone and 17-hydroxyprogesterone) when used in physiologic amounts in women with luteal phase defects do not increase the rate of fetal malformations (Andrews, 1979). Progesterone levels may be serially monitored (Ho Yuen *et al.*, 1981) to ensure that replacement treatment maintains acceptable plasma concentrations. The time course of the augmented progesterone levels after insertion of a single 25 mg vaginal suppository composed of polyethylene glycol (Jones, 1976) is shown in Figure 20.8.

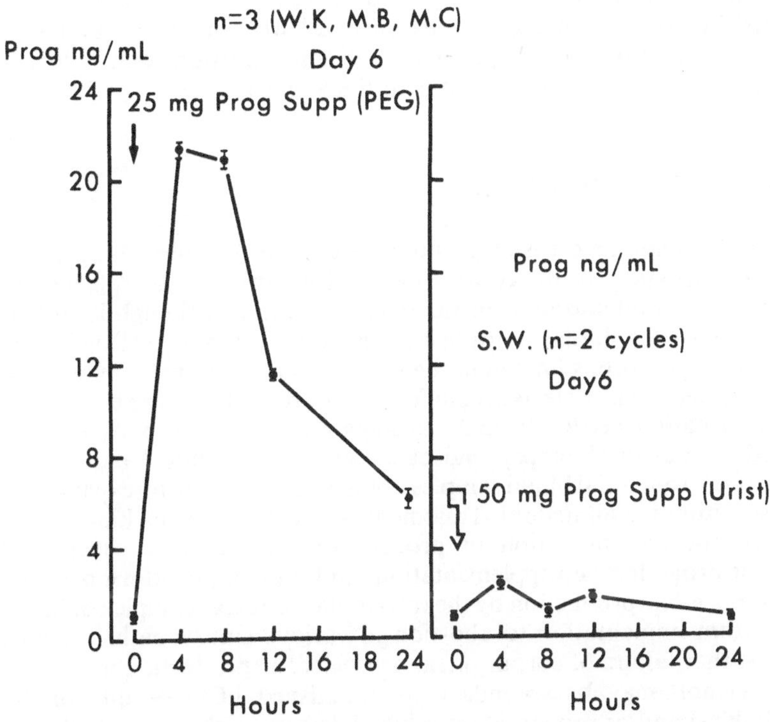

Figure 20.8 Plasma progesterone concentrations after insertion of a 25 mg progesterone suppository made up with polyethylene glycol (PEG), as described by Jones, 1976. Insertion of a 50 mg progesterone vaginal suppository not containing PEG as the base, purchased from another supplier (Urist), resulted in poor absorption and lower plasma levels of progesterone.

Clomiphene citrate

In patients with luteal defects and oligo-ovulatory cycles, clomiphene has the potential of restoring the luteal defect and the infrequent ovulations to a normal pattern. Seven of eight patients with luteal defects ultimately conceived when treated with clomiphene alone (Quagliarello and Weiss, 1979). Where the defect is not corrected or only inconsistently corrected, then supplemental therapy with progesterone may be commenced (Figure 20.2). Clomiphene followed by estrogen was successful in 55% of 268 patients (Grant, 1976). Clomiphene supplemented with hCG in the luteal phase may also be employed (Andrews, 1979). Patients receiving clomiphene therapy may also exhibit luteal phase defects (Van Hall and Mastboom, 1969).

Human gonadotropin therapy

Human gonadotropin therapy in patients with luteal defects has been shown to be helpful (Grant, 1976; Caspi and Hirsch, 1971). Nine of 12 patients treated by Grant conceived. Fourteen of 22 women treated by Caspi and Hirsch conceived; four pregnancies ended in abortion with mild ovarian hyperstimulation occurring in four of the women.

CONCLUDING REMARKS

The luteal phase defect is an identifiable clinical disorder which may result from disturbances in the control mechanisms involved in folliculogenesis, ovulation and luteinization of the ovarian follicle. Although its role in the pathogenesis of habitual abortion is not proven, current knowledge relating to the role of the corpus luteum in the maintenance of early pregnancy suggest that the luteal phase defects are clinically important. No single test provides all the information needed to make a diagnosis. The basal body temperature record, endometrial biopsy and calculation of the luteal index (for progesterone) from serial blood samples obtained from just before ovulation until menstruation are all helpful. Treatment is directed towards known etiologic factors, the administration of progesterone, clomiphene citrate with or without progesterone supplementation, and human gonadotropins. Studies on the hormone production by the trophoblastic-luteal-complex of individual cases from implantation to abortion in various embryopathic pregnancies suggest that failure of corpus luteal progesterone production and the rescue phenomenon may be secondary to diminished hCG production by the trophoblast and/or primary corpus luteal defects (with normal hCG production) in early pregnancy. Prospective studies of embryopathic pregnancies as a group (although in relatively small numbers) as compared to pregnancies with a normal outcome suggest that (1) decreased hCG and progesterone production are common findings in both growth disorganized pregnancies (i.e. pregnancies without an embryo or with severely malformed embryos) and in patients spontaneously aborting specimens containing embryos, and (2) growth disorganized pregnancies produced less estradiol from implantation to the time of abortion. In contrast, aborted specimens containing an embryo demonstrated essentially normal estradiol production during the same interval.

Acknowledgements

The authors wish to thank Wendy Cannon, Lydia Sy and Janet Livingston for their assistance throughout these studies. We are also grateful for the vaginal suppositories prepared by Penny Miller.

This study was supported in part by grants from the British Columbia Heart Foundation awarded to Dr Ho Yuen and grants from the Medical Research Council of Canada awarded to Dr Poland and Dr Ho Yuen.

References

Andrews, W. C. (1979). Luteal phase defects. *Fertil. Steril.*, **32,** 501

Apter, D. (1980). Serum steroids and pituitary hormones in female puberty: A partly longitudinal study. *Clin. Endocrinol.*, **12,** 107

Armstrong, D. T. (1980). Regulation of follicular steroid biosynthesis. In Tozzini, R. I., Reeves, G. and Pineda, R. L. (eds.) *Endocrine Physiopathology of the Ovary*, pp. 165–178. (New York: Elsevier)

Belchetz, P. E., Plant, T. M., Nakai, Y., Keogh, E. J. and Knobil, E. (1978). Hypophysial responses to continuous and intermittent delivery of hypothalamic gonadotropin-releasing hormone. *Science*, **202,** 631

Biggers, J. D. (1981). In vitro fertilization and embryo transfer in human beings. *N. Engl. J. Med.*, **304,** 336

Bohnet, H. G., Fiedler, K. and Leidenberger, F. A. (1981). Subclinical hypothyroidism and infertility. *Lancet*, **2,** 178

Bolt, D. J. (1979). Reduction by human chorionic gonadotropin of the luteolytic effect of prostaglandin $F_2\alpha$ in ewes. *Prostaglandins*, **18,** 387

Bosu, W. T. K. and Johansson, E. D. B. (1975). Implantation and maintenance of pregnancy in mated rhesus monkeys following bilateral oophorectomy or lutectomy with and without progesterone replacement. *Acta Endocrinol.*, **79,** 598

Botella Llusia, J. (1962). The endometrium in repeated abortion. *Int. J. Fertil.*, **7,** 147

Caspi, F. and Hirsch, H. (1971). Therapy of ovulatory sterility and corpus luteum insufficiency with human menopausal and chorionic gonadotropins. *Isr. J. Med. Sci.*, **7,** 1040

Cline, D. I. (1979). Unsuspected subclinical pregnancies in patients with luteal phase defects. *Am. J. Obstet. Gynecol.*, **134,** 438

Csapo, A. I., Pulkkinen, M. O., Ruttner, B., Sauvage, J. P. and Wiest, W. G. (1972). The significance of the human corpus luteum in pregnancy maintenance, I. Preliminary studies. *Am. J. Obstet. Gynecol.*, **112,** 1061

Csapo, A. I. and Pulkkinen, M. (1978). Indispensability of the human corpus luteum in the maintenance of early pregnancy lutectomy evidence. *Obstet. Gynecol. Survey.*, **33,** 69

Corenblum, B., Pairaudeau, N. and Shewchuk, A. B. (1976). Prolactin hypersecretion and short luteal phase defects. *Obstet. Gynecol.*, **47,** 486

Croxatto, H. B., Ortiz, M. E., Diaz, S., Hess, R., Balmaceda, J. and Croxatto, H.-D. (1978). Studies on the duration of egg transport by the human oviduct, II. Ovum location at various intervals following luteinizing hormone peak. *Am. J. Obstet. Gynecol.*, **139,** 629

Del Pozo, E., Wyss, H., Tolis, G., Alcaniz, J., Campana, A. and Naftolin, F. (1979). Prolactin and deficient luteal function. *Obstet. Gynecol.*, **53,** 282

Feicht Sanborn, C., Martin, B. J. and Wagner, W. W. (1982). Is athletic amenorrhea specific to runners? *Am. J. Obstet. Gynecol.*, **143,** 859

Fritz, M. A. and Speroff, L. (1982). The endocrinology of the menstrual cycle: The interaction of folliculogenesis and neuroendocrine mechanisms. *Fertil. Steril.*, **38,** 509

Grant, A. (1976). Clinical problems of ovulation defects. *Int. J. Gynaecol. Obstet.*, **14,** 123

Glass, R. H. and Golbus, M. S. (1978). Habitual abortion. *Fertil. Steril.*, **29,** 257

Hammerstein, J. (1974). Regulation of ovarian steroidogenesis: Gonadotropins, enzymes, prostaglandins, cyclic-AMP, luteolysins. In Guyton, A. C. and Horrobin, D. (eds.) *Reproductive Physiology*, pp. 279–311. (Baltimore: University Park Press)

Ho Yuen, B., Livingston, J. E., Poland, B. J., Wittmann, B. K., Sy, L. and Cannon, W. (1981).

Human chorionic gonadotropin, estradiol, progesterone, prolactin and B-scan ultrasound monitoring of complications in early pregnancy. *Obstet. Gynecol.*, **57**, 207

Ho Yuen, B. and Mincey, E. K. (1983). Role of androgens in menstrual disorders of non-hirsute and hirsute women and the effect of glucocorticoid therapy in hyperandrogenic women. *Am. J. Obstet. Gynecol.*, **145**, 152

Johansson, E. D. B. (1971). Depression of the progesterone levels in women treated with synthetic gestagens after ovulation. *Acta Endocrinol.*, **68**, 779

Jones, G. S. (1976). The luteal phase defects. *Fertil. Steril.* **27**, 351

Keller, D. W., Wiest, W. G., Askin, F. B., Johnson, F. W. and Strickler, R. C. (1979). Pseudocorpus luteum insufficiency: A local defect of progesterone action in endometrial stroma. *J. Clin. Endocrinol. Metab.*, **48**, 127

Kline, J., Stein, Z. A., Susser, M. and Warburton, D. (1977). Smoking: A risk factor for spontaneous abortion. *N. Engl. J. Med.*, **297**, 793

Kline, J., Stein, Z., Susser, M. and Warburton, D. (1980). Environmental influences on early loss in a current New York City study. In Porter, I. H. and Hook, E. B. (eds.) *Human Embryonic and Fetal Death*, pp. 225–240. (New York: Academic Press)

Knobil, E., Plant, T. M., Wildt, L., Belchetz, P. E. and Marshall, G. (1980). Control of the rhesus monkey's menstrual cycle: Permissive role of hypothalamic gonadotropin-releasing hormone. *Science*, **207**, 1371

Landgren, B. M., Unden, A. L. and Diczfalusy, E. (1980). Hormonal profile of the cycle in 68 normally menstruating women. *Acta Endocrinol.*, **94**, 89

Leyendecker, G., Wildt, L. and Hansmann, M. (1980). Pregnancies following chronic intermittent (pulsatile) administration of GnRH by means of a portable pump ('Zyklomat'): A new approach to treatment of infertility in hypothalamic amenorrhea. *J. Clin. Endocrinol. Metab.*, **51**, 1214

McNatty, K. P., Saywers, R. S. and McNeilly, A. S. (1974). A possible role for prolactin in control of steroid secretion by the human Graafian follicle. *Nature (Lond.)*, **250**, 653

Moon, Y. S., Tsang, B. K., Simpson, C. and Armstrong, D. (1978). 17β-estradiol biosynthesis in cultured granulosa and thecal cells of human follicles: Stimulation by follicle stimulating hormone. *J. Clin. Endocrinol. Metab.*, **47**, 263

Moon, Y. S., Leung, P. C. S., Ho Yuen, B. and Gomel, V. (1981). Prostaglandin-F in human endometriotic tissue. *Am. J. Obstet. Gynecol.*, **141**, 344

Naples, J. D., Batt, R. E. and Sadigh, H. (1981). Spontaneous abortion rate in patients with endometriosis. *Obstet. Gynecol.*, **57**, 509

Poland, B. J. and Ho Yuen, B. (1978). Embryonic development in consecutive specimens from recurrent spontaneous abortions. *Am. J. Obstet. Gynecol.*, **130**, 512

Poland, B. J., Miller, J. R., Harris, M. and Livingston, J. (1981). Spontaneous abortion: A study of 1,961 women and their conceptuses. *Acta Obstet. Gynaecol. Scand.*, **102**, 5

Prior, J., Ho Yuen, B., Clement, P., Bowie, L. and Thomas, J. (1982). Reversible luteal phase changes and infertility associated with marathon training. *Lancet*, **2**, 269

Quagliarello, J. and Weiss, G. (1979). Clomiphene in the management of infertility associated with shortened luteal phases. *Fertil. Steril.*, **31**, 373

Rodriguez-Rigau, L. J., Steinberger, E., Atkins, B. J. and Lucci, J. A. (1979). Effect of testosterone on human corpus luteum steroidogenesis in vitro. *Fertil. Steril.*, **31**, 448

Rosenberg, S. M., Luciano, A. A. and Riddick, D. H. (1980). The luteal phase defect: The relative frequency of, and encouraging response to, treatment with vaginal suppositories. *Fertil. Steril.*, **34**, 17

Ross, G. T., Cargille, C. M., Lipsett, M. B., Rayford, J. R., Marshall, J. R., Strott, C. A. and Rodbard, D. (1970). Pituitary and gonadal hormones in women during spontaneous and induced ovulatory cycles. *Rec. Prog. Hormon. Res.*, **26**, 1

Ross, G. T. (1979). Human chorionic gonadotropin and maternal recognition of pregnancy. In *Maternal Recognition of Pregnancy. Ciba Foundation Symposium (New Series)* Vol. 64, p. 196 (New York: Excerpta Medica)

Sarris, S., Swyer, G. I. M., Ward, R. H. T., Lawrence, D. M. and McCarrigle, H. H. (1978). The treatment of mild adrenal hyperplasia and associated infertility with prednisone. *Br. J. Obstet. Gynaecol.*, **85**, 251

Schulz, K. D., Geiger, W., Del Pozo, E. and Kunzig, H. J. (1978). Pattern of sexual steroids, prolactin and gonadotropin hormones during prolactin inhibition in normally cycling women. *Am. J. Obstet. Gvnecol.*, **132**, 561

Seron-Farre, M., Lawrence, C. C. and Jaffe, R. B. (1978). Role of hCG in the regulation of the fetal zone of the fetal adrenal gland. *J. Clin. Endocrinol. Metab.*, **46,** 834

Shangold, M., Freeman, R., Thysen, B. and Gatz, M. (1979). The relationship between long-distance running, plasma progesterone and luteal phase length. *Fertil. Steril.*, **31,** 130

Sherman, B. M. and Korenman, S. G. (1974). Measurement of plasma LH, FSH, estradiol and progesterone in disorders of the human menstrual cycle: The short luteal phase. *J. Clin. Endocrinol. Metab.*, **38,** 89

Sherman, B. M. and Korenman, S. G. (1975). Hormonal characteristics of the human menstrual cycle throughout life. *J. Clin. Invest.*, **55,** 699

Smith, K. D., Rodriguez-Ragau, L. J., Tcholakian, R. K. and Steinberger, E. (1979). The relation between plasma testosterone levels and the lengths of phases of the menstrual cycle. *Fertil. Steril.*, **32,** 403

Sotrel, G., Helvacioglu, A., Dowers, S., Scommegna, A. and Auletta, F. (1981). Mechanism of luteolysis: Effect of estradiol and prostaglandin F_2 on corpus luteum luteinizing hormone/human chorionic gonadotropin receptors and cyclic nucleotides in the rhesus monkey. *Am. J. Obstet. Gynecol.*, **139,** 134

Van Hall, E. V. and Mastboom, J. L. (1969). Luteal phase insufficiency in patients treated with clomiphene. *Am. J. Obstet. Gynecol.*, **103,** 165

Vande Wiele, R., Bogumil, J., Dyrenfurth, I., Ferin, M., Jewelewicz, R., Warren, M., Rizkallah, T. and Mikhail, G. (1970). Mechanisms regulating the menstrual cycle in women. *Rec. Prog. Horm. Res.*, **26,** 63

Vollman, R. F. (1977). *The Menstrual Cycle*, p. 127. (Toronto: Saunders)

Wentz, A. C. (1980). Endometrial biopsy in the evaluation of infertility. *Fertil. Steril.*, **33,** 124

Yen, S. S. C., Tsai, C. C., Naftolin, F., Vandenberg, G. and Ajabor, L. (1972). Pulsatile patterns of gonadotropin release in subjects with and without ovarian function. *J. Clin. Endocrinol. Metab.*, **34,** 671

21
Hormone patterns in early pregnancy disorders

I. GERHARD and B. RUNNEBAUM

In the course of an undisturbed pregnancy ultrasound examinations are usually performed only after the third month of gestation. Any additional determinations of hormones in serum are the exception and will normally be done only in cases of endangered pregnancy, e.g. when bleedings or contractions are observed (Eriksen and Philipsen, 1980; Hertz *et al.*, 1980*b*; Jouppila *et al.*, 1980*a,b*). This poses the question whether and when any hormone determinations in serum should be included in a clinical routine program to permit a prognosis with regard to the further course of pregnancy. Due to their different locations of synthesis the following hormones are suitable for testing the function of the pregnancy product: β-hCG and human placental lactogen (HPL) as placental parameters, 17-hydroxyprogesterone (17-OHP) which is almost exclusively produced by the corpus luteum. Progesterone (P) and estradiol (E_2), which are initially synthesized by the corpus luteum, increasing quantities of which are, however, from the second month of gestation onwards of placental origin. Finally estriol (E_3) needs to be mentioned which derives mainly from precursors of the fetal adrenal cortex and is synthesized by the placenta. Following the assessment of single and serial hormone determinations during normal pregnancy and in cases of impending abortion it is also the aim of this study to consider the special situation of pregnancies following sterility treatment.

METHODOLOGY

A prospective randomized study was carried out on 1125 pregnant women in order to evaluate the usefulness of hormone determinations in pregnancy. Immediately after detection of pregnancy (positive qualitative pregnancy test in urine) serial blood samples were collected at 1–4 week intervals. As the admission to this study was dependent on positive pregnancy tests in urine, no information could be obtained on hormonal changes in very early pregnancies (i.e. for periods before the 6th week of pregnancy). Several patients could not be followed up. They were under supervision of general practitioners and not all sets of serial controls were complete.

Of the 1125 women studied, 299 exhibited bleeding in the first trimester of pregnancy. All these women were hospitalized and had bed rest but no hormone therapy. After 3 days without bleeding the patients were mobilized. Weekly ultrasound examinations were performed. Negative ultrasonic results in the detection of fetal life signs after 8 weeks of gestation were followed by the evacuation of the uterus. The placentas underwent histological examination.

Of the 299 women with bleeding, 112 aborted before the 16th week of pregnancy (early abortion, e.a.), and 19 after the 16th week of pregnancy (late abortion, l.a.). 168 of the 299 women completed pregnancy and were delivered of a viable infant (threatened abortion, t.a.). During this study 229 women served as controls. They were chosen in accordance with the following criteria: uneventful course of pregnancy, no diseases, no drugs, delivery between weeks 37 and 41 of pregnancy, repeated normal ultrasound examinations, spontaneous delivery of a normal size baby (10th–90th birth weight percentile) without malformations. Apgar score 1 minute after birth >8, and normal postnatal development.

At each antenatal visit 10 ml blood was drawn from an antecubital vein between 8 a.m. and 10 a.m. Serum was separated and stored at $-20°C$ before analysis. After termination of pregnancy by delivery or abortion all data were computerized. Statistical evaluation was performed by SAS. χ^2 tests and Wilcoxon – as well as Kruskal Wallis – tests were performed. The level of significance was determined by $p < 0.01$.

An additional number of 132 sterility patients with bleeding before the 11th week of pregnancy was examined. Of those women, 29 had tubal pregnancies, 78 had abortions (week 5–7 of pregnancy: 24 patients, 8th week: 16 patients, weeks 9–11: 19 patients, weeks 12–15: 19 patients) and 25 of them continued pregnancy to term. As the prospective study had already demonstrated that β-hCG, P and E_2 were the most sensitive and specific endocrine parameters in early pregnancy, only these three hormones were routinely measured during each antenatal visit.

β-hCG was measured with the reagents of CIS. The detection limit was 4 miu/ml serum. The intra-assay precision was 7 %, the interassay precision was 8–15 %. The cross-reaction of the antiserum with luteinizing hormone (LH) was 0.16 %. While the antiserum cross-reacts with the entire hCG molecule in 100 %, this was only in 0.005 % the case with the α-subunit.

HPL was determined with the Amersham kit. The sensitivity of the assay was 10 ng HPL/ml serum. A sufficient accuracy of the method was however, only reached when the HPL content of the sample was above 50 ng. The intra-assay precision was below 4 %, the interassay precision between 6 and 8 %.

17-OHP was extracted from serum with petroleum ether and measured by radioimmunoassay with an antiserum against 17α-hydroxyprogesterone-3 (O-carboxymethyl)-oxime BSA. The sensitivity of the method was 0.3 ng/ml serum. The intra-assay precision was between 3 and 5 %, the interassay precision 7–11 %. The cross-reactions with P and desoxycortisol were 1 % and with 17-hydroxypregnenolone and 5α-pregnandione 0.5 %. The serum cross-reacted in less than 0.1 % with other steroids.

P was extracted with petroleum ether and determined radioimmunologically with an antiserum against 11α-hydroxyprogesterone-hemisuccinate BSA. The detection limit was 50–100 pg/sample. The intra-assay precision was 5–8 %, the interassay precision 8 %. The cross-reactions with different steroids were below 2 %.

E_2 was measured with the Travenol kit after extraction with diethylether. The detection limit was 2.5 pg/ml serum. The intra-assay precision was between 5 and 7 % depending on the E_2 concentration in the sample. The interassay precision was 8 %. The cross-reaction with estrone and estriol was 2 %, the cross-reactions with other steroids were below 0.1 %.

E_3 was extracted with diethylether and measured by radioimmunoassay with an antiserum against 6-oxo-estriol-carbomethoxime-BSA. The detection limit of the assay was 30 pg/ml serum. The intra-assay precision was below 6 %, the interassay precision between 5 and 8 %. Cross-reactions with different steroids were below 2 %.

ENDOCRINE PROFILES

In Figures 21.1–21.5 the serum hormone concentrations are shown for weeks 6–22 of pregnancy. Median, 10th and 90th percentiles are given for normal pregnancies, threatened abortion and abortion. The β-hCG concentrations (Figure 21.1) in women with threatened abortion showed a wider scattering of the individual values than was the case in normal pregnancies. The difference was not statistically significant. The β-hCG concentrations of women with abortion were significantly lower during weeks 6–13 of pregnancy.

The HPL concentrations (Figure 21.2) in women with threatened abortion did not differ from the normal controls. In women with abortion they were significantly lower during weeks 10–13 of pregnancy. The P concentrations (Figure 21.3) were normal in women with threatened abortion and significantly decreased in women with abortion during weeks 8–13 of pregnancy.

The E_2 concentrations (Figure 21.4) were mostly normal in women with threatened abortion. During weeks 12 and 15 of pregnancy they were, however, significantly lower. In women with abortion E_2 concentrations showed a significant decrease from weeks 8 through 14 of pregnancy.

Like E_2, the E_3 concentrations (Figure 21.5) significantly decreased in women with threatened abortion in weeks 13 and 15 of pregnancy, while women with abortion showed low E_3 concentrations from weeks 10–14.

On the basis of the 5th percentile of the hormone concentrations in the strictly defined normal controls the hormone values of each patient were classified as normal (i.e. > 5th percentile) or low (≤ 5th percentile). For Table 21.1, 425 women with apparently normal course of pregnancy were considered. They had two blood samples drawn at 1–2 week intervals before the 14th week of pregnancy. More than 90 % of the 350 women with regular delivery had normal β-hCG, P, E_2 and E_3 concentrations, while the HPL method produced no definite results. Of the 75 women with later abortion, 50 % had low or decreasing β-hCG, P, E_2 and E_3 values. In these cases HPL and E_2 were the most sensitive parameters.

At the time of uterine bleeding the assessment of pregnancy outcome was

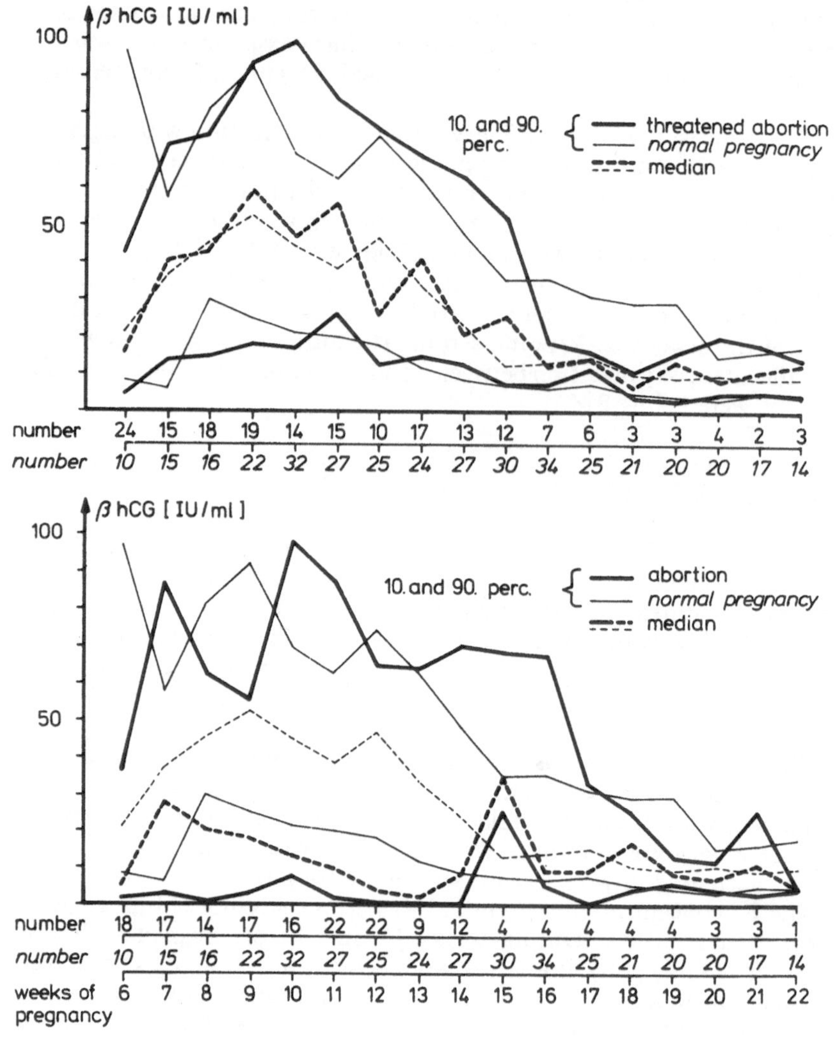

Figure 21.1 β-hCG concentrations in women with normal pregnancies ($n = 229$), threatened abortions ($n = 168$) and abortions ($n = 103$) during the first half of pregnancy. Median, 10th and 90th percentiles for each group are given.

easier through any of the hormones in question. As shown in Table 21.2 the specificity of β-hCG, HPL, P, E_2 and E_3 was above 90 %, and the sensitivity was highest for E_2 and β-hCG. To make a comparison between the different methods possible the relative risk was calculated. An increased risk could best be diagnosed by measuring E_2 (3.7) and β-hCG (3.2).

From Tables 21.1 and 21.2 it becomes evident that in case of e.a. the fetoplacental unit was usually irreversibly damaged at the time of bleeding, so

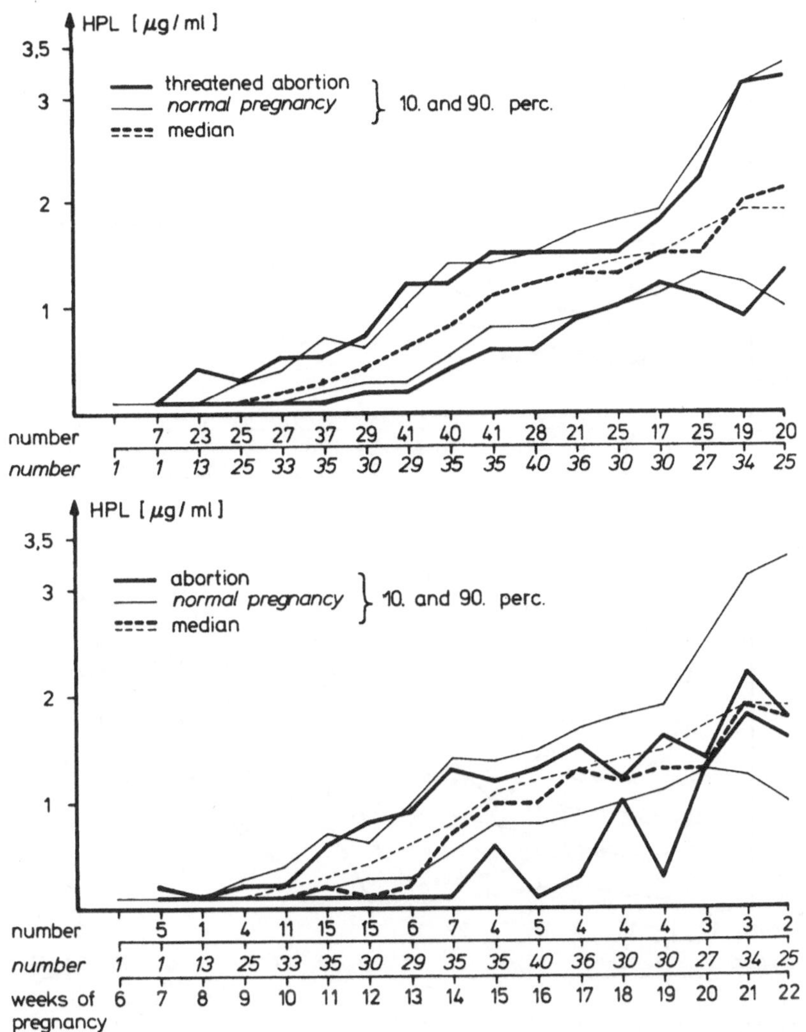

Figure 21.2 HPL concentrations in women with normal pregnancies ($n = 229$), threatened abortions ($n = 168$) and abortions ($n = 103$) during the first half of pregnancy. Median, 10th and 90th percentiles for each group are given.

that 90 % of these women had one or more decreased hormone values. The serial determinations in the 75 women with e.a. revealed that in 60 % of them one or several hormones decreased 1–5 weeks before bleeding occurred.

The frequency of low hormone concentrations was dependent on the week of pregnancy testing. Before the 6th week of pregnancy the determination of β-hCG proved to be most effective. From the 7th week onwards, E_2 and E_3 showed the highest percentage of low hormone values. The determination of

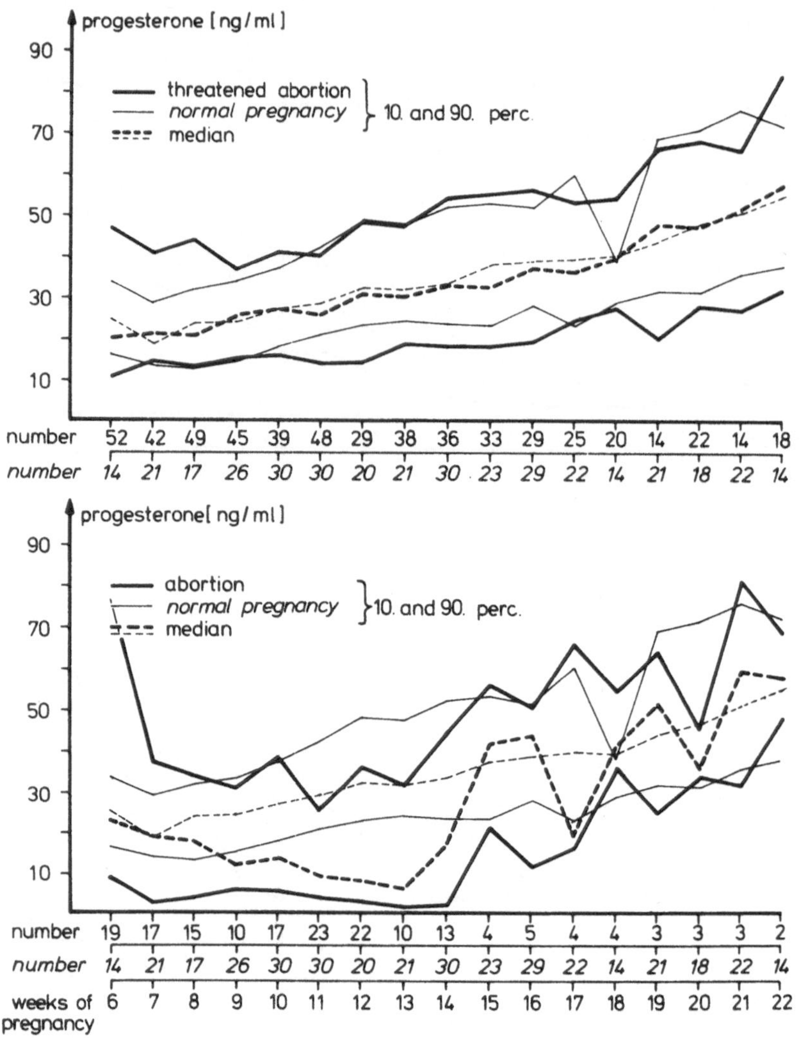

Figure 21.3 Progesterone concentrations in women with normal pregnancies ($n = 229$), threatened abortions ($n = 168$) and abortions ($n = 103$) during the first half of pregnancy. Median, 10th and 90th percentiles for each group are given.

HPL was appropriate only after the 9th week of pregnancy for substitution of the β-hCG measurement. In this normal population any isolated P-deficiency was not observed. However, the determination of P in addition to β-hCG gave better information from the 7th week onwards.

In the 19 women with l.a. serial hormone determinations showed a normal profile with the exception of four women who exhibited subnormal HPL or E_3 concentrations after the 14th week of pregnancy. The serial hormone

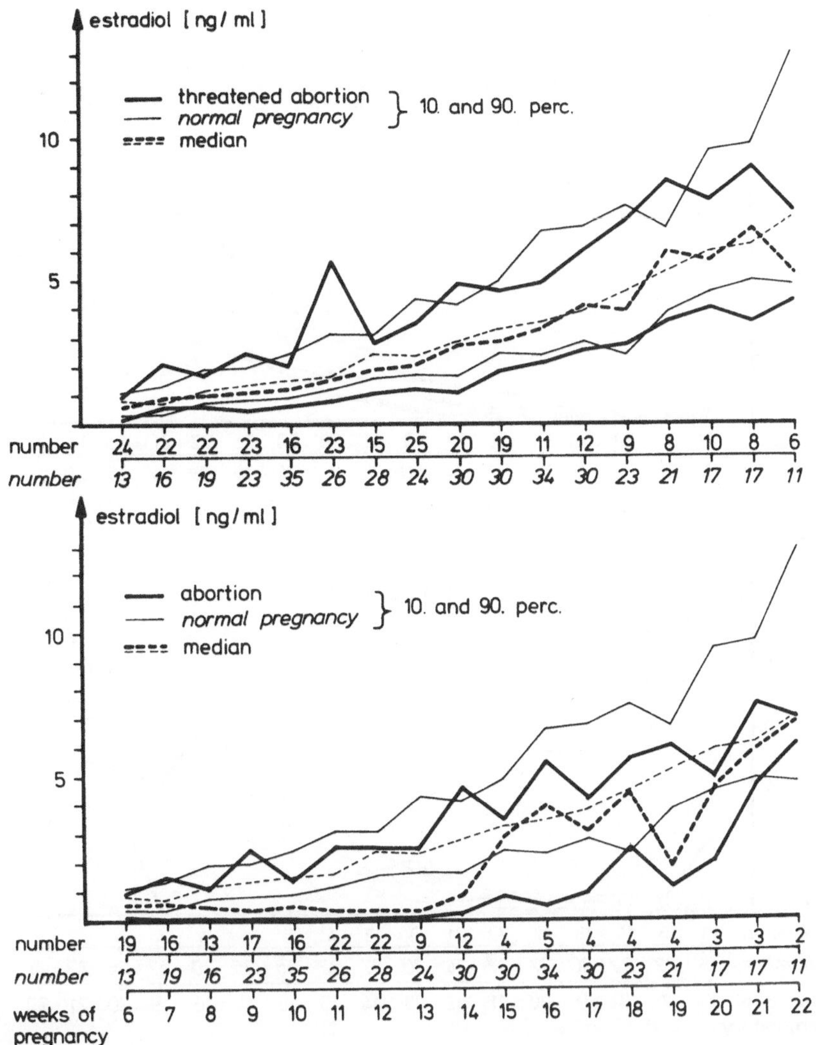

Figure 21.4 17β-estradiol concentrations in women with normal pregnancies ($n = 229$), threatened abortions ($n = 168$) and abortions ($n = 103$) during the first half of pregnancy. Median, 10th and 90th percentiles for each group are given.

determinations in women with t.a. demonstrated the normal increase of all parameters.

Serial determinations, as shown in Figures 21.6–21.11, were performed in 132 pregnant women after infertility treatment. As in some cases ovarian hyperstimulation was induced, P and E_2 concentrations appeared to be higher than normal during the first 2 months of pregnancy.

Of the 24 women who aborted during weeks 5–7 of pregnancy (Figure

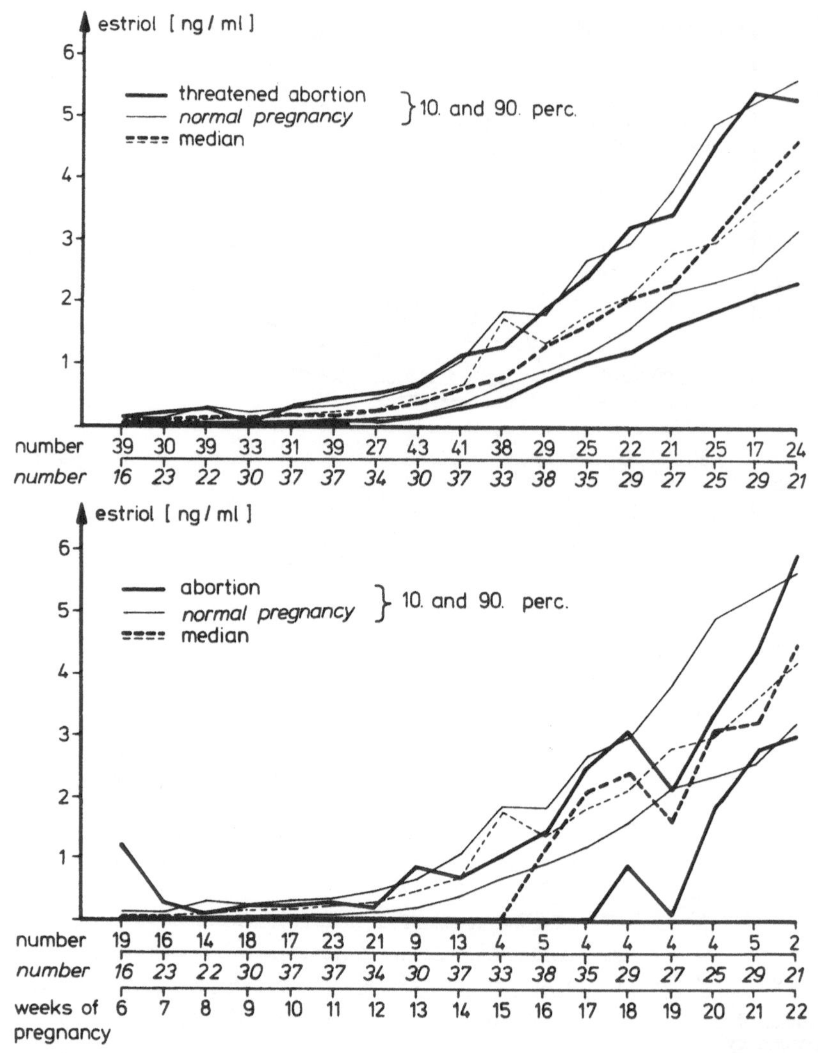

Figure 21.5 Estriol concentrations in women with normal pregnancies ($n = 229$), threatened abortions ($n = 168$) and abortions ($n = 103$) during the first half of pregnancy. Median, 10th and 90th percentiles for each group are given.

21.6), 88 % had decreased hormone concentrations (β-hCG 42 %, P 66 %, E_2 66 %). Only three women aborted despite normal hormone values. The determination of β-hCG which was necessary to prove pregnancy was completed by the P and E_2 measurement. Sixteen aborted in the 8th week of pregnancy (Figure 21.7); 15 of them exhibited decreased hormone concentrations (β-hCG 56 %, P 88 %, E_2 69 %). While eight women had simultaneous low hormone concentrations of β-hCG, P and E_2, we observed six women

Table 21.1 Distribution of normal (>5th percentile) and low (<5th percentile) hormone concentrations in the two first blood samples drawn at 1–2 week intervals during weeks 4–14 of pregnancy in 350 women with regular delivery (D) and 75 women with abortion (A)

Hormone	*Both values normal* (%)		*First value low; second normal* (%)		*First value normal; second low* (%)		*Both values low* (%)	
	A	*D*	*A*	*D*	*A*	*D*	*A*	*D*
β-HCG	52	94	8	3.7	16	1.2	24	1.1
HPL	24	53	12	33.0	24	3.0	40	11
Progesterone	50	93	4	4.0	15	1.0	31	2
17β-estradiol	45	93	4	3.7	12	2.7	39	0.6
Estriol	47	91	4	4.0	18	3.0	31	2

Table 21.2 Assessment of pregnancy outcome by various serum hormone tests at the first day of uterine bleeding in patients with abortion (n = 131) and threatened abortion (n = 106)

Test	*Sensitivity* (%)	*Specificity* (%)	*Predictive value* (%)	*Relative risk*
β-hCG	74.5	93.6	92.5	3.2
HPL	33.7	93.3	85.7	1.9
17-OHP	51.6	82.6	78.3	1.7
Progesterone	62.5	95.3	92.4	2.6
17β-estradiol	81.8	92.4	92.6	3.7
Estriol	65.1	93.1	91.5	2.6

Sensitivity was defined as the percentage of cases with abortion detected by the test
Specificity was defined as the percentage of cases with delivery and normal values
Predictive value concerns results out of normal range and describes the proportion of such results associated with abortion
Relative risk is the ratio of the percentage of positive results which were true positives to the percentage of negative results which were false negatives

whose drop of P and E_2 concentrations preceded a β-hCG decrease. All 19 women with abortion during weeks 9–11 of pregnancy (Figure 21.8) had decreased hormone concentrations (β-hCG 53 %, P 89 %, E_2 68 %). In eight of the women all hormones were found to be low, while in the majority of the remaining cases P or E_2 decreased before β-hCG.

Nineteen women aborted during weeks 12–15 of pregnancy (Figure 21.9), only one of them despite normal hormone values. The frequency of decreased concentrations was highest for P (β-hCG 42 %, P 84 %, E_2 63 %). 29 women had tubal pregnancies (Figure 21.10). Four of them had normal hormone concentrations prior to operation while the remaining had mostly low P concentrations (β-hCG 55 %, P 83 %, E_2 59 %).

Twenty-five women completed pregnancy to term (Figure 21.11) after bleeding occurred in early pregnancy. β-hCG concentrations were always above the 5th percentile, while two women showed transient low P concentrations and one additional woman persisting low E_2 values.

In Table 21.3 the results of the hormone determinations in women with

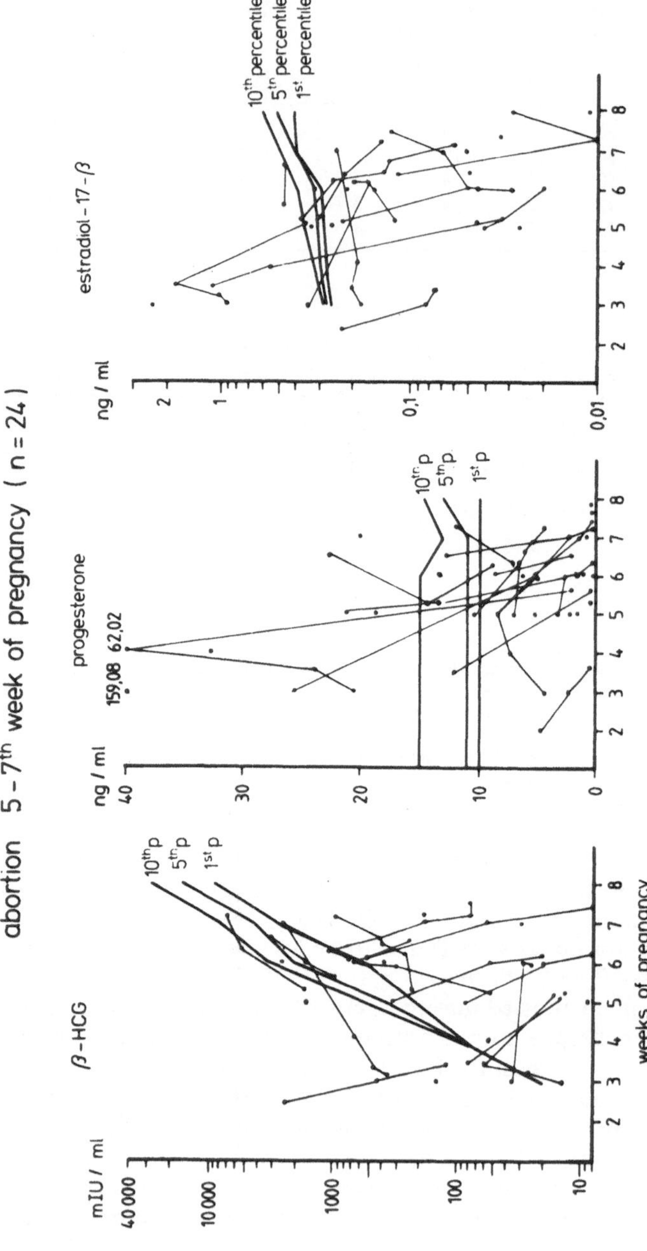

Figure 21.6 Serial determinations of β-hCG, P and E_2 in 24 women with abortions during weeks 5–7 of pregnancy after treatment of infertility. 1st, 5th and 10th percentiles of the hormone concentrations in normal pregnancies are given.

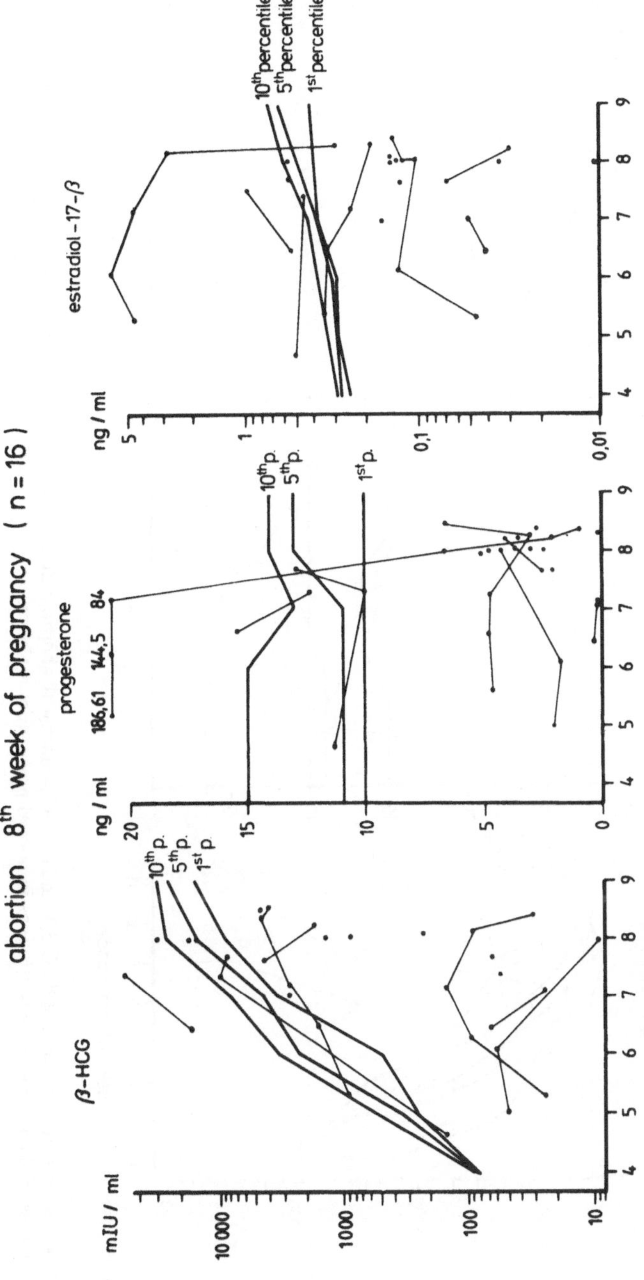

Figure 21.7 Serial determinations of β-hCG, P and E_2 in 16 women with abortion in the 8th week of pregnancy after treatment of infertility. 1st, 5th and 10th percentiles of the hormone concentrations in normal pregnancies are given.

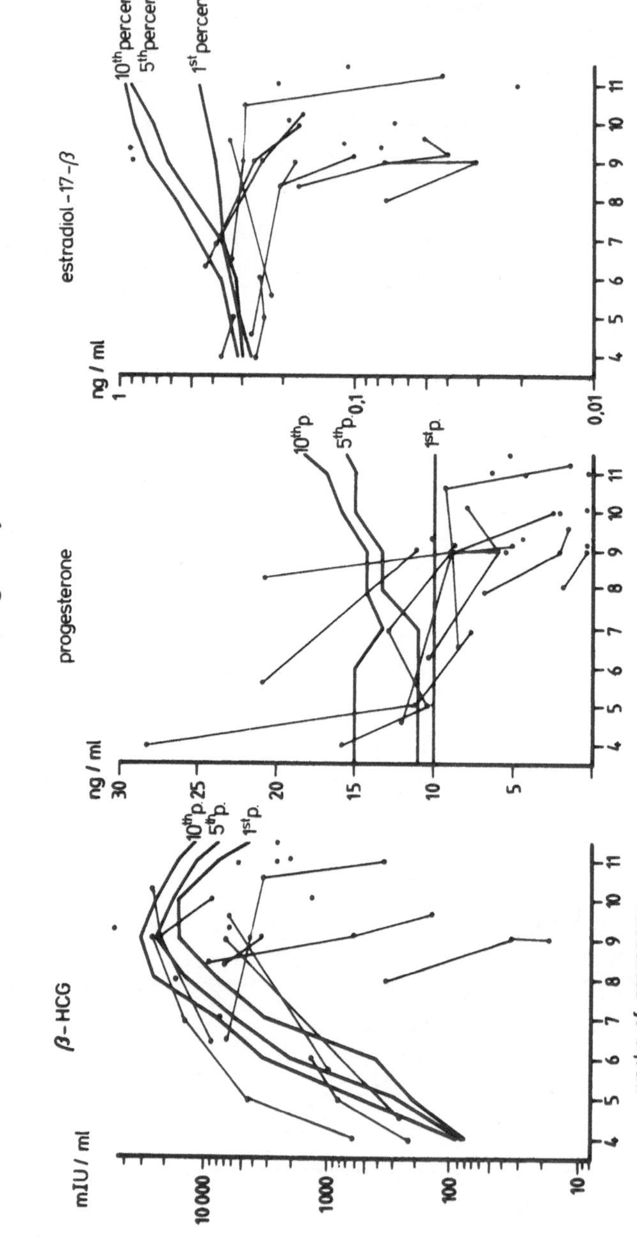

Figure 21.8 Serial determinations of β-hCG, P and E_2 in 19 women with abortions during weeks 9–11 of pregnancy after treatment of infertility. 1st, 5th and 10th percentiles of the hormone concentrations in normal pregnancies are given.

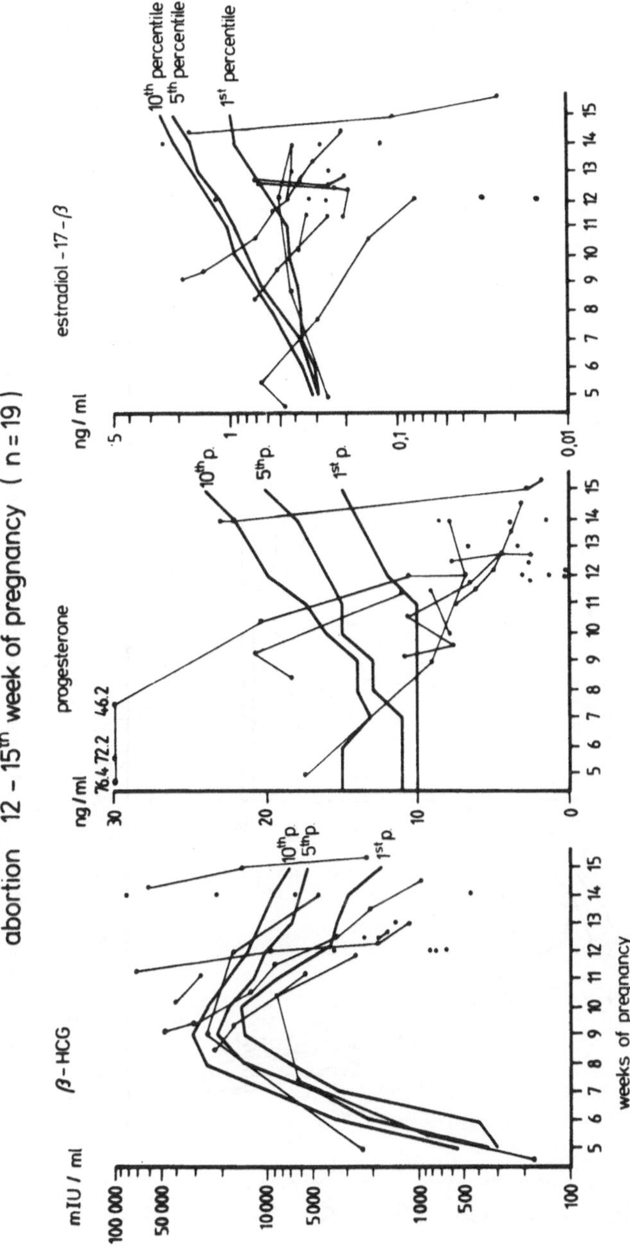

Figure 21.9 Serial determinations of β-hCG, P and E_2 in 19 women with abortions during weeks 12–15 of pregnancy after treatment of infertility. 1st, 5th and 10th percentiles of the hormone concentrations in normal pregnancies are given.

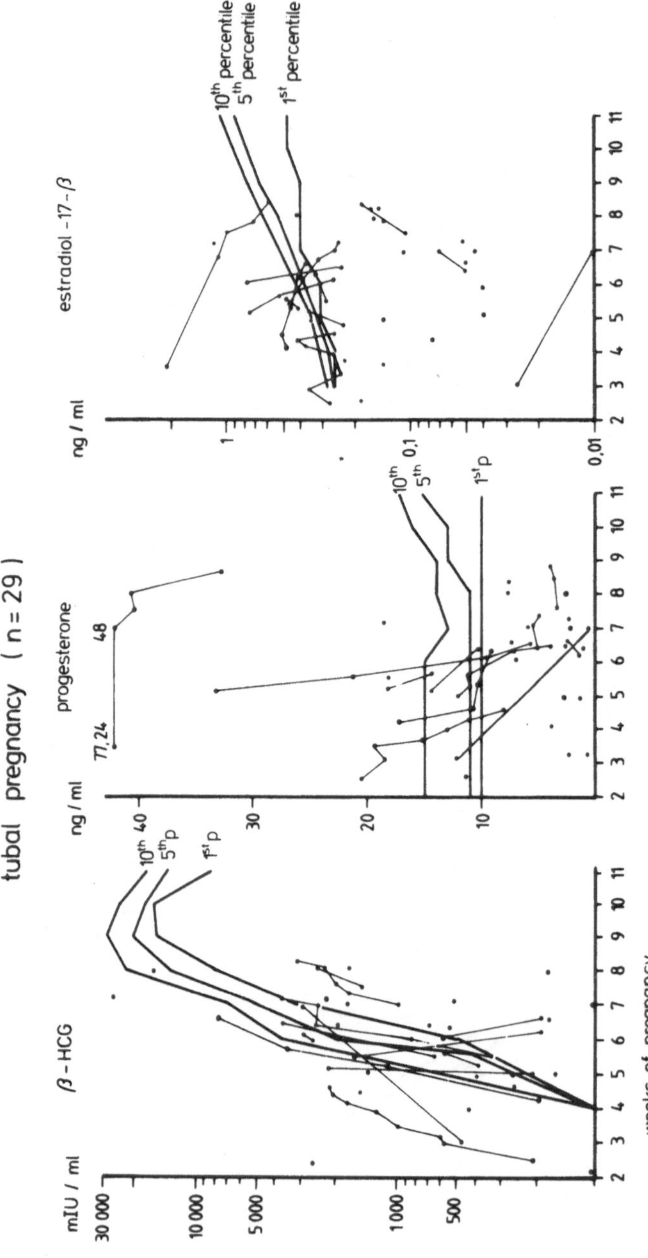

Figure 21.10 Serial determinations of *β*-hCG, P and E_2 in 29 women with tubal pregnancies after treatment of infertility. 1st, 5th and 10th percentiles of the hormone concentrations in normal pregnancies are given.

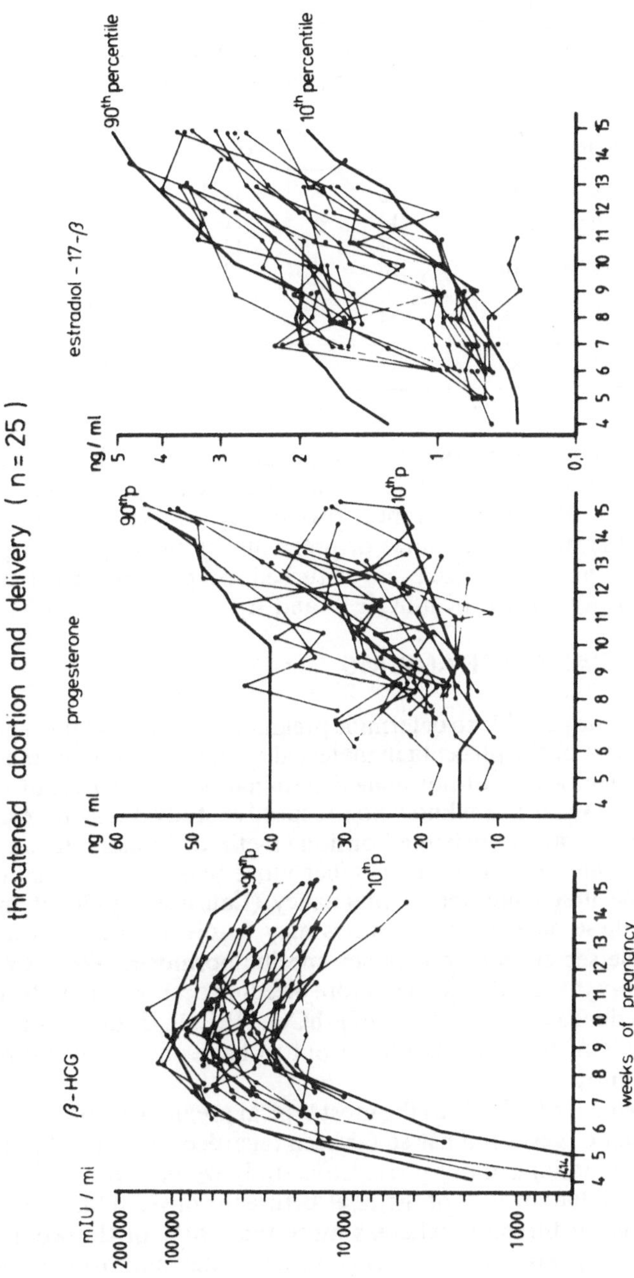

Figure 21.11 Serial determinations of β-hCG, P and E_2 in 25 women with threatened abortion and delivery after treatment of infertility. 1st, 5th and 10th percentiles of the hormone concentrations in normal pregnancies are given.

Table 21.3 Frequency of reduced hormone concentrations in 107 women with abortion following sterility treatment with reference date of abortion. Only the hormone that first showed reduced values was considered

Abortion/ weeks of pregnancy	*No. of patients*	*No. of patients with hormone concentrations ⩽ 5th percentile*				*All tests normal*
		β-hCG	*Progesterone (P)*	*17β-estradiol (E_2)*	*β-hCG+ P+E_2*	
5–7	24	11	16	16	6	3
8	16	9	14	11	8	1
9–11	19	12	17	13	8	–
12–15	19	10	16	12	7	1
Tubal pregnancy	29	16	24	17	8	4
Total	107	58	87	69	37	9

abortion after infertility treatment are summarized. While the measurement of β-hCG is an irreplacable method for pregnancy testing, in some cases the determination of P and sometimes also of E_2 enables a more precise assessment of the individual course of pregnancy. Only 8% of the patients with e.a. were not recognized as disturbed pregnancies by means of simultaneous measurement of β-hCG, P and E_2.

PHYSIOLOGICAL MECHANISMS

Since it has become possible to determine pregnancy specific products secreted by the trophoblast or the placenta in maternal serum, studies have repeatedly dealt with the significance of hormone determinations in the case of patients with signs of t.a. As far as we know no prospective study has so far examined the importance of various existing hormone methods in individual patients.

As chromosomal abnormalities number more than 50% of the abortion products in the first trimester of pregnancy (Lauritsen, 1976) it must be assumed that these deficient pregnancies may be distinguished by an early reduction in the secretion of pregnancy specific hormones. We proved in a prospective study that several weeks before bleeding occurred, half the women with e.a. had reduced concentrations of β-hCG, HPL, P, E_2 or E_3. At the time of bleeding 90% of the patients turned out to have one or several reduced hormone concentrations.

The measurement of β-hCG as the most typical pregnancy hormone during the first trimester of gestation has so far been regarded as the most important hormone determination. In our prospective study women with abortion had reduced β-hCG values in 40% of the cases before the onset of bleeding, and in 75% at the time of bleeding, whereas more than 90% of the women with regular delivery appeared to have normal values. Other authors have likewise reported a 60–80% share of reduced β-hCG concentrations in women with abortion compared to normal concentrations in 90–100% of the pregnancies with good prognosis (Nygren *et al.*, 1973; Kunz and Keller, 1976; Braunstein *et al.*, 1978; Gerhard and Runnebaum, 1978; Jouppila *et al.*, 1979, 1980, Crépin *et al.*, 1980; Gaspard *et al.*, 1980; Hertz *et al.*, 1980*a*; Scholler *et al.*, 1980; Kadar *et al.*, 1981). We observed in our patients who had undergone infertility treatment at first a decrease of β-hCG in 40–60 % of the cases with abortion depending on the week of gestation. The β-hCG decrease was sometimes accompanied by a decline in other hormone concentrations. Other authors stated similar results for β-hCG in patients following sterility treatment (Braunstein *et al.*, 1978; Scholler *et al.*, 1980; Batzer *et al.*, 1981). A correct prognosis of the further course of pregnancy was achieved in 80–90 % of the cases by interpreting the angle of ascent between two β-hCG values of samples taken at a 48 hour interval within the first 30 days of gestation (Chartier *et al.*, 1979; Batzer *et al.*, 1981; Kadar *et al.*, 1981).

Unlike the β-hCG method, the determination of HPL in women with bleeding did not allow an exact assessment in our study because the sensitivity of this method was too low when bleeding occurred before the 9th week of pregnancy. After the 9th week of pregnancy it was, however, possible to replace the determination of β-hCG by the one of HPL. Other authors reported reduced HPL values in 65–90 % of the cases with bleeding and following abortion, and in 2–25 % of the cases with good prognosis (Genazzani *et al.*, 1971; Karjalainen *et al.*, 1974; Garoff and Seppälä, 1975; Kunz and Keller, 1976; Gerhard and Runnebaum, 1978; Hertz *et al.*, 1979). In the two most extensive studies by Gartside and Tindall (1975) and Ylikorkala and Jouppila (1973) it has, however, been pointed out that this method reaches sufficient precision only after the 9th to 11th week of pregnancy.

In our study 17-OHP, a corpus luteum secretion product, was only measured at the time of bleeding in patients with abortion and t.a. No serial determination was followed through as both sensitivity (51.6 %) and specificity (82.6 %) as well as the relative risk (1.7) were much lower than in any of the other methods. Similarly unsatisfying results have been reported by other authors (Jovanovic *et al.*, 1978; Crépin *et al.*, 1980; Scholler *et al.*, 1980; Manganiello *et al.*, 1981).

In this prospective study no indication of the presence of a primary corpus luteum insufficiency could be obtained through the measurement of P in women with abortion. Reduced P concentrations were, however, discovered at a relatively early stage in the case of deficient pregnancy products. At the time of bleeding we observed this in 63 % of the patients. The specificity of P was remarkably high (95 %). Reduced P concentrations have been reported in 60–80 % of the women with bleeding and abortion while P was mainly within normal range in cases with good prognosis (Nygren *et al.*, 1973; Karjalainen *et al.*, 1974; Kunz and Keller, 1978; Jovanovic *et al.*, 1978; Radwanska *et al.*, 1978; Gerhard and Runnebaum, 1978; Crépin *et al.*, 1980; Jouppila *et al.*, 1980*b*; Hertz *et al.*, 1980*a*; Eriksen and Philipsen, 1980; Scholler *et al.*, 1980). In more than 80 % of our patients who had undergone infertility treatment, P was the first hormone to show decreased values. The P decrease was sometimes accompanied by a decline in other hormone concentrations. This confirms the results of various authors who found a relation between abortion after infertility treatment or repeated early abortion and luteal dysfunction in approximately 35 % (Jones, 1976; Karow and Gentry, 1976;

Horta *et al.*, 1977; Yip and Sung, 1977; Hensleigh and Fainstat, 1979). In all cases with P concentrations below 15 ng/ml before the 10th week of pregnancy Hensleigh and Fainstat (1979) observed an abortion. While Csapo and Pulkkinen (1978) postulated 10 ng P as a critical borderline before the 6th week of pregnancy, Radwanska *et al.* (1978) extended this limit up to the 12th week of pregnancy, which is in agreement with our results.

E_2 has been examined as a further test parameter, which is initially produced by the corpus luteum and later on in increasing quantities by the trophoblast. It could be demonstrated that this hormone makes a precise prognostication possible. More than half of the women with abortion had reduced E_2 concentrations before bleeding occurred. At the time of bleeding 82 % of the patients with abortion had reduced values and 92 % of the women with regular delivery showed normal values. The relative risk was highest for E_2 (3.7). Other authors also reported reduced E_2 values in 65–95 % of patients with abortion versus concentrations within normal ranges in women with good prognosis after bleeding had occurred (Nygren *et al.*, 1973; Kunz and Keller, 1976; Jovanovic *et al.*, 1978; Hertz *et al.*, 1979; Luyx *et al.*, 1979; Crépin *et al.*, 1980; Eriksen and Philipsen, 1980; Jouppila *et al.*, 1980*b*; Scholler *et al.*, 1980). E_2 was the first hormone to show a general decrease in 60–70 % of our patients who had undergone sterility treatment. This was sometimes accompanied by a decline in the concentration of one of the other hormones. An explanation for the significance of E_2 is given by Ho Yuen *et al.* (1981). These authors observed reduced E_2 concentrations from the beginning of all pregnancies without embryonic tissue, deriving in 80 % from chromosome anomalies. Their conclusion was that normal E_2 concentrations are dependent on a living fetus.

The determinations of serum E_3 as an operational test for the fetoplacental unit gains significance only after the 7th week of gestation. Of the patients with abortion, 49 % had reduced values even before bleeding occurred. At the time of bleeding this was the case in 65 % of the women. Only few other authors have determined E_3 levels in pregnant women with bleeding. They found reduced concentrations in 75–90 % of the women with abortion and values within normal range in more than 90 % of the women with good prognosis (Gerhard and Runnebaum, 1978; Hertz *et al.*, 1979; Luyx *et al.*, 1979).

The great significance of a determination of β-hCG, P, E_2 and E_3 in the first trimester becomes evident when summarizing the predictive value of the individual hormone parameters. There are not many studies comparing the efficiency of various hormones. Like ourselves, Hertz *et al.* (1979, 1980*b*) postulated the superiority of the E_2 measurement. Some authors who studied pregnancies at risk proposed the determination of β-hCG which was completed by the simultaneous E_2 and P determination (Crépin *et al.*, 1980; Scholler *et al.*, 1980). During the second trimester the hormone determinations in women with bleeding appear to be less important, a fact that is confirmed by results of the aforementioned authors.

Tubal pregnancy represents a special situation. While even the new and more sensitive pregnancy tests in urine reliably detect an existing pregnancy in only 80 % of the cases, this is almost in every case possible by means of β-hCG determination in serum. In the majority of studies a difference has only been marked between positive proof of pregnancy through β-hCG in extrauterine gravidity and negative proof in cases where the clinical symptoms were not caused by an actual pregnancy (Lorenz *et al.*, 1979; Jouppila *et al.*, 1980*a*; Schwartz and Da Pietro, 1980; Seppälä *et al.*, 1980; Forbes *et al.*, 1981; Massart *et al.*, 1981; Lindstedt *et al.*, 1981; Nilsson *et al.*, 1982).

Very often an early decline in the β-hCG concentration is observed in ectopic pregnancy due to insufficient trophoblast development. In our study this was the case in 55% of the patients. Other authors reported reduced β-hCG concentrations in 23–87% of extrauterine gravidities (Braunstein *et al.*, 1978; Jouppila *et al.*, 1980*a*; Sandvei *et al.*, 1981; Kadar *et al.*, 1982; Braunstein and Asch, 1983). With reference to this, Lundström *et al.* (1979) stressed that the actual β-hCG concentration correlated with the clinical finding. A remarkable result of our study was the fact that the concentration of P was often low even before β-hCG decreased. This could well point to corpus luteum insufficiency as original cause for the development of a tubal pregnancy. Radwanska *et al.* (1978) and Jouppila *et al.* (1980*a*) also observed significantly reduced P concentrations in extrauterine gravidities. Like the aforementioned authors we were also able to demonstrate the presence of reduced E_2 values in tubal gravidities.

Our experience with hormonal changes in women with undisturbed early pregnancy, with threatened abortion, after infertility treatment and in cases of ectopic pregnancy shows that the decision as to which hormone should be determined should be made on the basis of the individual clinical situation and the respective week of gestation. With regard to this we have worked out the following guidelines.

(1) In the case of an asymptomatic course of pregnancy a determination of β-hCG in the 6th–7th week of gestation is performed followed by one further control of β-hCG and simultaneous measurement of E_2 at the end of the second month of pregnancy. The hormone determinations should be repeated and an ultrasound examination should be performed if any of the values is not within normal range.

(2) β-hCG, P and/or E_2 should be determined in patients with bleeding during the first 2 months of pregnancy. If the values are within normal range, a favourable course of pregnancy may be assumed in more than 90% of the women. Should one of the hormone concentrations show a significant decline, a control of the hormone level and an ultrasound examination will be necessary after 1 week.

(3) When bleeding occurs after the 8th week of gestation a determination of β-hCG and E_2 in addition to an ultrasound examination will be sufficient for evaluation. In the women with an intact pregnancy a control of these three parameters is recommended after 2 weeks.

(4) Women with an increased risk of abortion (infertility treatment, habitual abortion, history of luteal insufficiency) should have frequent controls and weekly determinations of β-hCG, E_2 and also P as from the 5th week of gestation. This is to be followed by an ultrasound examination in

weeks 8–9 and determinations of P and E_2 at 2-weekly intervals from weeks 10–16 onwards.

(5) In the case of patients with suspected extrauterine gravidity before the 8th week of gestation P should be measured in addition to β-hCG.

When the methods suggested are employed at the times stated above, an early assessment of the individual condition of a pregnancy is possible. Application of these methods could improve the use of therapeutic procedures and recommendations and help to avoid long and unnecessary hospitalization.

CONCLUDING REMARKS

The significance of hormone determinations in maternal serum during early pregnancy was examined in a prospective study. After the onset of pregnancy β-hCG, HPL, progesterone (P), 17β-estradiol (E_2) and estriol (E_3) were radioimmunologically determined at regular intervals. In 299 women who suffered from bleeding, 17-hydroxyprogesterone (17-OHP) was also measured. In addition β-hCG, P and E_2 were repeatedly determined in a group of 132 patients who had previously undergone sterility treatment and had a history of threatened abortion before the 11th week of gestation. Twenty-nine of these women had a tubal pregnancy, 78 an early abortion, and 25 women suffering from bleeding had a normal delivery.

During the course of undisturbed asymptomatic early pregnancy 50% of those patients with following abortion had already reduced hormone concentrations, while more than 90% of the women with regular delivery showed normal values. At the time of bleeding, hormone concentrations in women with early abortion were reduced in 80–90% of the cases; E_2 and β-hCG proved to have the highest sensitivity. After the 9th week of gestation the determination of HPL and E_3 yielded exact results. The wide scattering of 17-OHP concentrations did not permit a reliable clinical interpretation. The majority of hormone determinations in women with late abortion, impending abortion and regular delivery was within normal range. In women who had undergone infertility treatment and in patients with tubal pregnancies, P showed frequent decreases before β-hCG concentrations declined. The choice of the hormone to be determined depending on the individual clinical symptoms and the week of gestation is described in detail.

References

Batzer, F. R., Schlaff, S., Goldfarb, A. and Corson, S. L. (1981). Serial β-subunit of human chorionic gonadotropin doubling time as a prognosticator of pregnancy outcome in an infertile population. *Fertil. Steril.*, **35**, 307

Braunstein, G. D., Karow, W. G., Gentry, W. C., Rasor, J. and Wade, M. E. (1978). First trimester chorionic gonadotropin measurements as an aid in the diagnosis of early pregnancy disorders. *Am. J. Obstet. Gynecol.*, **131**, 25

Braunstein, G. D. and Asch, R. H. (1983). Predictive values analysis of measurements of human chorionic gonadotropin, pregnancy specific beta 1-glycoprotein, placental lactogen, and cystine aminopeptidase for the diagnosis of ectopic pregnancy. *Fertil. Steril.*, **39**, 62

Chartier, M., Roger, M., Barrat, J. and Michelon, B. (1979). Measurement of plasma chorionic gonadotropin (hCG) and β-hCG activities in the late luteal phase: evidence of the occurrence of spontaneous menstrual abortions in infertile women. *Fertil. Steril.*, **31**, 134

Crépin, G., Delcroix, M., Querleu, D., Scholler, R. and Castanier, M. (1980). Les dosages hormonaux plasmatiques dans l'evaluation du pronostic des hémorrhagies du premier trimestre de la grossesse. *J. Gynecol. Obstet. Biol. Reprod.*, **9**, 67

Csapo, A. J. and Pulkkinen, M. (1978). Indispensability of the human corpus luteum in the maintenance of early pregnancy: luteectomy evidence. *Obstet. Gynecol. Survey*, **33**, 69

Eriksen, P. S. and Philipsen, T. (1980). Prognosis in threatened abortion evaluated by hormone assays and ultrasound scanning. *Obstet. Gynecol.*, **55**, 435

Forbes, K., Brennecke, A. M., Ho, P. C. and Jones, W. R. (1981). Human chorionic gonadotropin and pregnancy-specific beta-1 glycoprotein (SP-1) in ectopic pregnancy. *Aust. NZ J. Obstet. Gynecol.*, **21**, 177

Garoff, L. and Seppälä, M. (1975). Prediction of fetal outcome in threatened abortion by maternal serum placental lactogen and alpha fetoprotein. *Am. J. Obstet. Gynecol.*, **121**, 257

Gartside, M. W. and Tindall, V. R. (1975). The prognostic value of human placental lactogen (HPL) levels in threatened abortion. *Br. J. Obstet. Gynaecol.*, **82**, 303

Gaspard, V. J., Schaaps, J. P., Piront, E., Deville, J. L., Reuter, A. M., Vrindts-Gevaert, Y. and Franchimont, P. (1980). Pronostic et traitement de la menace d'avortement. *J. Gynecol. Obstet. Biol. Reprod.*, **9**, 62

Genazzani, A. R., Cocola, F., Casoli, M., Mello, G., Scarselli, G., Neri, P. and Fioretti, P. (1971). Human chorionic somatomammotrophin radioimmunoassay in evaluation of placental function. *J. Obstet. Gynaecol. Br. Commonw.*, **78**, 577

Gerhard, I. and Runnebaum, B. (1978). Aussagewert von hCG, HPL, Progesteron und Östriolbestimmungen bei Frauen mit drohender Fehlgeburt. *Geburtsh. Frauenheilk.*, **38**, 785

Hensleigh, P. A. and Fainstat, T. (1979). Corpus luteum dysfunction: serum progesterone levels in diagnosis and assessment of therapy for recurrent and threatened abortion. *Fertil. Steril.*, **32**, 396

Hertz, J. B., Larsen, J. F., Svenstrup, B. and Johnsen, S. G. (1979). Oestradiol, oestriol and human placental lactogen in serum in threatened abortion. *Acta Obstet. Gynecol. Scand.*, **58**, 365

Hertz, J. B., Larsen, J. F., Arends, J. and Nielsen, J. (1980*a*). Progesterone and human chorionic gonadotropin in serum and pregnandiol in urine in threatened abortion. *Acta Obstet. Gynecol. Scand.*, **59**, 23

Hertz, J. B., Mautoni, M. and Svenstrup, B. (1980*b*). Threatened abortion studied by estradiol-17 beta in serum and ultrasound. *Obstet. Gynecol.*, **55**, 324

Horta, J. L. H., Fernandez, J. G., De Leon, B. S. and Cortes-Gallegos, V. (1977). Direct evidence of luteal insufficiency in women with habitual abortion. *Obstet. Gynecol.*, **49**, 705

Ho Yuen, B. H., Livingstone, J. E., Poland, B. J., Wittmann, B. K., Sy, L. and Cannon, W. (1981). Human chorionic gonadotropin, estradiol, progesterone, prolactin, and B-scan ultrasound monitoring of complications in early pregnancy. *Obstet. Gynecol.*, **57**, 207

Jones, G. S. (1976). The luteal phase defect. *Fertil. Steril.*, **27**, 351

Jouppila, P., Tapanainen, J. and Huhtaniemi, I. (1979). Plasma hCG levels in patients with bleeding in the first and second trimesters of pregnancy. *Br. J. Obstet. Gynaecol.*, **86**, 343

Jouppila, P., Tapanainen, J. and Huhtaniemi, I. (1980*a*). Plasma hCG and ultrasound in suspected ectopic pregnancy. *Eur. J. Obstet. Gynaecol. Reprod. Biol.*, **10**, 3

Jouppila, P., Huhtaniemi, I. and Tapanainen, J. (1980*b*). Early pregnancy failure: study by ultrasonic and hormonal methods. *Obstet. Gynecol.*, **55**, 42

Jovanovic, L., Dawood, M. Y., Landesman, R. and Saxena, B. B. (1978). Hormonal profile as a prognostic index of early threatened abortion. *Am. J. Obstet. Gynecol.*, **130**, 274

Kadar, N., Caldwell, B. V. and Romero, R. (1981). A method of screening for ectopic pregnancy and its indications. *Obstet. Gynecol.*, **58**, 162

Kadar, N., De Cherney, A. H. and Romero, R. (1982). Receiver operating charateristic (ROC) curve analysis of the relative efficacy of single and serial chorionic gonadotropin determinations in the early diagnosis of ectopic pregnancy. *Fertil. Steril.*, **37**, 452

Karjalainen, O., Stenman, U., Wichman, K. and Widholm, O. (1974). Evaluation of the outcome of pregnancy in threatened abortion by biochemical methods. *Ann. Chir. Gynaecol. Fenn.*, **63**, 457

Karow, W. G. and Gentry, W. C. (1976). Corpus luteum function during pregnancies of previously infertile women. *Obstet. Gynecol.*, **48**, 503

Kunz, J. and Keller, P. J. (1976). HCG, HPL, oestradiol, progesterone and AFP in serum in patients with threatened abortion. *Br. J. Obstet. Gynaecol.*, **83**, 640

Lauritsen, J. G. (1976). Aetiology of spontaneous abortion. A cytogenetic and epidemiological study of 288 abortuses and their parents. *Acta Obstet. Gynecol. Scand. Suppl.*, **52**, 1

Lindstedt, G., Janson, P. O. and Thorburn, J. (1981). Sensitivity of serum-chorionic gonadotrophin assays for ectopic pregnancy. *Lancet*, **1**, 781

Lorenz, R. P., Work, B. A. and Menon, K. M. (1979). A radioreceptor assay for human chorionic gonadotropin in normal and abnormal pregnancies: A clinical evaluation. *Am. J. Obstet. Gynecol.*, **134**, 471

Lundström, V., Bremme, K., Eneroth, P., Nyg'ard, I. and Sundvall, M. (1979). Serum beta-human chorionic gonadotrophin levels in the early diagnosis of ectopic pregnancy. *Acta Obstet. Gynecol. Scand.*, **58**, 231

Luyx, A., De Hertogh, R., Foldesi, A. and Rousseau, P. (1979). Corrélation entre la morphologie échographique et les dosages plasmatique d'oestradiol et d'oestriol en début de grossesse. *J. Gynecol. Obstet. Biol. Reprod.*, **8**, 131

Manganiello, P. D., Nazian, S. J., Ellegood, J. O., Mc Donough, P. G. and Mahesh, V. B. (1981). Sequential serum determinations of prolactin, 17α-hydroxyprogesterone, progesterone and β-human chorionic gonadotropin during early pregnancy. *Fertil. Steril.*, **35**, 237

Massart, C., Le Pogamp, C., Mention, J. E., Grall, J. Y., Toulouse, R. and Nicol, M. (1981). Application d'un dosage rapide de la beta-hCG sérique à la détection précoce des grossesses extrautérines. *J. Gynecol. Obstet. Biol. Reprod.*, **10**, 675

Nilsson, C. G., Laehteenmaeki, P. and Haukkamaa, M. (1982). Diagnostic value of a rapid hCG-beta-subunit radioimmunoassay in cases of suspected ectopic pregnancies. *Int. J. Fertil.*, **27**, 36

Nygren, K. G., Johannson, E. D. B. and Wide, L. (1973). Evaluation of the prognosis of threatened abortion from the peripheral plasma levels of progesterone, estradiol and human chorionic gonadotropin. *Am. J. Obstet. Gynecol.*, **116**, 916

Radwanska, E., Frankenberg, J. and Allen, E. I. (1978). Plasma progesterone levels in normal and abnormal early pregnancy. *Fertil. Steril.*, **30**, 398

Sandvei, R., Stra, K. F. and Ulstein, M. (1981). Radioimmunoassay of human chorionic gonadotropin beta-subunit as an early diagnostic test in ectopic pregnancy. *Acta Gynecol. Scand.*, **60**, 389

Seppälä, M., Tontti, K., Ranta, T., Stenman, U. H. and Chard, T. (1980). Use of a rapid hCG-beta-subunit radioimmunoassay in acute gynaecological emergencies. *Lancet*, **1**, 165

Scholler, R., Chartier, M., Barrat, J., Roger, M., Castanier, M. and Avidor, R. (1980). Profil de hCG et des steroides dans les avortements spontanes du ler trimestre. *J. Gynecol. Obstet. Biol. Reprod.*, **9**, 79

Schwartz, R. O. and Di Pietro, D. L. (1980). β-hCG as a diagnostic aid of suspected ectopic pregnancy. *Obstet. Gynecol.*, **56**, 197

Yip, S. K. and Sung, M. L. (1977). Plasma progesterone in women with a history of recurrent early abortion. *Fertil. Steril.* **28**, 151

Ylikorkala, O. and Jouppila, P. (1973). Human placental lactogen (HPL) in serum in complicated early pregnancy. *J. Obstet. Gynaecol. Br. Commonw.*, **80**, 1040

22
Predictive value of hormone measurements in threatened abortion

J. B. HERTZ

Threatened abortion is the most frequently encountered complication in early human pregnancy. The exact incidence is unknown, but an incidence of vaginal bleeding before the 28th week of pregnancy of 16 % has been reported (South and Naldrett, 1973). The study, however, only included singleton pregnancies carried beyond the 28th week and not pregnancies with vaginal bleeding ending in spontaneous abortion. With reference to incidences of spontaneous abortion from about 27–28 % (Stickle, 1968; Hertig, 1975) to 43 % (Miller *et al.*, 1980) an estimated incidence of 20–30 % of all pregnancies recognized clinically and/or biochemically seems reasonable.

In cases of vaginal bleeding in early pregnancy the fetus may have been dead for some time. When parts of the chorionic tissue are still functioning the pregnancy test may remain positive for several days and if spontaneous termination of the threatened pregnancy is awaited, many days of unnecessary delay and anxiety may result. Only when parts of or the entire conceptus are visible through the os, or may be examined after expulsion, can the diagnosis of spontaneous abortion be made with certainty on clinical grounds alone. Clinical examination alone (the amount of vaginal bleeding, the uterine size) only proved to be 62.3 % correct in the prediction of the outcome of threatened abortion, the prediction of abortion being the more accurate (Duff *et al.*, 1980).

In order to identify the failing gestations and thus avoid prolonged anxiety, and in cases of hospitalization to minimize the costly stay in hospital, reliable indicators of the viability of the conceptus in early threatened pregnancy are needed. A number of diagnostic tests have been applied to the evaluation of threatened abortion. The karyopyknotic index of vaginal smears reflecting the status of hormonal production and ultrasound examination with the recording of the size and contents of the uterus are dealt with in other chapters. The aim of this chapter is to review the current knowledge of the predictive value of hormone measurements in threatened abortion.

CRITERIA FOR HORMONAL PARAMETERS

The levels of the hormonal products of the fetoplacental unit in maternal blood and urine are dependant on the amount produced and on maternal metabolism and clearance. This should be taken into account when tests of fetal well-being are evaluated. The speed and convenience of the methods of analysis developed during recent years favor assays on plasma rather than those on urine, but urinary measurements provide information about the sum of events during a certain period of time, whereas measurements on plasma only provide information about the moment the blood was sampled. This chapter, however, will deal only with the hormonal measurements on plasma.

Several hormonal parameters have been tested as indices of the outcome in cases of threatened abortion; some of the more commonly evaluated and the ones to be dealt with here include progesterone, 17β-estradiol, estriol, human chorionic gonadotropin (hCG), human placental lactogen, pregnancy-specific β_1-glycoprotein, α-fetoprotein, relaxin and 17α-hydroxyprogesterone. Before these hormones are evaluated, some general considerations and criteria for the clinical use of tests of fetal well-being have to be mentioned.

Ranges of normality should be established on an adequate number of individuals and samples and each laboratory should define its own normal range. The calculation of ranges should be uniform, e.g. mean $\pm$ two standard deviations, making the comparison of the results of different workers possible (Figure 22.1). In most tests such ranges are not normally distributed. They tend to be skewed at the upper end due to the occurrence of a few high values. Thus ranges should be calculated after logarithmic transformation of the data. By plotting hormone values from patients with threatened abortion into such reference curves it is possible to calculate the predictive value of abortion and successful outcome from the formulas:

(1) Predictive value of a positive test (i.e. prediction of abortion):

$$\frac{\text{true positives}}{\text{true positives} + \text{false positives}}$$

(2) Predictive value of a negative test (prediction of successful outcome):

$$\frac{\text{true negatives}}{\text{true negatives} + \text{false negatives}}$$

(See Figure 22.1.)

Variation. Any analysis will show some degree of variation – biological, due to differences between individuals or within the same individual – or technical, due to the assay applied. The greater the variation, the more likely is an overlap between normal and abnormal values, making the test of less clinical value. The majority of plasma hormone assays are nowadays carried out by radioimmunoassays possessing low assay variation due to the simplified sampling techniques and standardized methods of analysis. The precision of any radioimmunoassay, however, is dependent upon the point on the standard curve at which the measurements are made. Values from the extremes of the

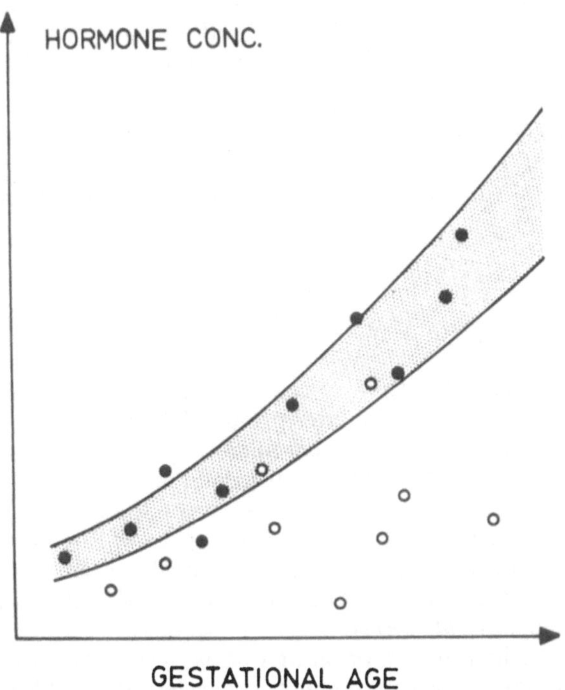

Figure 22.1 An example of a reference curve with ranges calculated as mean ± 2 SD (shaded area) after logarithmic transformation of the data. The variation of the exemplified analysis is small, making the range narrow. Hormone values from patients with threatened abortion have been plotted on the curve. From this the predictive values of abortion and successful outcome can be calculated as explained in the text. ●= patients with successful outcome of the threatened pregnancy. ○= patients with pregnancies ending in spontaneous abortion.

standard curve show much greater variability than those from the central and steep part of the curve. (For further details, see Chard, 1977).

Hormonal parameters used in the evaluation of early threatened pregnancy should fulfil certain criteria.

(1) The test should clearly separate pregnancies that will end in abortion from those that will precede to delivery, i.e. no overlapping between the abortive and non-abortive cases. The diagnostic specificity must be very high, i.e. the prediction of abortion must be reliable. False results predicting unfavourable outcome where the pregnancy, however, continues until delivery must not occur since they imply the risk of terminating an otherwise normal pregnancy by evacuation. The diagnostic sensitivity, i.e. the prediction of successful outcome, should be reliable as well. But false results indicative of successful outcome where the pregnancy ends in spontaneous abortion are not that important because of the minor therapeutic consequences.

(2) The method of analysis should be simple, inexpensive, reliable and rapid, with a low analytical error. These criteria are met by the radioimmunoassays. Moreover the day-to-day and diurnal variation should be minimal.

(3) The half-life of the estimated hormones should be sufficiently short (minutes or a few hours) that any deterioration in placental and/or fetoplacental function is rapidly reflected in the liquid analysed.

PLACENTA

Steroid hormones

Progesterone (P) is a 21 carbon steroid, which in early pregnancy is mainly produced in the corpus luteum, later presumably solely in the placenta with maternal cholesterol as the predominant precurser in the synthesis (Scommegna *et al.*, 1972). The 'luteo-placental shift' in the site of steroidogenesis takes place around the 7th week, the corpus luteum being indispensable before this gestational week (Csapo *et al.*, 1973). Accordingly a transient fall in plasma progesterone has been found around the 7th week, and the functional life span of the corpus luteum has been reported to be 8–10 weeks (Yoshimi *et al.*, 1969; Holmdahl *et al.*, 1971).

The biological half-life of progesterone is very short, about 6 minutes (Fylling, 1970), making measurements of progesterone suitable for recognition of deteriorations in the placental function. However, in a study of 32 healthy pregnant women a large spread, great individual variations and large but non-systematic diurnal variations were reported (Lindberg *et al.*, 1974). In another study the progesterone levels remained constant and only slightly above luteal phase levels between the 5th and 10th weeks of pregnancy in healthy women (Tulchinsky and Hobel, 1973). Consequently steady or decreasing levels of progesterone are not necessarily pathological, but they may result in the misjudgment of the prognosis and could lead to the evacuation of a normal pregnancy. Due to a great deal of overlapping in the levels of progesterone between aborters and women carrying to term, 'progesterone rendered an uncertain prediction' in cases of threatened abortion (Nygren *et al.*, 1973). In another study the mean plasma levels of progesterone in patients that subsequently aborted were found to be significantly lower ($p < 0.001$) than mean levels in patients continuing pregnancy after the threatened abortion. Several patients, however, aborted in spite of normal progesterone levels, indicating a greater diagnostic and prognostic value of low rather than normal progesterone levels in cases of threatened abortion (Radwanska *et al.*, 1978). Other investigators have reported on the predictive value of progesterone measurements in threatened abortion (Table 22.1). The low values for prediction of successful outcome in some of the studies are due to the above-mentioned overlap, i.e. many aborters presented normal progesterone levels.

The estrogens include the derivates estrone (E_1), estradiol (E_2) estriol (E_3) and estetrol (E_4) of which especially measurements of E_2 and E_3 (mostly the unconjugated forms) have been used as diagnostic tools in the evaluation of

Table 22.1 The predictive values (%) of placental steroid hormone, hCG and β-subunit hCG measurements in maternal plasma in threatened abortion

Parameter & reference	*No. of patients examined*	*Prediction* of abortion*	*successful outcome*
Progesterone			
Kunz & Keller (1976)	65	89	60
Gerhard & Runnebaum (1978)	187	100	52
Duff *et al.* (1980)	69	100	79
Hertz *et al.* (1980*a*)	64	100(96)	76(85)
Jouppila *et al.* (1980)	188	93	73
Estradiol			
Kunz & Keller (1976)	65	92	68
Hertz *et al.* (1979)	64	92(100)	87(92)
Duff *et al.* (1980)	69	93	88
Hertz *et al.* (1980*b*)	100	93(90)	80(80)
Jouppila *et al.* (1980)	188	77	79
Estriol			
Gerhard & Runnebaum (1978)	182	83	35
Hertz *et al.* (1979)	64	89(96)	87(89)
hCG			
Kunz & Keller (1976)	65	79	71
Gerhard & Runnebaum (1978)	67	94	47
Hertz *et al.* (1980*a*)	64	100(96)	88(89)
Sande *et al.* (1980)	104	100	79
β-hCG			
Duff *et al.* (1980)	69	96	57
Jouppila *et al.* (1980)	188	93	74

* The predictive values after serial determinations are in parentheses

complicated pregnancy. Only these two derivatives are to be dealt with in this content.

In the first few weeks of pregnancy E_2 is synthesized partly in the placenta and partly in the corpus luteum. This leaves the possibility of estimating the function of the early placenta and the corpus luteum by measurements of E_2. The E_2 levels in serum rise steadily from the 3rd week of pregnancy to levels which in the 6th–8th weeks are significantly above the highest levels found in the menstrual cycle (Tulchinsky and Hobel, 1973). In the non-pregnant woman, and presumably in the first few weeks of pregnancy too, E_3 is derived primarily by conversion from circulating E_1 and E_2. 'Genuine' E_3 synthesis demands development and function of the fetoplacental unit and in studies of early normal pregnancies, E_3 became detectable (> 50 pg/ml) in all the studied women after the 11th week of pregnancy (Tulchinsky and Hobel, 1973) and the 13th week (Harrison and Kitchin, 1980). With a detection limit of 30 pg/ml we found E_3 measurements to be valid after the 8th gestational week in patients with threatened abortion (Hertz *et al.*, 1979). Placental E_2 and E_3 are synthesized mainly, if not entirely, from dehydroepiandrosterone sulfate (DHA-S) of fetal and maternal origin and the synthesis involves enzymatic processes in the fetal and maternal liver and the placenta (Diczfalusy, 1974).

In the first study to examine the evaluation of the prognosis in threatened abortion from E_2 levels in plasma, overlapping of E_2 values was found between aborters and non-aborters and it was concluded that assays of E_2 rendered a more uncertain prediction than hCG assays and that they did not add further information for the evaluation of the prognosis (Nygren *et al.*, 1973). Since then several studies have been carried out to investigate the value of E_2 and E_3 measurements in cases of threatened abortion (Table 22.1).

The half-life of both E_2 and E_3 seems to follow a two-compartment model with mean $T_{\frac{1}{2}}$ for E_2 of 22 minutes and 7 hours (Tulchinsky and Korenman, 1971) and for E_3 of 22 minutes and 9 hours (Tulchinsky and Abraham, 1971). The short first half-life of both hormones is in favour of early recognition of a deterioration in the conceptional status.

Protein hormones

The detection of human chorionic gonadotropin (hCG) in urine or blood has traditionally been the method of choice in the diagnosis of pregnancy. Measurements of this glycoprotein hormone produced in the syncytiotrophoblast in the placenta (Leznoff and Davis, 1963) have also been used to assess the condition and viability of the conceptus in cases of threatened abortion (Table 22.1). Due to the cross-reaction between hCG and the pituitary luteinizing hormone (LH) measurements of hCG are only to be interpreted with safety after the levels of hCG have exceeded the highest physiological concentrations of LH. The problems arising from these cross-reactions have been overcome by the development of a highly sensitive and hormone specific β-subunit hCG (β-hCG) radioimmunoassay, which has also been used in the evaluation of early threatened pregnancy (Table 22.1). Using a specific radioreceptor assay for hCG, spontaneous abortion could be predicted as early as 8–10 days after conception (Rosal *et al.*, 1975). In another prospective study serial measurements of β-hCG gave an 88.9% correct prediction of the spontaneous abortions (Braunstein *et al.*, 1978).

While all other hormonal parameters discussed in this chapter show steadily increasing levels throughout pregnancy until at least the 36th gestational week, hCG displays a trend of concentration reaching peak levels between the 8th and 12th weeks of pregnancy. After this an abrupt fall is seen to minimum values at about the 20th–24th weeks. Decreasing levels of hCG might thus be a normal phenomenon. In the evaluation of threatened abortion the gestational age must be known with certainty, otherwise decreasing hCG values might suggest that the pregnancy is incapable of continuing and result in the evacuation of a normal pregnancy. The interpretation of serial hCG measurements must thus be undertaken with caution.

The disappearance rate of hCG has been a matter of debate but it seems to follow a double exponential curve with an initial disappearance rate with $T_{\frac{1}{2}}$ about 11 hours and a second rate with $T_{\frac{1}{2}}$ about 23 hours (Yen *et al.*, 1968).

Human placental lactogen (*HPL*) is a polypeptide hormone exclusively produced in the syncytiotrophoblast of the placenta (Sciarra *et al.*, 1963).

Pregnancy-specific-β_1-glycoprotein (SP_1 or PSβG) is produced in the same part of the chorionic tissue (Horne *et al.*, 1976) and both are thus markers of the placental function. A certain gestational age is to be expected before these two protein hormones become detectable in the maternal plasma, but SP_1 has been detected in plasma as early as 7 days after ovulation (Grudzinskas *et al.*, 1977), levels rising steadily thereafter. HPL is first detectable at a later gestational age and is first to be interpreted with safety after approximately the 9th gestational week (Garoff and Seppälä, 1975; Hertz and Schultz-Larsen, 1983).

The prognostic value of HPL and SP_1 measurements in threatened abortion have been thoroughly evaluated (Table 22.2). Beyond this a single HPL determination proved to be a sufficiently reliable index of the outcome of the threatened pregnancy from the 9th week. Before this gestational week serial samples were needed (Niven *et al.*, 1972). Gartside and Tindall (1975) found a single reading of HPL between 9 and 19 weeks of pregnancy to give the correct immediate prognosis in 86% of threatened abortions, an equivocal prognosis in 11% of cases and a wrong prognosis in 3%.

The greater amount of SP_1 in serum in very early pregnancy compared to the amount of HPL and the highly significant positive correlation between these two hormones found in cases of threatened abortion (Hertz and Schultz-Larzen, 1983) suggest that SP_1 might replace HPL in the evaluation of early threatened pregnancy. An argument against such replacement is the half-lives of the hormones, 13 minutes in the case of HPL and 21–22 hours in that of SP_1 (Klopper *et al.*, 1978).

Table 22.2 The predictive values (%) of HPL, SP_1 and AFP measurements in maternal plasma in threatened abortion

Parameter & reference	*No. of patients examined*	*Prediction* of abortion*	*Prediction* of successful outcome*
HPL			
Garoff & Seppälä (1975)	86	100	60
Kunz & Keller (1976)	65	81	61
Gerhard & Runnebaum (1978)	84	92	45
Hertz *et al.* (1979)	64	89(100)	89(92)
Duff *et al.* (1980)	69	91	52
Hertz & Schultz-Larsen (1983)	109	92(100)	69(83)
SP_1			
Jandial *et al.* (1978)	64	87	75
Schultz-Larzen & Hertz (1978)	59	89(100)	94(94)
Duff *et al.* (1980)	69	72	83
Karg *et al.* (1981)	64	75(90)	81(87)
Hertz & Schultz-Larsen (1983)	82	76(83)	74(82)
AFP			
Garoff & Seppälä (1975)	112	80	39
Kunz & Keller (1976)	65	38	30
Lidbjörk *et al.* (1977)	77	91	75
Duff *et al.* (1980)	69	77	64
Hertz & Schultz-Larsen (1983)	97	82(100)	65(81)

* The predictive values after serial determinations are in parentheses

FETUS

α-Fetoprotein (AFP) is an embryonic glycoprotein produced in the fetal liver and yolksac (Gitlin *et al.*, 1972) and thus reflects the fetal condition. It is probably transported to maternal serum either transplacentally from fetal serum or via a transmembrane route from the amniotic fluid (Editorial, *Lancet*, 1979). An elevated AFP in maternal serum might result from neural tube defects or other fetal anomalies like congenital nephrosis or exomphalos or from gemelli. Elevated levels of AFP have also been reported in connection with fetal death, levels declining thereafter due to the clearance from the maternal circulation, and in cases of feto-maternal bleeding. Low levels of AFP may be attributed to anembryonic gestations (Bennett *et al.*, 1978) or a dead fetus when the AFP has been cleared from the maternal plasma.

Since Seppälä and Ruoslahti (1972*a*) reported abnormal levels of AFP in maternal serum in patients with spontaneous abortion several studies have been carried out in order to evaluate the prognostic value of AFP determinations in cases of threatened abortion (Table 22.2). The results are rather divergent: some investigators found the test most valuable (Lidbjörk *et al.*, 1977), others (Garoff and Seppälä, 1975; Kunz and Keller, 1976; Hertz and Schultz-Larsen, 1983) found it to be of no or limited value, one of the reasons being the uncertain interpretation in early pregnancy (i.e. before the 10th–12th gestational weeks). The half-life of maternal AFP has been estimated to be approximately 5 days (Seppälä and Ruoslahti, 1972*b*) which is a further disadvantage as regards the usefulness of the test.

THE CORPUS LUTEUM

Relaxin is a peptide hormone produced by the corpus luteum of pregnancy (Weiss *et al.*, 1976) and is thus a specific index of the luteal function in early human pregnancy. It can be detected in serum as early as 10 days after conception and is usually detectable around the time of the missed menses (Quagliarello *et al.*, 1979). In a recent study serum relaxin levels were found subnormal in only nine of 18 cases of first trimester spontaneous abortions, whereas β-subunit hCG was subnormal in 14 of these patients. In seven patients who subsequently aborted 2–6 weeks later serum relaxin was normal in all, β-hCG was subnormal in five. Accordingly it was suggested that decreases in placental activity seem to precede a decrease in luteal activity (Quagliarello *et al.*, 1981). Serum relaxin measurements thus seem to be of limited value in the evaluation of threatened abortion.

17α-hydroxyprogesterone (17-OHP) is probably also exclusively produced by the corpus luteum since the placenta has no, or at the most very limited, capability for 17-hydroxylation. The levels of 17-OHP rise gradually until the 5th–6th weeks of pregnancy, then fall to a plateau which at the 13th gestational week is significantly lower than that observed in the 5th week. This lower level then remains constant for the rest of pregnancy (Tulchinsky and Hobel, 1973; MacNaughton, 1976). In seven healthy women whose dates of conception were carefully monitored with the use of artificial inseminations, the individual 17-OHP values showed considerable day-to-day variability. By the 5th gestational week 17-OHP levels were significantly elevated compared to levels during the luteal phase, levels remaining constant or slightly decreasing thereafter. In one of the women aborting spontaneously 17-OHP values declined progressively; the levels, however, remained inside the 95% confidence range. It was concluded that the range of normal 17-OHP values limits its use in evaluating corpus luteum function during early pregnancy (Manganiello *et al.*, 1981)

SINGLE VERSUS SERIAL DETERMINATIONS

A single measurement of any hormonal parameter represents just a glimpse of the endocrine status. Serial measurements, e.g. analyses daily or twice weekly, may add further information in demonstrating the changing of hormonal levels, but it has to be kept in mind that the changes registered might just reflect random variation, biological or technical, and not necessarily an important change in the status of the conceptus. For hormonal parameters showing high day-to-day variation (e.g. placental steroid hormones, especially progesterone and unconjugated E_3) even apparently large changes in the hormonal levels can hardly be called abnormal. In serial measurements, however, the patient will act as her own control, and serial values may give added confidence to the relationship between results in an individual patient and those in the population as a whole (Chard, 1977).

The value of serial measurements in the monitoring of threatened abortion has only been evaluated in a limited number of the quoted studies (values in parenthesis in Tables 22.1 and 22.2). Only in some of these studies the prediction of the outcome of the threatened pregnancy seems to improve when it is based on serial measurements.

COMBINATION OF HORMONAL PARAMETERS

The main purpose of introducing measurements of hormonal parameters in cases of threatened abortion is to identify the failing gestations and thus accelerate a definite treatment. Serial measurements are, in this respect, time-wasting. Consequently some investigators have established the value of the combination of different hormonal parameters (Table 22.3). Apparently the best results are achieved by the combination of hormonal parameters of different origin, e.g. E_2 and progesterone or E_2 and hCG instead of hormones of pure trophoblastic origin.

CONCLUDING REMARKS

When the predictive values in the Tables are compared it has to be emphasized once again that the different investigators and their laboratories do not use the same standardized analyses, and that the normal ranges have been calculated

Table 22.3 The predictive values (%) when pathological low hormone levels are combined (single measurements)

Parameters & reference	*Outcome of pregnancy* abortion	*successful outcome*
hCG + estradiol		
Kunz & Keller (1976)	97	3
Jouppila *et al.* (1980)	97	3
Hertz (unpublished results)	100	0
hCG + progesterone		
Kunz & Keller (1976)	90	10
Jouppila *et al.* (1980)	98	2
Hertz (unpublished results)	100	0
estradiol + progesterone		
Kunz & Keller (1976)	94	6
Jouppila *et al.* (1980)	100	0
Hertz (unpublished results)	100	0
estradiol + HPL		
Kunz & Keller (1976)	94	6
Hertz *et al.* (1979)	96	4
HPL + progesterone		
Kunz & Keller (1976)	88	12
Hertz (unpublished results)	100	0
HPL + hCG		
Kunz & Keller (1976)	84	16
Hertz (unpublished results)	100	0
HPL + SP_1		
Hertz & Schultz-Larsen (1983)	93	7
HPL + estriol		
Hertz *et al.* (1979)	93	7
estradiol + SP_1		
Hertz (unpublished results)	100	0

differently (mean ± SD, mean ± 2 SD or percentiles). Too direct comparison is thus meaningless. With a few exceptions the prediction of abortion proves to be more accurate than that of successful outcome, i.e. the diagnostic specificity is more accurate than the diagnostic sensitivity, which is the desired aim, as has been stated at the beginning of this chapter. The lower diagnostic sensitivity can probably in part be explained by the so-called 'live-abortions', where the pregnancy apparently seems normal until the expulsion of the conceptus, as confirmed by ultrasound (Hertz *et al.*, 1980*b*). The etiology of these, often late, abortions remains obscure, but factors like cervical incompetence and submucosal leiomyomas of the uterus might be an explanation. Until now no simple diagnostic procedure has been able with certainty to distinguish these pregnancies from those proceeding to delivery. Another explanation of the lower sensitivity is the greater amount of overlapping between abortive and non-abortive cases in some analyses, e.g. progesterone.

Hormonal parameters of purely placental origin may continue to be normal for some time after fetal death or in anembryonic gestations in cases where the trophoblastic tissue, or parts of it, continues its hormonal production. Some of the parameters reviewed in this chapter demand a certain gestational age to be detectable in plasma (e.g. HPL and E_3), others to exceed normal non-pregnant values (e.g. progesterone). Despite these objections two hormones of purely placental origin (HPL and hCG) and progesterone are the only ones to show 100% correct prediction of abortion in some of the studies. With all three hormones, however, the prediction of successful outcome in some of the studies is rather low due to overlapping between aborters and non-aborters.

The perfect hormonal test which predicts abortion and successful outcome accurately in 100% of cases remains to be detected. A hormonal marker of fetoplacental origin or of maternal-fetoplacental origin like E_2 seems to be the best choice since it to some extent marks the function of all three compartments. The results of E_2 determinations (Table 22.1), however, are somewhat disappointing, but if this parameter is combined with measurements of progesterone or hCG excellent results are achieved (Table 22.3).

Studies combining ultrasound examination with measurements of different hormonal parameters have shown that the combination of ultrasound without fetal life and low E_2 (Hertz *et al.*, 1980*b*) or low levels of hCG, progesterone and/or E_2 (Jouppila *et al.*, 1980) is unavoidably followed by miscarriage in 100% of cases from the 6th week of pregnancy onwards. With the development of highly sensitive real-time scanning equipment, hormonal measurements alone thus seem to be obsolete in the evaluation of the prognosis in threatened abortion.

References

Bennett, M. J., Grudzinskas, J. G., Gordon, Y. B. and Turnbull, A. C. (1978). Circulating levels of alpha-fetoprotein and pregnancy specific β_1 glycoprotein in pregnancies without an embryo. *Br. J. Obstet. Gynaecol.*, **85**, 348

Braunstein, G. D., Karow, W. G., Gentry, W. C., Rasor, J. and Wade, M. E. (1978). First-trimester chorionic gonadotropin measurements as an aid in the diagnosis of early pregnancy disorders. *Am. J. Obstet. Gynecol.*, **131**, 25

Csapo, A. I., Pulkkinen, M. O. and Wiest, W. G. (1973). Effects of luteectomy and progesterone replacement therapy in early pregnant patients. *Am. J. Obstet. Gynecol.*, **115**, 759

Chard, T. (1977). Placental function. In Stallworthy, J. and Bourne, G. (eds.) *Recent Advances in Obstetrics and Gynaecology, No. XII*, pp. 105–125. (Edinburgh, London, New York: Churchill Livingstone)

Diczfalusy, E. (1974). Endocrine functions of the human fetus and placenta. *Am. J. Obstet. Gynecol.*, **119**, 419

Duff, G. B., Evans, J. J. and Legge, M. (1980). A study of investigations used to predict outcome of pregnancy after threatened abortion. *Br. J. Obstet. Gynaecol.*, **87**, 194

Editorial (1979). Origin of maternal serum AFP. *Lancet*, **2**, 999

Fylling, P. (1970). Disappearance rate of progesterone following simultaneous removal of the corpus luteum and the foeto-placental unit in women. *Acta Endocrinol.*, **65**, 284

Garoff, L. and Seppälä, M. (1975). Prediction of fetal outcome in threatened abortion by maternal serum placental lactogen and alpha fetoprotein. *Am. J. Obstet. Gynecol.*, **121**, 257

Gartside, M. W. and Tindall, V. R. (1975). The prognostic value of human placental lactogen (HPL) levels in threatened abortion. *Br. J. Obstet. Gynaecol.*, **82**, 303

Gerhard, I. and Runnebaum, B. (1978). Aussagewert von HCG-, HPL-, progesteron- und östriol-bestimmungen bei frauen mit drohender fehlgeburt. *Geburtsh. Frauenheilk.*, **38**, 785

Gitlin, D., Perricelli, A. and Gitlin, G. M. (1972). Synthesis of α-fetoprotein by liver, yolk sac, and gastrointestinal tract of the human conceptus. *Cancer Res.*, **32,** 979

Grudzinskas, J. G., Jeffrey, D., Gordon, Y. B. and Chard, T. (1977). Specific and sensitive determination of pregnancy-specific β_1-glycoprotein by radioimmunoassay. *Lancet,* **1,** 333

Harrison, R. F. and Kitchin, Y. (1980). Maternal plasma unconjugated oestrogens in early human pregnancy. *Br. J. Obstet. Gynaecol.,* **87,** 686

Hertig, A. T. (1975). Implantation of the human ovum. In Behrman, S. J. and Kistner, R. W. (eds.) *Progress in Infertility.* 2nd Edn., pp. 411–438. (Boston: Little, Brown)

Hertz, J. B., Larsen, J. F., Svenstrup, B. and Johnsen, S. G. (1979). Estradiol, estriol and human placental lactogen in serum in threatened abortion. *Acta Obstet. Gynecol. Scand.,* **58,** 365

Hertz, J. B., Larsen, J. F., Arends, J. and Nielsen, J. (1980*a*). Progesterone and human chorionic gonadotrophin in serum and pregnandiol in urine in threatened abortion. *Acta Obstet. Gynecol. Scand.,* **59,** 23

Hertz, J. B., Mantoni, M. and Svenstrup, B. (1980*b*). Threatened abortion studied by estradiol-17β in serum and ultrasound. *Obstet. Gynecol.,* **55,** 324

Hertz, J. B. and Schultz-Larsen, P. (1983). Human placental lactogen, pregnancy-specific β_1-glycoprotein and α-fetoprotein in serum in threatened abortion. *Int. J. Gynaecol. Obstet.,* **21,** 111

Holmdahl, T. H., Johansson, E. D. B. and Wide, L. (1971). The site of progesterone production in early pregnancy. *Acta Endocrinol.,* **67,** 353

Horne, C. H. W., Towler, C. M., Pugh-Humphreys, R. G. P., Thompson, A. W. and Bohn, H. (1976). Pregnancy specific β_1-glycoprotein – a product of the syncytiotrophoblast. *Experientia,* **32,** 1197

Jandial, V., Towler, C. M., Horne, C. H. W. and Abramovich, D. R. (1978). Plasma pregnancy-specific β_1-glycoprotein in complications of early pregnancy. *Br. J. Obstet. Gynaecol.,* **85,** 832

Jouppila, P., Huhtaniemi, I. and Tapanainen, J. (1980). Early pregnancy failure: Study by ultrasonic and hormonal methods. *Obstet. Gynecol.,* **55,** 42

Karg, N. J., Csaba, I. F., Than, G. N., Vereczkey, G. and Szalmásy, M. (1981). The diagnostic value of maternal pregnancy-specific β_1-glycoprotein in threatened abortion. *Z. Geburtsh. Perinatol.,* **185,** 38

Klopper, A., Buchan, P. and Wilson, G. (1978). The plasma half-life of placental hormones. *Br. J. Obstet. Gynaecol.,* **85,** 738

Kunz, J. and Keller, P. J. (1976). HCG, HPL, oestradiol, progesterone and AFP in serum in patients with threatened abortion. *Br. J. Obstet. Gynaecol.,* **83,** 640

Leznoff, A. and Davis, B. A. (1963). The cytological localization of human chorionic gonadotropin. *Can. J. Biochem. Physiol.,* **41,** 2517

Lidbjörk, G., Kjessler, B. and Johansson, S. G. O. (1977). Alpha-fetoprotein (AFP) in maternal serum and human chorionic gonadotrophin (hCG) in urine in 77 patients with vaginal bleeding in early pregnancy. *Acta Obstet. Gynecol. Scand. Suppl.,* **69,** 54

Lindberg, B. S., Nilsson, B. A. and Johansson, E. D. B. (1974). Plasma progesterone levels in normal and abnormal pregnancies. *Acta Obstet. Gynecol. Scand.,* **53,** 329

MacNaughton, M. C. (1976). Hormone assays in early pregnancy. In Klopper, A. (ed.) *Plasma Hormone Assays in Evaluation of Fetal Wellbeing,* pp. 36–47. (Edinburgh, London, New York: Churchill Livingstone)

Manganiello, P. D., Nazian, S. J., Ellegood, J. O., McDonough, P. G. and Mahesh, V. B. (1981). Serum progesterone, 17α-hydroxyprogesterone, human chorionic gonadotropin, and prolactin in early pregnancy and a case of spontaneous abortion. *Fertil. Steril.,* **36,** 55

Miller, J. F., Williamson, E., Glue. J., Gordon, Y. B., Grudzinskas, J. G. and Sykes, A. (1980). Fetal loss after implantation. *Lancet,* **2,** 554

Niven, P. A. R., Landon, J. and Chard, T. (1972). Placental lactogen levels as guide to outcome of threatened abortion. *Br. Med. J.,* **3,** 799

Nygren, K.-G., Johansson, E. D. B. and Wide, L. (1973). Evaluation of the prognosis of threatened abortion from the peripheral plasma levels of progesterone, estradiol, and human chorionic gonadotropin. *Am. J. Obstet. Gynecol.,* **116,** 916

Quagliarello, J., Steinetz, B. G. and Weiss, G. (1979). Relaxin secretion in early pregnancy. *Obstet. Gynecol.,* **53,** 62

Quagliarello, J., Szlachter, N., Nisselbaum, J. S., Schwartz, M. K., Steinetz, B. and Weiss, G. (1981). Serum relaxin and human chorionic gonadotropin concentrations in spontaneous abortions. *Fertil. Steril.,* **36,** 399

Radwanska, E., Frankenberg, J. and Allen, E. I. (1978). Plasma progesterone levels in normal and abnormal early human pregnancy. *Fertil. Steril.*, **30**, 398

Rosal, T. P., Saxena, B. B. and Landesman, R. (1975). Application of a radioreceptorassay of human chorionic gonadotropin in the diagnosis of early abortion. *Fertil. Steril.*, **26**, 1105

Sande, H. A., Reiertsen, O., Fønstelien, E. and Torjesen, P. (1980). Evaluation of threatened abortion by human chorionic gonadotropin levels and ultrasonography. *Int. J. Gynaecol. Obstet.*, **18**, 123

Sciarra, J. J., Kaplan, S. L. and Grumbach, M. M. (1963). Localization of anti-human growth hormone serum within the human placenta: Evidence for a human chorionic growth hormone-prolactin. *Nature (Lond.)*, **199**, 1005

Schultz-Larsen, P. and Hertz, J. B. (1978). The predictive value of pregnancy-specific β_1-glycoprotein (SP_1) in threatened abortion. *Eur. J. Obstet. Gynecol. Reprod. Biol.*, **8**, 253

Scommegna, A., Burd, L., Bieniarz, J., Seals, C. and Wineman, C. (1972). Progesterone and pregnenolone sulfate in pregnancy plasma. *Am. J. Obstet. Gynecol.*, **113**, 60

Seppälä, M. and Ruoslahti, E. (1972*a*). Alpha-fetoprotein in abortion. *Br. Med. J.*, **4**, 769

Seppälä, M. and Ruoslahti, E. (1972*b*). Radioimmunoassay of maternal serum alpha fetoprotein during pregnancy and delivery. *Am. J. Obstet. Gynecol.*, **112**, 208

South, J. and Naldrett, J. (1973). The effect of vaginal bleeding in early pregnancy on the infant born after the 28th week of pregnancy. *J. Obstet. Gynaecol. Br. Commonw.*, **80**, 236

Stickle, G. (1968). Defective development and reproductive wastage in the United States. *Am. J. Obstet. Gynecol.*, **100**, 442

Tulchinsky, D. and Abraham, G. E. (1971). Radioimmunoassay of plasma estriol. *J. Clin. Endocr.*, **33**, 775

Tulchinsky, D. and Korenman, S. G. (1971). The plasma estradiol as an index of fetoplacental function. *J. Clin. Invest.*, **50**, 1490

Tulchinsky, D. and Hobel, C. J. (1973). Plasma human chorionic gonadotropin, estrone, estradiol, estriol, progesterone, and 17α-hydroxyprogesterone in human pregnancy. *Am. J. Obstet. Gynecol.*, **117**, 884

Weiss, G., O'Byrne, E. M. and Steinetz, B. G. (1976). Relaxin: A product of the human corpus luteum of pregnancy. *Science*, **194**, 948

Yen, S. S. C., Llerena, O., Little, B. and Pearson, O. H. (1968). Disappearance rates of endogeneous luteinizing hormone and chorionic gonadotropin in man. *J. Clin. Endocrinol.*, **28**, 1763

Yoshimi, T., Strott, C. A., Marshall, J. R. and Lipsett, M. B. (1969). Corpus luteum function in early pregnancy. *J. Clin. Endocrinol.*, **29**, 225

23
Ultrasound in early pregnancy

M. BULIĆ

Diagnostic ultrasound is now accepted as a significant method in early pregnancy diagnosis and as a leading tool in the differential diagnosis of disturbed early pregnancy. Its characteristics are simplicity of technique, the speed with which immediate precise diagnostic information is obtained and the complete absence of maternal and fetal mortality and morbidity.

In this chapter we have tried to describe firstly the ultrasonic morphology of normal early pregnancy and secondly the various forms of disturbed or failed early pregnancy.

NORMAL EARLY PREGNANCY

Ultrasound detection of the gestational sac

Present-day ultrasound technology allows intrauterine pregnancy to be visualized after 5 weeks of amenorrhea, an annular formation known as the gestational sac (Donald and Abdulla, 1967) being a reliable and representative indicator of intrauterine pregnancy in the first trimester.

The gestational sac may be detected by echoes from the chorionic membrane which encloses the cavity filled with other products of conception: extra-amniotic and amniotic fluid, amnion, embryo, yolk sac and allantois. Some of these structures are subsequently visualized by characteristic echoes.

The gestational sac can be of normal size, large or small-for-dates, single or multiple, and implanted in any part of the uterine cavity. Its form is initially spherical (Figure 23.1a) and subsequently mainly oval, reniform or completely irregular. The growth and development of the gestational sac and the appearance of the characteristic fetal echoes indicate a regular development of pregnancy.

Fetal echoes are observed from the 7th to 8th week of pregnancy as a solitary or bipolar echo (Figure 23.2). One pole is the echo of the fetal head and the other of the fetal body. The two poles can be differentiated and identified by means of a pulsating precordium, which together with fetal body movement is a sign of fetal life with no false positive findings. A growing fetus assumes human appearance (Figure 23.1b,c).

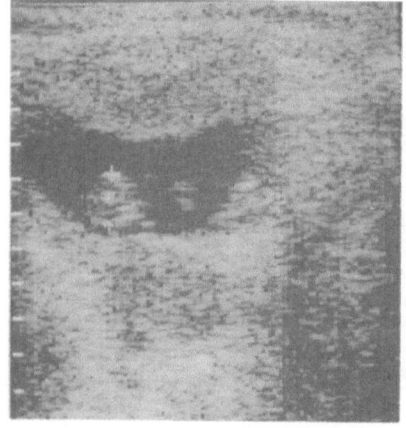

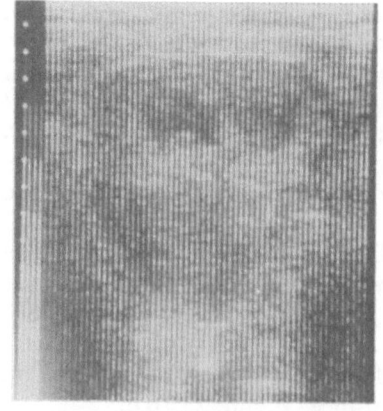

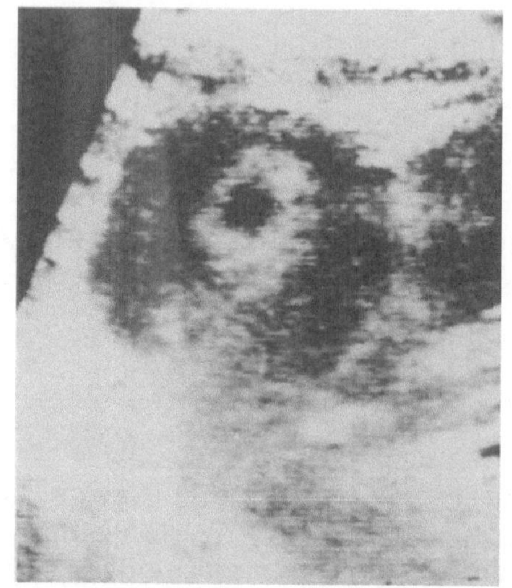

a

b

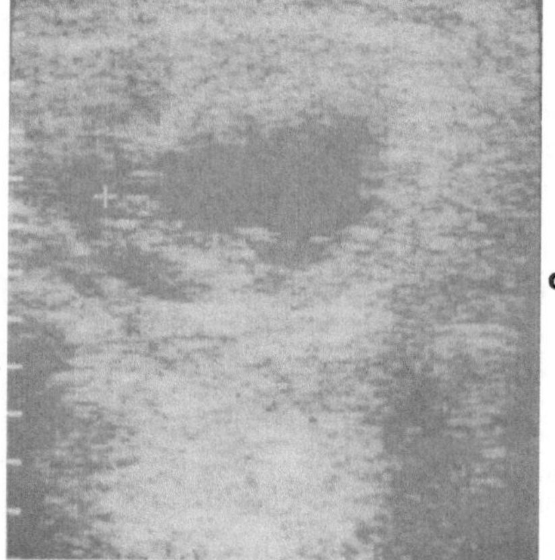

c

d

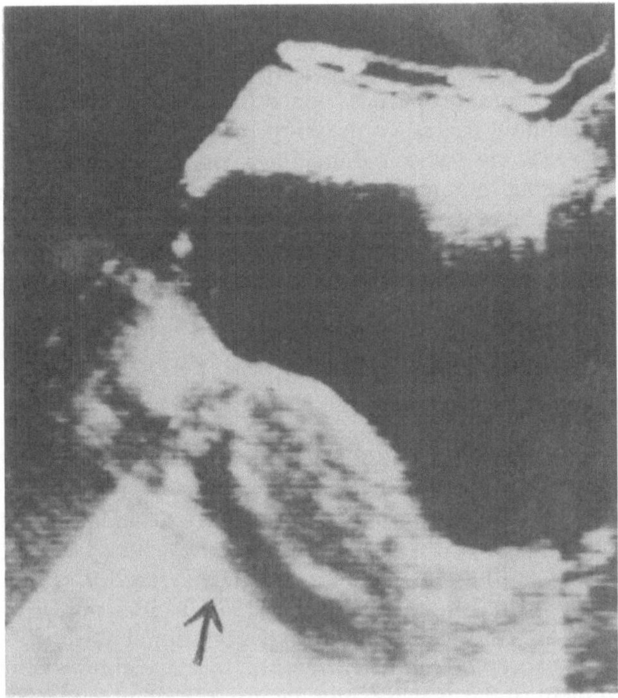

Figure 23.2 Grey-scale compound scan. 'C' form gestational sac without fetal echo, small for a 12-week pregnancy. Anembryonal pregnancy.

As the chorion differentiates into chorion frondosum and chorion laeve and grows, the base of the placenta is projected on the spot of implantation (Figure 23.1b,c). The remainder of the gestational sac expands, filling the uterine cavity and fully obstructing it by fusion with the decidua basalis. The typical shape of the gestational sac is thus lost. The critical moment of gestational sac 'disappearance', as identified by B scan, was said to to be the 12th week; its contours can, however, be seen for a much longer period, up to the 16th week.

The yolk sac and, occasionally, part of the thin amniotic membrane are also observed (Sauerbrei *et al.*, 1980).

The identification of two or more gestational sacs is a sign of multiple pregnancy, confirmed by the identification of two or more live fetuses (Figure 23.1d). In cases involving monozygotic-monochorionic twins (about 10% of cases), a double gestational sac is not identified, but there are echoes of two fetuses in a single gestational sac (Mantoni and Pedersen, 1981).

Figure 23.1 **a**, Grey-scale compound scan. Six-weeks gestation. Typical image of gestational sac in the uterus. **b**, Real-time scan. Pregnancy of 10 weeks – typical image of fetal calotte with midline echo. Biparietal diameter 15 mm. **c**, The same case, whole embryo, CRL 31 mm, well visible head, body, all limbs and funicular cord. Placenta anterior. **d**, Real-time scan. Two gestational sacs with two embryo echoes. Twin pregnancy at 8 weeks.

Not infrequently, particularly in older pregnant women, pregnancy is identified in a fibromyomatous uterus. Like the uterus, the fibroma also actively increases in the first trimester. A hyperemic fibromyoma partly changes its echosonic properties, hence the possible substitution for cystic tumor. Occasionally partial contraction of the uterus can imitate fibroma.

Smaller ovarian cysts with a diameter of up to 5 cm and of constant form and size, i.e., corpus luteum cysts, are not rare in pregnancy and may persist up to the 20th week. They do not pose a major clinical problem. Conversely, large cysts, and cysts with a partly solid content, should be surgically removed.

The existence of pregnancy in the uterus bicornis or duplex is detected by establishing pregnancy in one horn, whereas the second horn is empty.

Early fetal biometry

Accurate knowledge of gestational age is important in pregnancy management to reduce perinatal risk. Early pregnancy is the period of the most constant fetal growth, minor biological variations and fastest rate of increase in measured structures and is, therefore, the best time for fetal biometry.

Measuring of gestational sac diameter (Hellman *et al.*, 1969), area (Bulić and Vrtar, 1978) or volume (Robinson, 1975*a*), does not yield satisfactory results for the accurate determination of gestational age.

A universally accepted biometric method for determining gestational age is the measurement of the crown–rump length (CRL) introduced by Robinson, who visualized the embryo along its length from crown to rump and measured it between 8 and 14 weeks. He achieved an accuracy of ±4.7 days (Robinson, 1973).

The real-time technique opens up new possibilities in fetal biometry, embryometry in particular (Adams and Robinson, 1980). The alteration of numerous planes helps to overcome the difficulties presented by a mobile fetus and CRL is shown in the optimum plane, the image is frozen and measured accurately by multidirectional callipers.

The real-time technique allows for the easy distinction of the fetal head and body using morphologic or dynamic (precordium pulsation) criteria. Once the head is shown and positively identified, there is no reason why it should not be measured for biometric purposes (Bovicelli *et al.*, 1981). We measured the diameter of a uniformly spherical head or completely definable biparietal diameter of the head (Figure 23.1b,c). The mean values and deviations are shown in Table 23.1.

Table 23.1 Mean head diameter weekly values and variables in millimeters for 8–13 gestational weeks ($n = 153$)

Week	8	9	10	11	12	13
Number	13	38	26	25	24	27
Mean	6.8	10.5	14.6	18.1	20.0	25.2
2 SD	1.3	2.5	2.9	1.9	4.1	4.0

The correlation between head diameter values and CRL is very high ($r = 0.96$).

Early cephalometry as a biometric tool may be used in addition to CRL measurement or as a fully independent biometric method in early pregnancy.

ABNORMAL EARLY PREGNANCY

Major or minor episodes of vaginal bleeding in early pregnancy, sometimes associated with abdominal pain as well, are common clinical symptoms but still do not show whether we have a regularly continuing, failed or ectopic pregnancy. Numerous reports of less recent (Jouppila, 1977; Drumm, 1977; Bulić and Vrtar, 1977) and more recent (Jouppila, 1980; Eriksen and Philipsen, 1980) date present nearly identical general dates obtained by ultrasound in this population. Failed pregnancy is detected in 50–60% of cases, and a live fetus in the remaining cases where such pregnancy is most frequently sustained and, in about 90% of cases, concluded by a successful delivery. It may, therefore, be concluded that ultrasonic demonstration of the live fetus represents a most significant diagnostic and prognostic finding in abortion diagnostics and management.

Ultrasound differentiation of a failed pregnancy may indicate: anembryonal pregnancy, incomplete or missed abortion, a hydatidiform mole and directly or indirectly demonstrable ectopic pregnancy.

Anembryonal pregnancy

Anembryonal pregnancy (syn: blighted ovum (Donald, *et al.*, 1972); hydrovum (Bulić and Singer, 1980)) is a unique biological entity, characterized by the absence of embryoblast differentiation, where only trophoblast products develop but no embryo forms.

Ultrasonic evidence of anembryonal pregnancy includes a well- or poorly-defined gestational sac echo, of circular or 'C' form, but without any fetal echoes (Figure 23.2). The size of the gestational sac is usually small-for-dates, increases slowly or does not grow at all at repeated examination, but is, rather, reduced to almost complete collapse of the gestational sac image. The diagnostic problem consists only in excluding later conception by subsequent examination.

An anembryonal pregnancy is usually a single one, although twin forms have also been reported. A combination of a normal and anembryonic ovum is possible. The absorption of the latter does not influence the development of the normal conceptus.

In clinical terms this form of pregnancy may have a long asymptomatic course, occasionally even up to the 20th week, with positive pregnancy tests, although abortion is inevitable. The main clinical symptom is repeated bleeding of shorter or longer duration and zero uterine growth. Histological examination shows hydropic, avascularized chorionic villi, similar to hydatidiform mole, but with atrophic trophoblast. It is difficult to say that this form of pregnancy may be the precursor to hydatidiform mole. There are cases where a direct transition from blighted ovum to hydatidiform mole have been described (Kurjak and Jouppila, 1981).

Cytogenetic studies of the evacuated sample of anembryonal pregnancy point to the frequent underlying genetic factors of this pregnancy disorder (Bulić and Singer, 1980).

Abortion

The period of intrauterine fetus retention between fetal death and expulsion of fetus disintegration products is known to be very long. Hence the different ultrasound manifestations are found in spontaneous abortion, depending on the stage of the abortion process. Thus a retained gestational sac may be found, although small-for-dates and not quite sonolucent, with fetal echo but without signs of life. In most cases structureless echoes are found in the uterus, due to the disintegrated partial residues of the fetus in incomplete abortion.

Cases where the patient has aborted soon after a live fetus was demonstrated were called 'early live abortion' (Robinson, 1975*b*) and ultrasound criteria for anticipating such an outcome, e.g. the relatively smaller volume of the gestational sac according to gestational age and fetus size, were laid down. The septation of the gestational sac has recently been described as the consequence of intrauterine hematoma (Mantoni and Pedersen, 1981) and a sign heralding the unfavorable outcome of pregnancy.

Hydatidiform mole

Hydatidiform mole diagnosis is based on a characteristic ultrasound picture: snowstorm-like echoes filling the entire cavity are found, whereas other identifiable structures, e.g. the gestational sac or fetus, are missing (Figure 23.3). Nevertheless, it should be noted that this typical picture is encountered in the second trimester of pregnancy simultaneously with the onset of trophoblast disease symptoms. In the first trimester it is difficult to distinguish between hydatidiform mole and incomplete abortion by means of ultrasound. At that stage the hydatids are small, microscopic, whereas incomplete abortion is associated with hydropic alteration of the placenta. Partial moles with a coexistent fetus appear at a later stage of pregnancy (Munyer *et al*., 1981).

Finally, it should be stressed that a timely ultrasound diagnosis of pathological early pregnancy forms and their timely evacuation prevent the clinical manifestation of the hydatidiform mole and other trophoblast disease forms.

Ectopic pregnancy

Chronic forms of ectopic pregnancy pose a diagnostic problem, particularly in relation to imminent abortion.

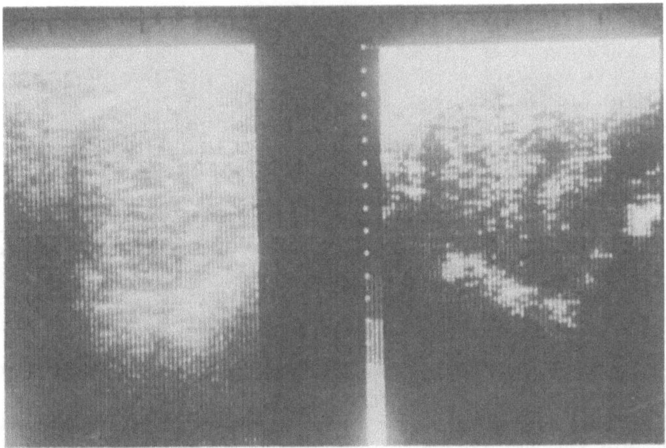

Figure 23.3 *Left*: Real-time scan. Eleven-week pregnancy. Enlarged uterus filled with snowstorm-like, highly transonic echoes. *Right*: Same case. The number of echoes is reduced with a lower output of ultrasound intensity. Hydatidiform mole.

Ultrasound diagnosis of ectopic pregnancy as confirmed by the identification of the extrauterine gestational sac is virtually exceptional, although the real-time technique does offer this opportunity as well. The true value of ultrasound within the overall scope of ectopic pregnancy diagnosis is to be found in the practical exclusion of ectopic pregnancy by the demonstration of intrauterine pregnancy. At any rate, a positive pregnancy test and negative ultrasound evidence of intrauterine pregnancy, associated with non-typical parauterine findings, is highly indicative of ectopic pregnancy and requires additional diagnostic steps to be taken.

CONCLUSIONS

It may be concluded that diagnostic ultrasound has a broad range of clinical applications in early pregnancy.

Ultrasonic examinations in the first trimester of pregnancy:

(1) confirm pregnancy (single or multiple) in the uterus,

(2) establish the presence of the fetus and signs of fetal life,

(3) provide estimates of gestational age,

(4) detect possible pathological conditions in the pelvis associated with pregnancy,

(5) identify failed pregnancy.

The advantages offered to the clinician through the use of ultrasound in early pregnancy diagnosis open up unprecedented opportunities in management.

References

Adam, A. H. and Robinson, H. P. (1980). An evaluation of real-time scanning in the first trimester of pregnancy. In Benett, M. J. and Campbell, S. (eds.), *Real-Time Ultrasound in Obstetrics*, p. 39. (Oxford, London, Edinburgh, Melbourne: Blackwell)

Bovicelli, L., Orsini, L. F., Razzo, N., Michelacci, L., Calderon, P. and Pazzaglia, F. L. (1981). Estimation of gestational age during the first trimester by real-time measurement of fetal crown–rump and biparietal diameter. *J. Clin. Ultrasound*, **9**, 71

Bulić, M. and Vrtar M. (1977). Clinical significance of gestational sac planimetry. In White, D. and Brown, R. E. (eds.) *Ultrasound in Medicine*. Vol. 3A, p. 603. (New York, London: Plenum)

Bulić, M. and Vrtar, M. (1978). Ultrasonic planimetry of the gestational sac as a biometric method in early pregnancy. *J. Clin. Ultrasound*, **6**, 228

Bulić, M. and Singer, Z. (1980). Blighted ovum (Hydrovum) – ultrasonic, clinical and cytogenetical aspect. In Kurjak, A. (ed.) *Recent Advances in Ultrasound Diagnosis 2*, p. 528. (Amsterdam, Oxford, Princeton: Excerpta Medica)

Donald, J. and Abdulla, U. (1967). Ultrasonics in obstetrics and gynaecology. *Br. J. Radiol.*, **40**, 604

Donald, J., Morley, P. and Barnett, E. (1972). The diagnosis of blighted ovum by sonar. *J. Obstet. Gynaecol. Br. Commonw.*, **79**, 304

Drumm, J. E. (1977). Pulsed ultrasound in the management of first trimester bleeding. In White, D. and Brown, R. E. (eds.) *Ultrasound in Medicine*. Vol. 3A, p. 611. (New York, London: Plenum)

Eriksen, P. S. and Philipsen, T. (1980). Prognosis in threatened abortion evaluated by hormone assays and ultrasound scanning. *Obstet. Gynecol.*, **55**, 435

Hellman, L. M. Kobayashi, M., Fillisti, L. and Lavenhar, M. (1969). Growth and development of human fetus prior to the twentieth week of gestation. *Am. J. Obstet. Gynecol.*, **103**, 789

Jouppila, P. (1977). Diagnostics in a threatened abortion. A study by ultrasound, hormonal and histological methods. In White, D. and Brown, R. E. (eds.) *Ultrasound in Medicine*. Vol. 3A, p. 595. (New York, London: Plenum)

Jouppila, P. (1980). Clinical and ultrasonic aspect in diagnosis and follow-up of patients with early pregnancy failure. *Acta Obstet. Gynecol. Scand.*, **59**, 405

Kurjak, A. and Jouppila, P. (1981). Ultrasonic, biochemical and histopathological assessment of blighted ovum. *J. Fet. Med.*, **1**, 54

Mantoni, M. and Pedersen, J. F. (1980). Monoamniotic twins diagnosed by ultrasound in the first trimester. *Acta Obstet. Gynecol. Scand.*, **59**, 555

Mantoni, M. and Pedersen, J. F. (1981). Intrauterine haematoma. An ultrasonic study of threatened abortion. *Br. J. Obstet. Gynaecol.*, **88**, 47

Munyer, T. P., Callen, P. W., Filli, R. A., Braga, C. A. and Jones, H. W. III (1981). Further observation on the sonographic spectrum of gestational trophoblastic disease. *J. Clin. Ultrasound*, **9**, 349

Robinson, H. P. (1973). Sonar measurement of fetal crown–rump length as a means of assessing maturity in first trimester of pregnancy. *Br. Med. J.*, **4**, 83

Robinson, H. P. (1975*a*). 'Gestation sac' volumes as determined by sonar in the first trimester of pregnancy. *Br. J. Obstet. Gynaecol.*, **82**, 100

Robinson, H. P. (1975*b*). The diagnosis of early pregnancy failure by sonar. *Br. J. Obstet. Gynaecol.*, **82**, 849

Sauerbrei, E., Cooperberg, P. L. and Poland, B. J. (1980). Ultrasonic demonstration of the normal fetal yolk sac. *J. Clin. Ultrasound*, **8**, 217

24
Ultrasonic examination of early fetal dynamics and congenital defects

J. W. WLADIMIROFF

Diagnostic ultrasound has greatly contributed to the present views on both normal and abnormal embryonic differentiation and growth. Grey-scale and real-time imaging have considerably raised the accuracy and speed of scanning procedures in this period of pregnancy.

FETAL DYNAMICS

Using a real-time scanner fetal heart action can be observed in about 50% between 6 and 7 weeks and in 100% after 7 weeks. Fetal heart rate shows a rise from about 130 beats/min at 7 weeks to approximately 180 beats/min at 9 weeks, which is followed by a gradual decrease to about 140 beats/min at 15 weeks (Wladimiroff, 1972). The changes which have been observed after 9 weeks are compatible with the development of fetal vagal function. Fetal movements seldom occur before 8 weeks of menstrual age. From 9 weeks episodes of slow and abrupt movements can be seen. These movements are gradually becoming more differentiated and provide a fascinating object of study for those who want to assess early development of the fetal central nervous system. Fetal stomach and urinary bladder filling become apparent at 14–15 weeks. We can also observe occasional breathing and swallowing movements. A few weeks later eye movements can be seen. The various parts which constitute the heart can be analysed (Wladimiroff, 1981).

THE ROLE OF ULTRASOUND WITH RESPECT TO THE TECHNIQUE OF ABORTION

Real-time ultrasound is useful in monitoring procedures like suction evacuation or curettage. Constant visualization of the suction device or curet relative to the location of the pregnancy and uterine wall clearly diminishes the chance of uterine damage, which may lead to infection, haemorrhage, shock or even death (Figure 24.1a). In case of bicornuate uterus, it is possible to differentiate the pregnant from the non-pregnant horn. Ultrasonic monitoring is of additional value during the evacuation of a molar pregnancy (Figure 24.1b). The ultrasonic presence of a sharply delineated inner uterine wall over the entire uterus virtually ensures that total removal of molar tissue has been achieved.

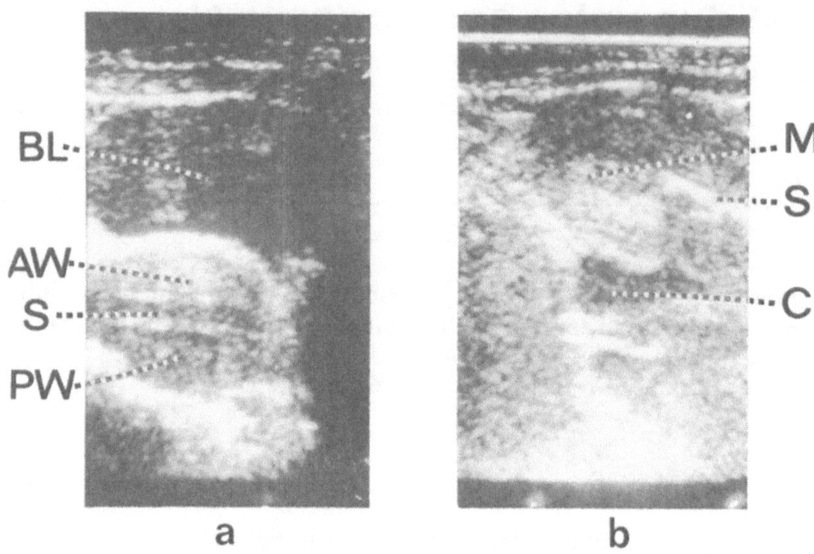

Figure 24.1 Suction cannula inside uterine cavity in a case of missed abortion (**a**) and molar pregnancy (**b**). S = suction cannula, BL = maternal urinary bladder, AW and PW = anterior and posterior uterine wall, C = lutein cyst, M = molar tissue.

PREDICTION OF FETAL ABNORMALITY

Diagnostic ultrasound particularly plays an increasingly important part in the diagnosis of fetal congenital disorders.

Indirect role of ultrasound

Ultrasound primarily plays an important role in early amniocentesis. Jahoda *et al.* (1981), using a linear-array real-time scanner for establishing placental location and fetal position, experienced only two abortions in 500 consecutive cases, that is within 4 weeks following the procedure.

When a raised amniotic fluid α-fetoprotein (AFP) level is found, an ultrasonic examination should be carried out in order to identify structural abnormalities such as open neural tube defects, omphalocele, cystic hygroma

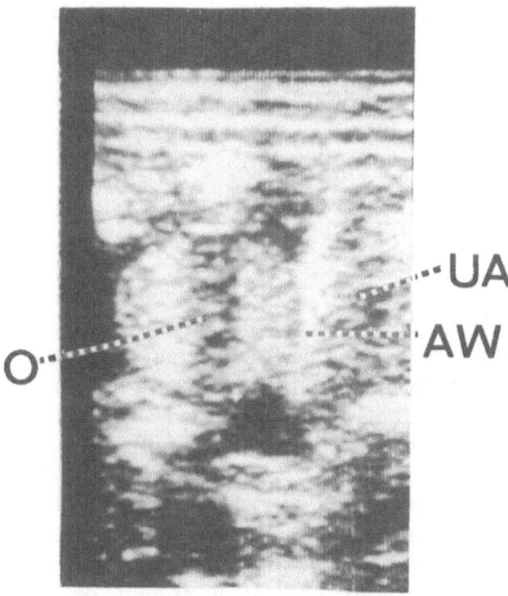

Figure 24.2 Omphalocele (O) at 25 weeks of gestation. UA = transverse cross-section of upper abdomen, AW = anterior abdominal wall.

or duodenal atresia. An omphalocele is recognized as a bulge in the anterior abdominal wall (Figure 24.2). Careful longitudinal and particularly cross-sectional scanning of the spinal column should reveal the presence of a spina bifida (Figure 24.3) (Campbell, 1979; Sabbagha, 1980). The determination of acetylcholine esterase concentration in amniotic fluid has further improved the accuracy of diagnosing open neural tube defects.

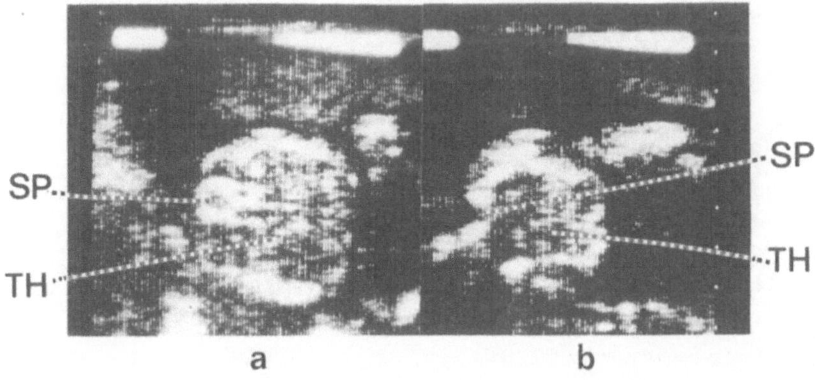

Figure 24.3 Transverse cross-section of upper abdomen at the upper lumbar region with normal spine (**a**) and at the lower thoracic region with open spina bifida (**b**). TH = fetal trunk, SP = spine.

Another application of ultrasound is the detection of an abnormal amniotic fluid volume. Only gross changes in amniotic fluid volume will be detectable. In case of polyhydramnios a careful search should be made for fetal cardiac abnormalities, skeletal abnormalities, neural tube defects, esophageal atresia. Oligohydramnios may be caused by severe growth retardation due to placental malfunction or renal agenesis.

Direct role of ultrasound

Renal tract abnormalities

Although functionally the presence of an intact renal tract can be established as from 16–17 weeks of gestation by observing fetal urinary bladder filling, morphological evidence can only be obtained as from 19–20 weeks onwards. Cystic renal changes may be diagnosed (Figure 24.4). A measurable fetal urinary production rate starts at 22–23 weeks during which period a few milliliters of urine are produced every hour (Wladimiroff, 1978). This makes early diagnosis of renal agenesis more difficult. Moreover, an empty fetal bladder may also be observed in fetal growth retardation. Distinction between poor placental function and renal agenesis may be made on the basis of maternal intravenous administration of 60 mg of the diuretic agent frusemide (Lasix), which will result in a measurable fetal bladder filling in the former and absence of any filling in the latter case.

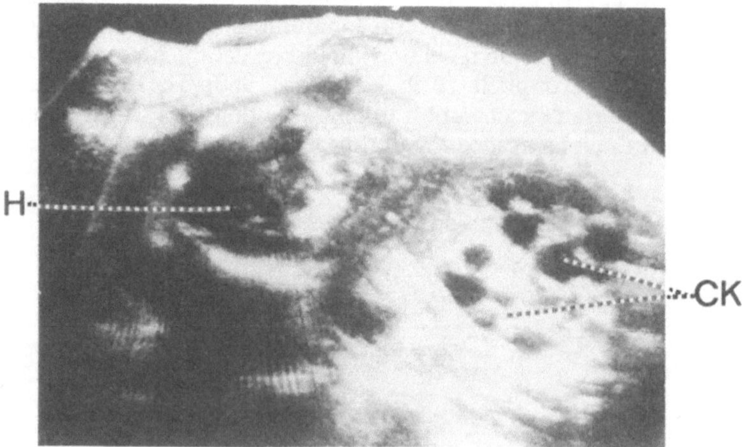

Figure 24.4 Longitudinal cross-section of fetal head (H) and upper abdomen at 26 weeks of gestation, demonstrating grossly enlarged cystic kidneys (CK).

Hydrocephaly

Hydrocephaly is not associated with raised amniotic fluid (AFP) levels and can therefore only be diagnosed by ultrasound. An ultrasonic scan should be made of a transverse plane of the fetal head at the level of the cavum septum pellucidum. This particular plane will also demonstrate a midline or falx cerebri and the lateral margin of the anterior horn of the lateral ventricle (Figure 24.5a,b). We calculated according to Campbell (1979) the ventricle–hemisphere ratio which expresses the relationship between the distance from the lateral margin of the anterior horn of the lateral ventricle to the midline and the maximal width of the cerebral hemisphere at that particular level. Normal curves of this particular ratio (Figure 24.6a) and the fetal head circumference (Figure 24.6b) demonstrate that the ventricle–hemisphere ratio in an affected fetus may be well above the normal limit, whereas the fetal head circumference at the stage has no predictive value (Egmond-Linden *et al.*, 1981).

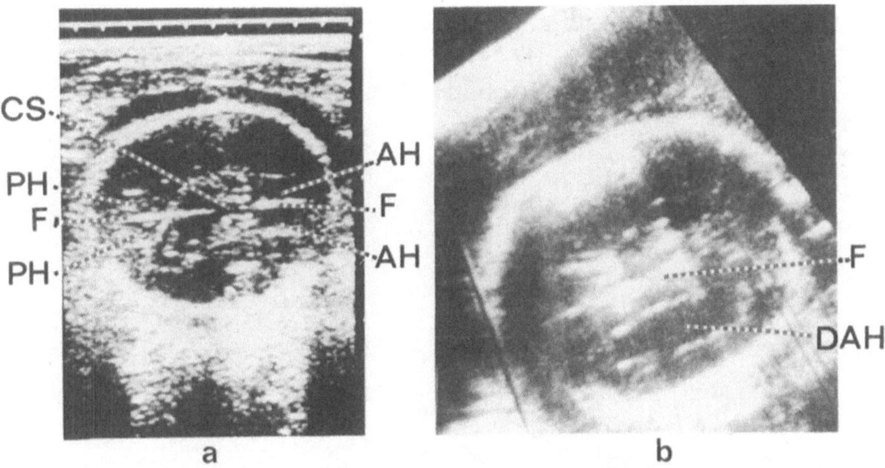

Figure 24.5 **a**, Transverse cross-section through normal fetal head at 18 weeks, F = falx cerebri, CS = cavum septum pellucidum, AH = anterior horn of lateral ventricles, PH = posterior horn of lateral ventricles. **b**, Transverse cross-section through hydrocephalic head at 20 weeks, DAH = dilated anterior horn of lateral ventricle.

Limb bone deformities

Limb bone deformities are receiving increasing attention (Figure 24.7a,b). Several reports have recently appeared on early prenatal diagnosis of limb bone deformities (Mahoney and Hobbins, 1977; Queenan *et al.*, 1980; O'Brien *et al.*, 1981; Salvo, 1981; Mantagos *et al.*, 1981; Frijns *et al.*, 1981; Wladimiroff *et al.*, 1981). We diagnosed a Majewski-like syndrome at 17 weeks of gestation in a patient who had a previous infant with the same syndrome, that is a short limb short rib syndrome without polydactyly. The length of all four fetal extremities was well below the lower limit of our normal curve (Figures 24.8, 24.9) (Wladimiroff *et al.*, 1981). The head-to-chest ratio revealed a relatively small chest (Wladimiroff *et al.*, 1978). Termination of pregnancy was requested, the syndrome was confirmed (Figure 24.10).

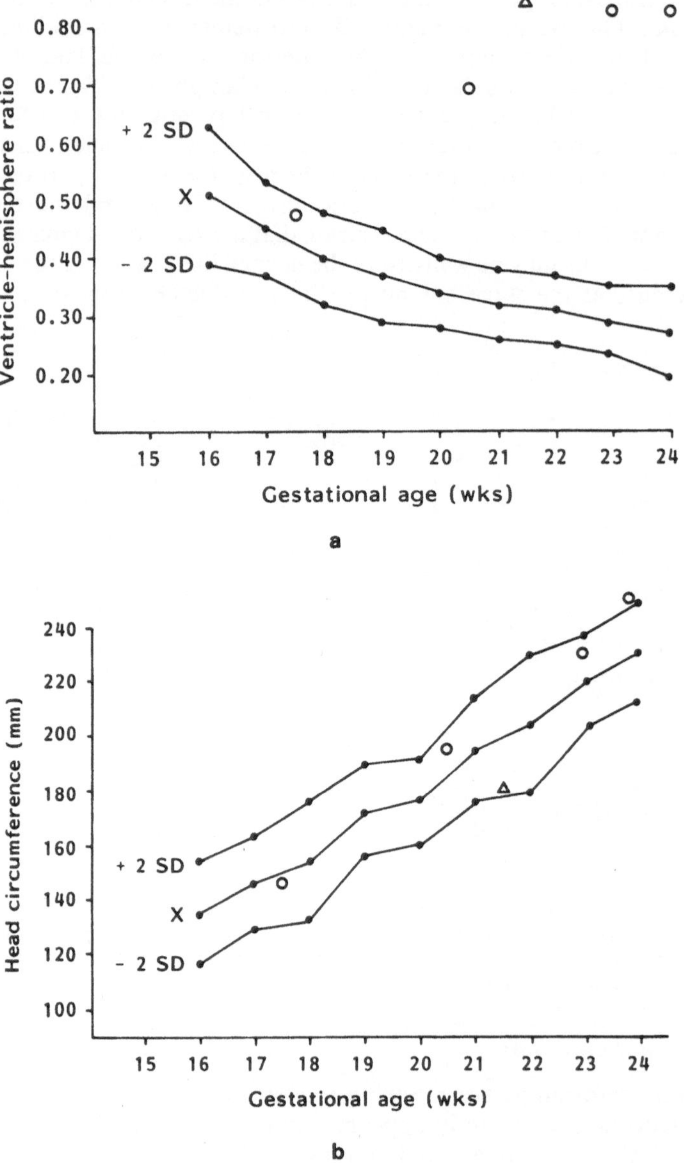

Figure 24.6 Normal curve of ventricle/hemisphere ratio (**a**) and head circumference (**b**), are relative to gestational age. Note the two hydrocephalic cases.

Cardiac abnormalities

Marked improvement of real-time imaging and the introduction of M-mode recording and pulsed Doppler systems have provided valuable information on

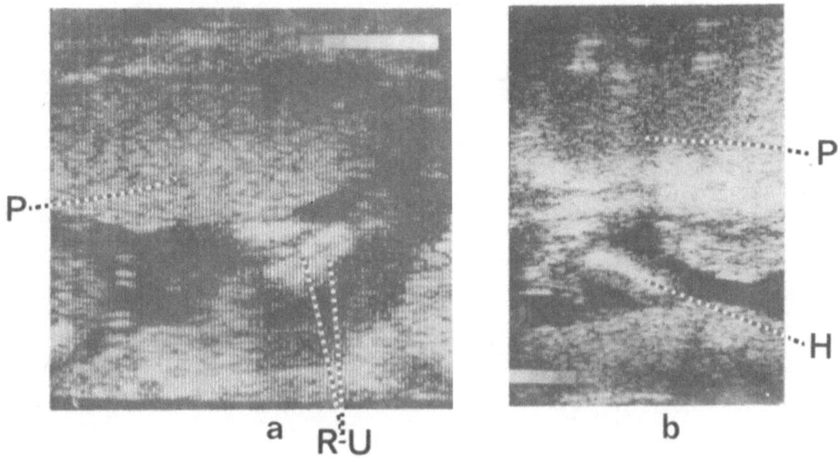

Figure 24.7 Fetal radius–ulna complex (R–U) (a) and humerus (H) (b) at 17 weeks.

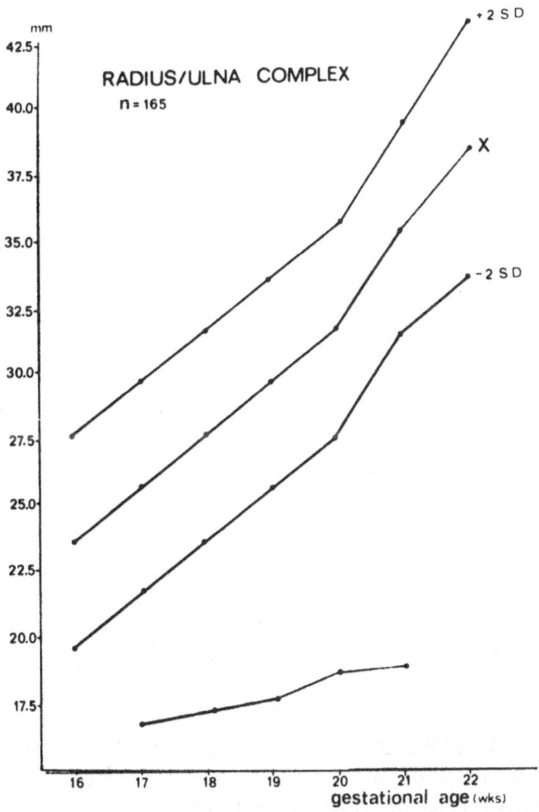

Figure 24.8 Normal curve of radius–ulna complex relative to gestational age. Note very reduced values for fetus with Majewski-like syndrome.

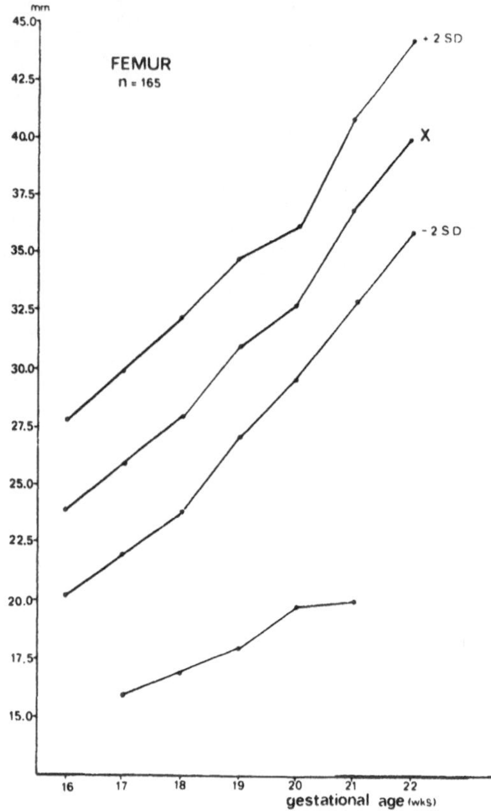

Figure 24.9 Normal curve of femur length relative to gestational age. Note very reduced values for fetus with Majewski-like syndrome.

the geometry and function of the fetal cardiovascular system (Figure 24.11). Data on fetal left ventricular function (Wladimiroff and McGhie, 1981*a*,*b*) and absolute blood flow in the fetal descending aorta and umbilical vein have been collected (Gill and Kossoff, 1979; Eik-Nes *et al.*, 1980; Wladimiroff and McGhie, 1981*a*,*b*). Ultrasound is also a useful adjunct in the diagnosis of fetal cardiac abnormalities (Allan *et al.*, 1980, 1981; Kleinman *et al.*, 1980). The combination of structural analysis and dynamic information of the heart by means of M-mode recording systems will provide us with a full picture of the anatomy and function of the fetal cardiovascular system in cases of suspected cardiac abnormalities (Wladimiroff and McGhie, 1981*c*). Since most cardiac abnormalities are amenable to surgical correction, the value of diagnosing this category of abnormalities lies not so much in the possibility of early pregnancy termination, but in careful antenatal monitoring and close cooperation with the neonatologist and pediatric cardiologist.

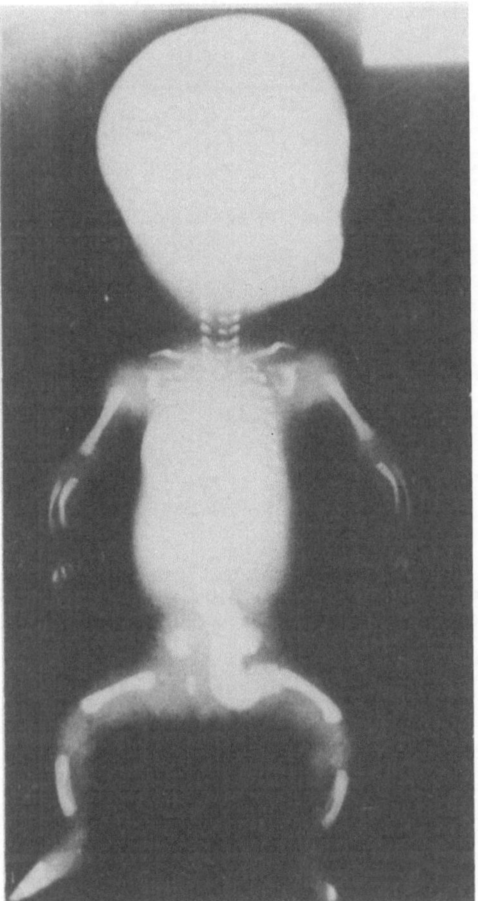

Figure 24.10 X-ray picture of fetus with Majewski-like syndrome following pregnancy termination. Note very short extremities.

Termination of midtrimester pregnancies

Prostaglandins by local intra- or extra-amniotic administration offer the best prospect in mid trimester induced abortion. In the case of intra-amniotic administration of prostaglandins, real-time ultrasound may help to make this procedure safer and more effective. One should ensure that the tip of the amniocentesis needle is correctly situated in the amniotic fluid cavity. Further evidence that the prostaglandins are properly instilled into the cavity may be obtained from the turbulent fluid changes which occur around the needle exit during the instillation (Figure 24.12) and can be visualized by ultrasound.

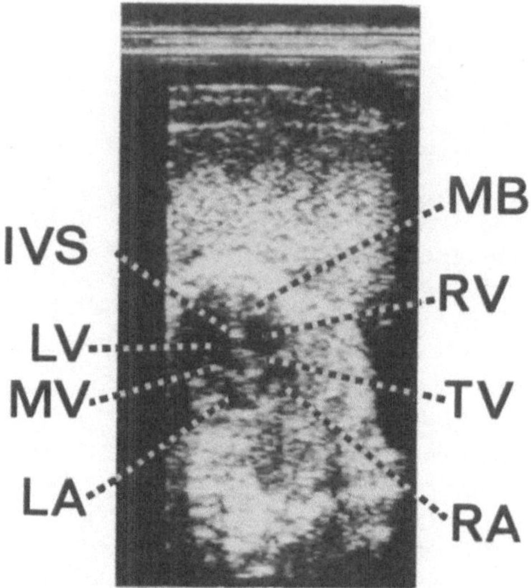

Figure 24.11 Four-chamber view of fetal heart at 24 weeks of gestation. LV and RV = left and right ventricle, IVS = interventricular septum, MB = moderator band in right ventricle, MV and TV = mitral and tricuspid valves, LA and RA = left and right atrium.

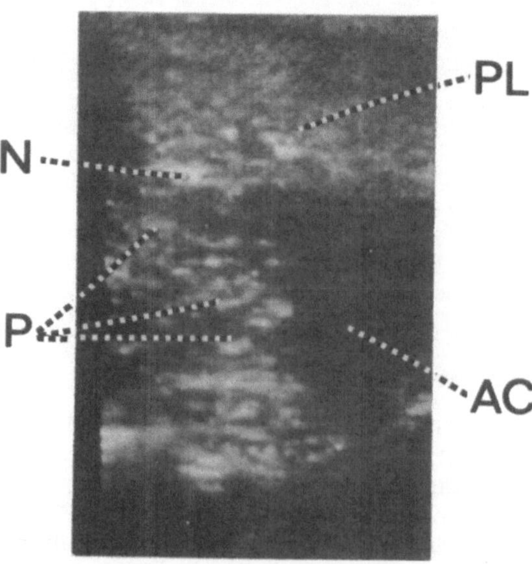

Figure 24.12 Prostaglandin ($F_2\alpha$) instillation into the amniotic cavity (AC). Note the tip of the needle (N) and turbulence (P) in cavity. PL = anterior placenta.

CONCLUSIONS

Ultrasound must now be considered as a major tool in first and second trimester obstetric problems. It has deepened our insight into embryonic morphological and dynamic development. It has also contributed to the change in attitude towards clinical problems such as vaginal blood loss. Ultrasound is a useful adjunct in the diagnosis of genetic abnormalities. Accurate assessment of gestational age and real-time monitoring of fetal and placental location during amniocentesis has greatly improved the effectiveness and safety of this procedure. Recognition of structural abnormalities is becoming increasingly successful with further improvement of image resolution. Ultrasound should be employed more often during evacuation procedures. Both suction devices and curets can be easily visualized relative to surrounding structures, achieving a twofold purpose: reduction of complications such as bleeding and perforation and more effective emptying of the uterine cavity.

References

Allan, L. D., Tynan, M. J., Campbell, S., Wilkinson, J. W. and Anderson, R. H. (1980). Echocardiographic and anatomical correlates in the fetus. *Br. Heart J.*, **44,** 444

Allan, L. D., Tynan, M., Campbell, S. and Anderson, R. H. (1981). Normal fetal cardiac anatomy. A basis for the echocardiographic detection of abnormalities. *Prenat. Diagn.*, **1,** 131

Campbell, S. (1979). Diagnosis of fetal abnormalities by ultrasound. In Milunski, A. (ed.) *Genetic Disorders and the Fetus. Diagnosis, Prevention and Treatment*, p. 431. (New York, London: Plenum)

Egmond-Linden, A. van, Wladimiroff, J. W., Jahoda, M. G. J. and Laar-van Sabben, J.(1981). Second trimester study of intracranial anatomy. In *Abstract Book of 4th European Congress on Ultrasonics in Medicine*, Dubrovnik, p. 32

Eik-Nes, S. H., Brubakk, A. O. and Ulstein, H. K. (1980). Measurement of human fetal blood flow. *Br. Med. J.*, **1,** 283

Frijns, J. P., Vandenberghe, K., van Assche, A. and Vandenberghe, H. (1981). Prenatal diagnosis of campomelic dwarfism. *Clin. Genet.*, **19,** 199

Gill, R. W. and Kossoff, G. (1979). Pulsed Doppler combined with B-mode imaging for blood flow measurement. *Contrib. Gynaecol. Obstet.*, **6,** 139

Jahoda, M. G. J. and Sachs, E. S. (1981). Follow up of 500 consecutive cases after amniocentesis for prenatal diagnosis in a series of 3500 patients. In *Abstract Book of the 6th International Congress of Human* Genetics, Israel, p. 303

Kleinman, C. S., Hobbins, J. C., Iaffe, C. C., Lynch, D. C. and Talner, N. S. (1980). Echocardiographic studies of the human fetus. Prenatal diagnosis of congenital heart disease and cardiac dysrhythmics. *Pediatrics*, **65,** 1059

Mahoney, M. J. and Hobbins, J. C. (1977). Prenatal diagnosis of chondroectodermal dysplasia (Ellis van Creveld Syndrome) with fetoscopy and ultrasound. *N. Engl. J. Med.*, **297,** 258

Mantagos, S., Weiss, R. R., Mahoney, M. and Hobbins, J. C. (1981). Prenatal diagnosis of diastrophic dwarfism. *Am. J. Obstet. Gynecol.*, **139,** 111

O'Brien, G. D., Queenan J. T. and Campbell, S. (1981). Assessment of gestational age in the second trimester by real-time ultrasound measurement of the femur length. *Am. J. Obstet. Gynecol.*, **139,** 540

Queenan, J. T., O'Brien, G. D. and Campbell, S. (1980). Ultrasound measurement of fetal limb bones. *Am. J. Obstet. Gynecol.*, **138,** 297

Sabbagha, R. E. (1980). Ultrasonic evaluation of fetal congenital anomalies. In Gerbie, E. B. (ed.) *Clinics in Obstetrics and Gynaecology*, Vol. 7, no. 1, p. 103. (London, Philadelphia, Toronto: Saunders)

Salvo, A. F. (1981). In utero diagnosis of Kleeblatt Schädel (Cloverleaf skull). *Prenat. Diagn*, **1**, 141

Wladimiroff, J. W. (1972). Fetal heart action in early pregnancy. Development of fetal vagal function. *Eur. J. Obstet. Gynecol.*, **2**, 55

Wladimiroff, J. W. (1978). Studies of fetal physiology by sonography. In M. de Vlieger, (ed.) *Handbook of Clinical Ultrasound*, p. 103. (New York, Chichester, Brisbane, Toronto: Wiley)

Wladimiroff, J. W. (1981). Ultrasound in normal and high-risk pregnancy. In Mulunski, A. Friedman, E. and Gluck, L. (eds.) *Advances in Perinatal Medicine*. Vol. 1, p. 165. (New York: Plenum)

Wladimiroff, J. W., Bloemsma, C. A. and Wallenburg, H. C. S. (1978). Ultrasonic assessment of fetal head and body sizes in relation to normal and retarded fetal growth. *Am. J. Obstet. Gynecol.*, **131**, 857

Wladimiroff, J. W., Beemer, F. A. and Hemmes, A. M. (1981). Early diagnosis of skeletal dysplasia by real-time ultrasound. *Lancet*, **1**, 661

Wladimiroff, J. W. and McGhie, J. (1981*a*). Ultrasonic assessment of cardiovascular geometry and function in the human fetus. *Br. J. Obstet. Gynaecol.*, **88**, 870

Wladimiroff, J. W. and McGhie, J. (1981*b*). M-mode ultrasonic assessment of fetal cardiovascular dynamics. *Br. J. Obstet. Gynaecol.*, **88**, 1241

Wladimiroff, J. W. and McGhie, J. (1981*c*). M-mode and pulsed Doppler ultrasound assessment of severe bradycardia, a case report. *Br. J. Obstet. Gynaecol.*, **88**, 1246

Part IV

Clinical Parameters

25
Spontaneous abortion due to cervical insufficiency

D. BARSOUM, K. I. EL-LAMIE and E. S. E. HAFEZ

Spontaneous abortion due to cervical incompetence is caused by dilatation of the cervix which allows the fetal sac to bulge down and protrude into the vagina. With this condition abortion occurs within a matter of days and/or weeks. This sequence of events is frequently seen repeatedly in the same patients and usually occurs between the 18th and 24th week of gestation.

Cervical incompetence was first reported by Gream (1865). This report was followed by extensive studies of effective therapy by several pioneer investigators (Palmer and Lacomme, 1948; Lash and Lash, 1950; Shirodkar, 1955; McDonald, 1957).

The incidence of cervical incompetence relative to all pregnancies varies from 0.05% to 1% (Jennings, 1972). There are other causes of midtrimester abortions, such as fetal abnormalities; however, as many as 16% of second trimester pregnancy losses are due to cervical incompetence (Stromme and Haywa, 1963). Kuhn and Pepperell (1977) point out that comparison of the incidence of this problem in different obstetrical populations is difficult based on variation in the laws governing termination of pregnancy and selective referral of high risk patients to special institutions.

ETIOLOGY

Several congenital and acquired (gynecological and obstetric) factors are responsible for incompetent cervix (Table 25.1). Various causes have changed significantly from previous reports due to changing trends of gynecological and obstetrical practices.

Acquired factors

Gynecological

Laceration to the cervix due to D & C

In most cases, cervical incompetency may be due to the splitting of tissue at the fibro-muscular junction (Forster, 1967). A split cervix is often held responsible

Table 25.1 Summary of etiology of the incompetent cervix

Parameters		*Mechanism*	*Reference*
Congenital			
With uterine anomaly	Septate uterus	Accompanied by incompetent os	
Without uterine anomaly	DES induced	Caudal displacement of isthmic stroma	
		The ratio of muscular element to connective tissue increases, causing decrease in cervical resistance	
	Muscular cervix	Increase in the muscular component causing a decrease in functional capacity of the cervix	Herbst, 1978 Cousins, 1980 Danforth and Buckingham, 1962
	Inherent weakness	Disturbance in the normal structural changes in connective tissue	Roddick *et al*, 1961
		Premature triggering of normal mechanism of dilation and effacement	Forster, 1967
Acquired			
Gynecological	Dilatation of cervix as in curettage, dysmenorrhea or termination of pregnancy Conization of cervix Amputation of cervix	Mechanical disruption of fibrous ring	Lees and Sutherst, 1974 Moinian and Andersch, 1982 Forster, 1967 Johnstone *et al.*, 1976 Hulka *et al.*, 1974
Obstetrical	Precipitate labor, forceps or vacuum	Mechanical disruption of fibrous ring	Dumont and Poizat, 1974 Danforth and Buckingham, 1962
	Multiple gestation	Premature distension of the uterus	Barter *et al.*, 1958

for late abortion and premature labor (Lees and Sutherst, 1974). An incorrectly performed dilatation for primary spasmodic dysmenorrhea is usually responsible.

The nulliparous cervix is especially at risk and may begin to tear when dilated with No. 8 Hegar dilator. This dilatation is usually synonymous with rupture.

Maximal resistance to dilatation of the internal os in the first trimester of pregnancy occurs at 9 mm. Dilatation to 11 or 12 mm may represent tearing of the internal os rather than true dilatation (Hulka *et al.*, 1974).

Dilatation of the cervix to 12 mm or above, at suction termination of pregnancy, may result in abnormally high cervical measurements in some patients and hence may increase the possibility of second trimester abortion or premature labor from cervical incompetence. No such association is found when the cervix is dilated to 10 mm or less (Johnstone *et al.*, 1976).

In patients with an incompetent cervix, a tissue defect or a split can very often be palpated in its upper part. This is commonly situated anterolaterally, and is easily felt when the cervix is dilated and the bladder is reflected upwards (Forster, 1967).

Conization

In a series of 414 patients who underwent cervical conization because of cancer *in situ* of the cervix, it was found that after conization the incidence of late spontaneous abortion was seven times higher than before conization. However, a series of 50 extensive conization failed to reveal an increased risk of incompetent cervix in subsequent pregnancies (McLaren *et al.*, 1974). Moinian and Andersch (1982) reported that 20% of the women who conceived following cone biopsy required cervical cerclage because of suspected cervical insufficiency.

Amputation

High amputation of the cervix in the treatment of uterine prolapse could be a cause of cervical incompetence (Lees and Sutherst, 1974; Fisher, 1951).

Obstetric causes

An incompetent cervix may be caused by rapid delivery, with the use of forceps or vacuum extractor before dilatation is complete, by child-birth with difficult presentation (Dumont and Poizat, 1974), and placenta praevia from tissue loss.

Cervical incompetence in relation to multiple gestation was first demonstrated by Barter *et al.* (1958). Dennerstein (1971) reviewed ten cases of twin gestation and reported a case of triplets with relative cervical incompetence successfully treated with cerclage (Cousins, 1980). This type of cervical incompetence may be qualified as relative because gravidas with cervical incompetence during a multiple pregnancy have demonstrated normal cervical function in previous and subsequent pregnancies.

DIAGNOSIS

There is no diagnostic method which will confirm precisely the presence of an incompetent cervix. The diagnosis is made based on the current condition and past obstetrical history (Table 25.2).

Diagnosis during pregnancy

The history of previous pregnancies is most important for accurate diagnosis. Patients with one or more spontaneous midtrimester abortions with early rupture of membranes, usually before the onset of labor without significant hemorrhage, short and relatively painfree labor with delivery of a live fetus is indicative of an incompetent cervix. Repeated middle-term spontaneous abortions at similar gestational age are significant (Barter *et al.*, 1958; Gibbs, 1973; Cousins, 1980). There are some incompetent cervix subjects (25–50 %) who will carry pregnancies beyond 19 weeks (Gibbs, 1973; Jennings, 1972, McDonald, 1957; Weingold *et al.*, 1968). Although lower uterine segment distension, cervical effacement and dilatation can occur silently over several weeks, there are instances in which the evacuation of the uterus is not totally painless. Therefore, the presence of uterine contractions does not eliminate the diagnosis of cervical incompetence.

Incompetent cervix during a current pregnancy is associated with several indications: (1) mucus discharge; (2) a sensation of retropubic or lower abdominal pressure from partial cervical dilatation; (3) presence of urinary urgency without urinary tract infection; (4) presence of a bag of forewaters in the cervix or upper vagina causing a sensation of fullness in the vagina (Toaff and Toaff, 1974; Toaff and Toaff, 1977). The diagnosis is confirmed by visualization of a partly dilated cervix or bulging membranes on speculum examination.

If the diagnosis is suspected in a pregnant patient, vaginal examinations should be performed on a weekly basis to identify premature cervical effacement and dilatation (Barter *et al.*, 1963; Gibbs, 1973; Cousins, 1980).

Ultrasonography is a valuable diagnostic technique during pregnancy (Sarti *et al.*, 1979). Thus it is possible to visualize a dilated cervix, and other causes of midtrimester spontaneous abortions such as fetal abnormalities and aberrations of uterine shape can be excluded.

A width of the internal os of 19 mm or more is suggestive of cervical incompetence (Brook *et al.*, 1981). Nevertheless, every unit should establish its own normal values, taking into account differences in instruments and calibrations.

A midterm finding of the amniotic fluid in the endocervical canal should alert the physician to the possibility of an incompetent cervix. A patient with a previous history of spontaneous abortion, but without actual physical confirmation of bulging membranes, or cervical effacement can now undergo diagnostic ultrasonography early in pregnancy and be followed periodically (Sarti *et al.*, 1979).

Table 25.2 Summary of some of the diagnostic approaches for the incompetent cervix

Diagnostic	*During pregnancy*		*During non-pregnancy*	
History	Previous pregnancy	recurrent painless midtrimester abortion	Of previous pregnancy	recurrent painless midtrimester abortion
	Current pregnancy	mucus discharge retropubic pressure urinary urgency and frequency		
Exam	Cervical effacement and dilatation Bulging bag of membranes	felt by gentle digital exam and seen by speculum examination	Patulous os Hegar's test	passage of No. 8 Hegar
Investigation	Ultrasonography	a width of the internal os of 19 mm or more is suggestive	Intracervical balloon	a diameter of 6 mm balloon withdrawn easily
			Foley's catheter traction test	visualization of cervical canal wider than 8 mm
			Hysterogram	

Diagnosis during non-pregnancy

Hegar test

The easy passage of a No. 8 Hegar dilator through the non-gravid cervix is diagnostic for cervical incompetence (Palmer, 1961; Lash, 1960).

Hysterography

With a water soluble contrast medium a cannula is introduced 5 mm into the cervical canal, which is kept tightly closed by the use of one or more tenaculum forceps to prevent leakage of the contrast medium. Steady traction on the cervix allowed visualization of the entire uterocervical cavity. Cervical incompetence was diagnosed by the disappearance of the normal uterocervical angle and by an abnormally wide isthmico-cervical canal. A cervical canal wider than 8 mm at the level of the internal os proves cervical incompetence.

Traction test

In this test, the mechanical ability of the cervix is evaluated. A Foley catheter (No. 16) is inserted into the uterus, and the balloon is filled with 1 ml of water to reach a diameter of 6 mm. In cases of incompetent cervix, the catheter can be easily and painlessly withdrawn (Soihet, 1974; Peterson and Keifer, 1973; Bergman and Svennerund, 1957; Cousins, 1980).

MANAGEMENT

Several procedures are employed in the management of the incompetent cervix during pregnancy and non-pregnancy (Table 25.3). The objective of management is to enhance the resistance of the cervix to effacement and dilatation.

Ligature of the cervix is better inserted in pregnancy for several reasons. Patients with an incompetent cervix appear to be more fertile than others and hence, if the cervix is closed in the non-gravid state, it may impede conception. Also, first trimester abortion may occur due to imperfect development of the ovum or its faulty implantation. If the cervix is already ligated, evacuation of the product of conception will be difficult. Furthermore, only few patients come into premature labor, immediately after ligation of the cervix (Ritter, 1978).

Selection of patients

Contraindications to operation

A patient with a history of persistent bleeding during pregnancy or signs of toxemia or polyhydramnios is unsuitable for cervical cerclage. Vesicular mole, fetal abnormalities or fetal death *in utero* must be excluded. Ultrasonography

Table 25.3 Different methods of management of cervical incompetence

Method	*Stage*	*Procedure*	*Advantages*	*Disadvantages and/or complications*	*Reference*
1. *Surgical* (a) *Cerclage* (i) Vaginal route		Placement of a band – originally fascia lata, now 5 mm Mersilene – in the submucosa via anterior and posterior	Effective, infant survival after operation 82%	Difficult to remove stitch need general anesthesia cesarean section rate 53–82%	Shirodkar, 1955 Raphael *et al.*, 1958
Shirodkar's procedure	Pregnant	Incisions originally tied anteriorly now tied posteriorly to reduce canal to 3–5 mm (Figure 25.2)		Infection	Strand, 1963
McDonald cerclage	Prègnant	A pursestring suture of 4 Mersilene band is inserted around the cervix 4 or 5 bites, the knot made anteriorly (Figure 25.3)	Effective infant survival after operation 73% Cesarean section rate same after operation Easier to remove Can be done on a dilated cervix Technically easy	Failure of procedure Infection Cervical fibrotic ring causing prolonged labor Cervical lacerations	McDonald, 1957 McDonald, 1978 Naver, 1968 Picot *et al.*, 1959 Toaff and Toaff, 1977
In a dilated cervix	Pregnancy	Patient steep Trendelenburg, deep anesthesia, tocolytic drug reposition of bulging membrane by Foley's catheter ligature inserted, Foley's catheter withdrawn, suture firmly tied	Effective in cases of dilated cervix when other methods fail	Difficult, failure rate high Rupture of membranes	Olatunbosum and Dyck, 1981 Orr, 1973
(ii) Abdominal route: transabdominal cerclage	Pregnancy	Abdomen is opened and a tunnel made between uterine isthmus medialy and uterine vessels laterally. A 15 cm Merseline ribbon 0.5 cm wide is passed on each side and tied anteriorly (Figure 25.4)	Effective when other methods fail or impossible e.g. congenitally short cervix or amputated, marked scarring, deep cervical defects, forniceal lacerations Advanced cervical effacement Infant survival after procedure 85%	Two abdominal operations, the second for cesarean section High complication rate Increased risk of maternal morbidity and potential mortality	Novy, 1982 Ritter, 1978 Watkins, 1972

Table 25.3 (*Contd.*)

Method	*Stage*	*Procedure*	*Advantages*	*Disadvantages and/or complications*	*Reference*
(b) *Reconstruction of cervix*	Non-pregnant				
(ii) Lash procedure		Removal of anterior rhomboid segment of uterocervical muscle. Suturing the deficiency to narrow canal at internal os (Figure 25.1)	Infant survival improves after treatment	45% sterility after operation Cannot be done during pregnancy Of value if defect is present	Lash and Lash, 1950 Lash, 1960 Lees and Sutherst, 1974
(iii) Palmer and Lacomme	Non-pregnant	Removal of a wedge of cervix Reconstitution of canal			Palmer and Lacomme, 1948
(iv) McDonald modification of abdominal cerclage	Non-pregnant	Uterosacral and cardinal ligament visualized by sharp and blunt dissection. A 5 mm merseline band or polyvinyl tubing Portex 2 placed above the uterosacral ligament	Effective method used when other methods fail or difficult	Ligature is permanent Delivery by cesarean section	McDonald, 1980 Ritter, 1978
(c) Electrocautery	Non-pregnant	Electrocauterization at level of internal os	Outpatient procedure	Result less than other methods Cervical stenosis Cervical lacerations Limited to non-pregnant state	Ranney, 1963 Vogel, 1972
2. *Mechanical vaginal pessary*					
(a) *Smith-Hodge Pessary*	Pregnancy	Pessary inserted in outpatient causing displacement of the cervix posteriorly, relieving direct pressure on the internal os. Fetal head, elevated by the sling-like action of pessary	Effective method Infant survival rate 90% No operative or anesthetic risk Quick outpatient procedure	More results are needed	Vitsky, 1961, 1963, 1968 Oster and Javert, 1966 Javert, 1962
(b) *Mayer Pessary*	Pregnancy	As above	Can be used with dilated cervix up to 3 cm		Bayer, 1977

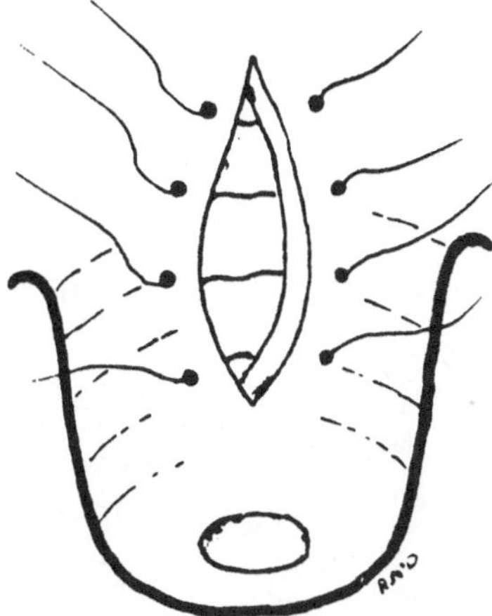

Figure 25.1 The original Lash operation. A diamond-shaped area of tissue at the cervico-vaginal junction is excised and the deficiency repaired with sutures (McDonald, 1980).

is useful when selecting patient for ligature. Patients with spontaneous ruptured membranes, serious pelvic infection, in established labor or when the cervix is far too dilated are not candidates for the cerclage procedure.

Indications

Toaff and Toaff, (1977) have suggested the following indications:

(1) Elective indications:
  (a) typical history of one pregnancy loss in the second trimester,
  (b) history of two or more second trimester pregnancy losses,
  (c) history of one second trimester pregnancy loss with prior cervical trauma, dilatation and currettage, cone biopsy, cervical laceration, or Duhressen incision,
  (d) history of premature labor in the third trimester,
  (e) history of painless cervical dilatation in the second trimester of a previous pregnancy,
  (f) history of a successful cerclage in a previous pregnancy.

(2) Emergency indications. The dilatation and/or effacement of the cervix is noticed on digital examination during the second trimester without uterine contraction, or with uterine contraction after suppression of contractions.

(3) Other indications: Twin primapara, multiple births after the use of human gonadotropins, and in pregnancies where the uterus is unihorned or malformed (Henry-Suchet, 1977)

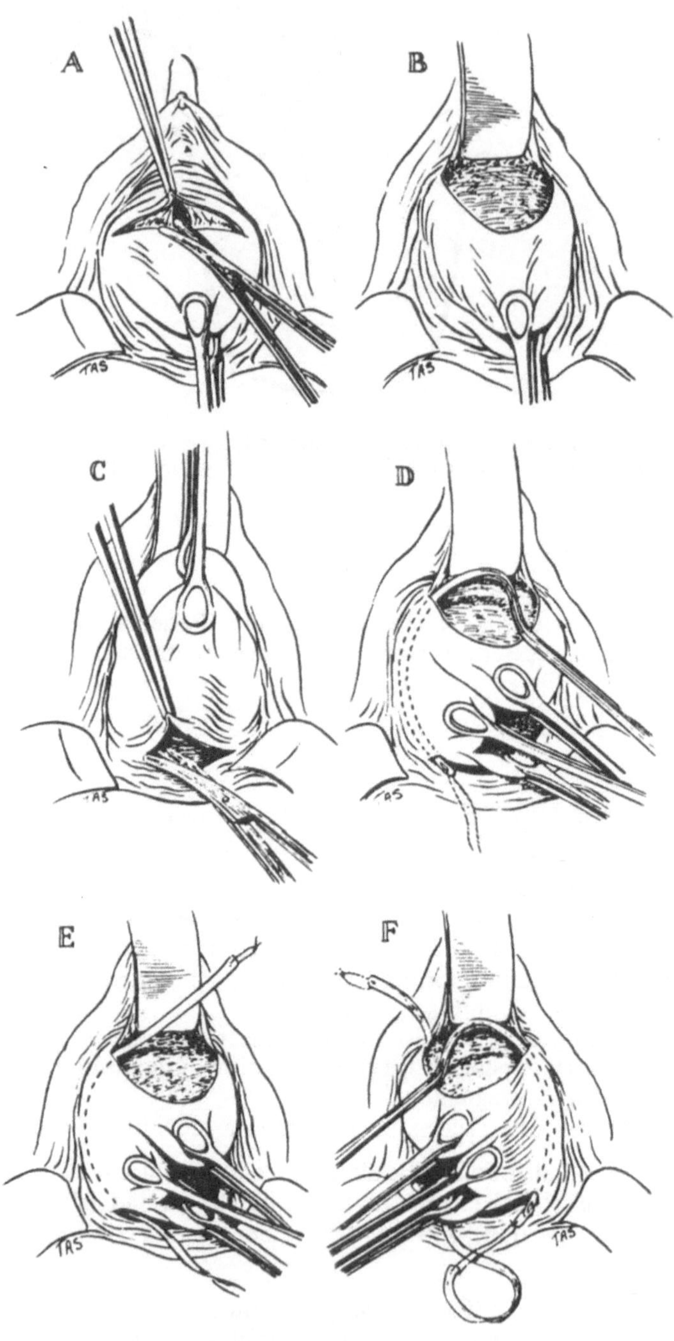
A
B
C
D
E
F
TAS
TAS
TAS
TAS
TAS
TAS

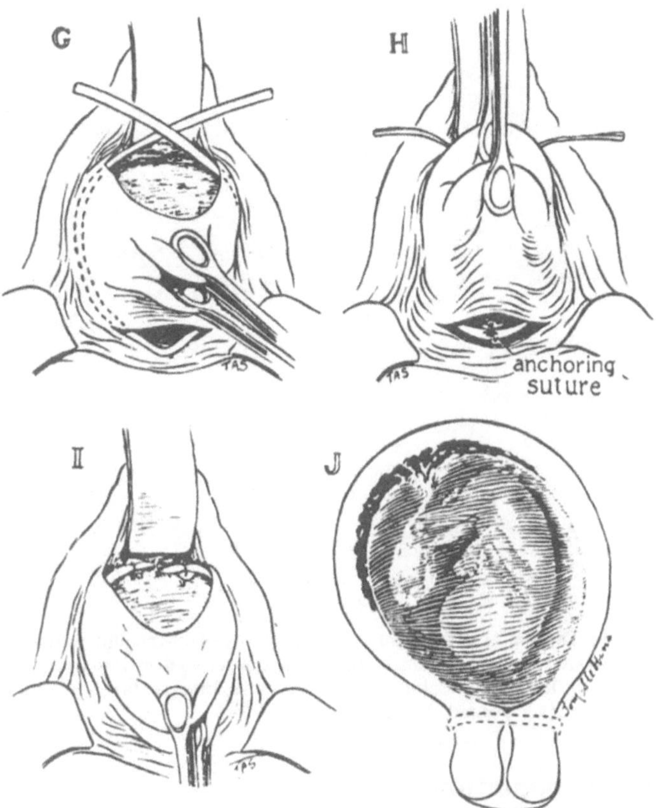

Figure 25.2 A, the anterior vaginal mucosa is being opened transversely by scissors dissection. B, The bladder has been advanced to the level of the internal os of the cervix. C, The posterior vaginal mucosa is being opened transversely 5 cm (2 inches) above the external os. D, The special aneurysm needle has been passed through the anterior incision, under the vaginal mucosa, and out through the incision in the posterior mucosa. The fascial strip is now attached to the needle. E, One end of the fascial strip has been drawn out through the anterior mucosal incision on the right side of the cervix. F, The other aneurysm needle has been passed through the anterior mucosal incision, under the vaginal mucosa, and has emerged through the posterior incision. The other end of the fascial strip has been attached to the needle by means of a silk suture. G, The fascial strip now completely encircles the cervix. H, The fascial strip is anchored to the posterior cervix by a silk suture, to prevent the fascial graft from slipping over the posterior lip of the cervix. I, The fascial strip has been pulled tightly around the cervix, tied, and sutured to the anterior cervix. J, Diagram showing the level at which the fascial strip should lie at the conclusion of the operation (Barter *et al.*, 1958).

In present practice the fascia lata is being replaced by 5 mm Mersilene band. The knot is tied posteriorly instead of anteriorly.

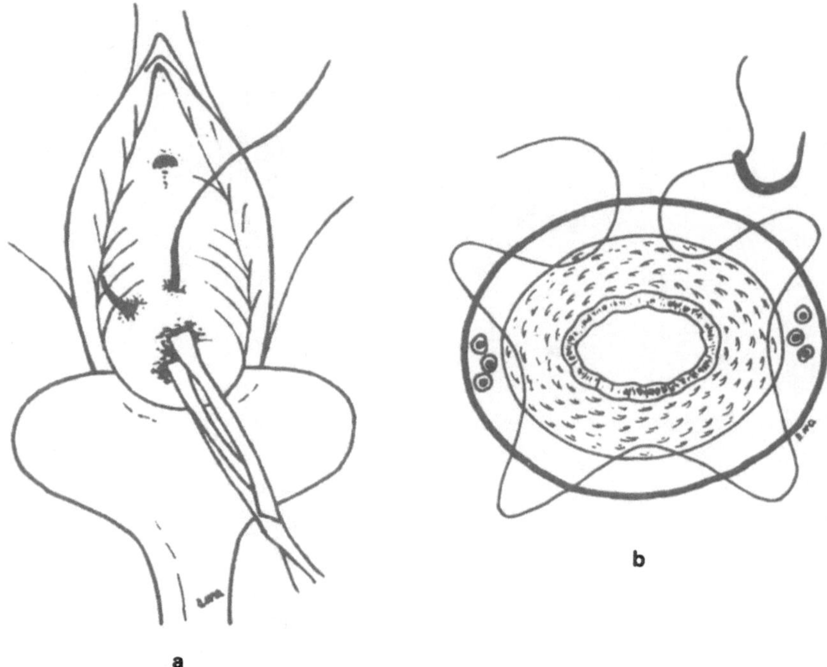

Figure 25.3 **a**, McDonald's suture. A purse string ligature of 4 Mersiline commences in front of the cervix at the cervicovaginal junction. **b**, The suture is inserted deep into the musculature of the cervix and underruns the blood vessels laterally. Four or five bites are taken. A knot is made firmly in front of the cervix (McDonald, 1980).

Timing of the operation

The optimal time of surgery is between the 12th and the 16th week of pregnancy. The reasons for this are:

(1) exclusion of the spontaneous abortions of the first trimester,
(2) greater placental hormonal activity which makes the ovum sound, and
(3) easier surgical performance from the practical point of view (Robboy, 1973; Kaskeralis, 1976).

Cerclage may be done late or on an emergent basis between the 16th and the 26th week because of:

(1) when probability of cervical incompetence was known, but for some reason, no treatment was done,
(2) an alarming shortening or opening of the cervix without any previous history of similar occurrence, and without any apparent contractions,
(3) threatened premature birth with uterine hypercontractility and shortening of the cervix as soon as the acute phase is controlled,
(4) placenta praevia because of tissue loss and weakness of the cervix (Henry-Suchet, 1977), or

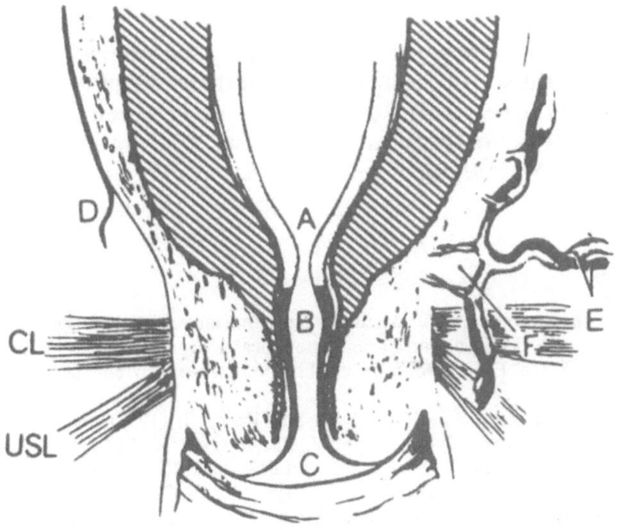

Figure 25.4 Anatomy of the uterine cervicoisthmic junction. Hatched zone depicts arrangement of smooth muscle, most of which is in the corpus and the isthmus. The stippled area represents endometrium, and the dark zone is cervical glandular tissue. In the region of the internal os (A) there is a junction (i.e., the isthmus), between the predominantly muscular tissue of the corpus uteri and the predominantly fibrous tissue of the cervix. There is no constant relationship between the position of the internal os. (4). The endocervical-endometrial junction (histologic internal os) (B) and the fibromuscular junction (C) indicate the external cervical os; D, the peritoneal reflection; E, the uterine artery and vein; and F, the 'free space' for placement of the Mersilene band in the cervicouterine vasculature near the isthmus. CL is the cardinal ligament; USL is the uterosacral ligament. (Modified from Novy, M. J. (1982). Managing reproductive failure by transabdominal isthmic cerclage. *Contemp. Obstet. Gynecol.*, **10**, 17.

(5) twin or multiple birth especially after use of gonadotropins (Henry-Suchet, 1977).

Aftercare

The patient remains in the hospital for at least 5 days. It is noticed (McDonald, 1980) that failure occurs most likely in the first few days. Apart from routine narcotic analgesics, broad spectrum antibiotics are provided for 5 days. Ambulation is encouraged before the patient is discharged. Uterine muscle relaxants, i.e. progesterone (Savarese and Chang, 1964), isoxuprine (Jennings, 1972), alcohol (Seppälä and Vara, 1970) and ephedrine (Smith and Seragg, 1969) may be administered to inhibit uterine contractions. β-Sympathomimetic drugs such as salbutamol and orciprenaline are recommended in cases when cervical effacement has commenced. Patients are kept under close observation and are examined biweekly with speculum and careful palpation. If the ligature seems to be cutting through, it is easily removed and replaced with little trauma. When the pregnancy is progressing normally, the ligature is divided at 38 weeks of maturity.

Mode of delivery

Most patients with cervical cerclage deliver by the vaginal route. A fibrotic ring may form at the site of the ligature, but it rarely seems to be an obstacle to full dilatation of the cervix. If a cesarean section has been made, a shirodkar suture may be left *in situ* for future pregnancies. If an abdominal ligature has been inserted, a lower segment cesarean section may be difficult.

References

Ásplund (1952). The uterine cervix and isthmus under normal and pathological conditions; *Acta Radiol. (Suppl.)*, **91**, 3 Clinical and roentgenological study.
Baden, W. F. and Baden, E. E. (1960). Cervical incompetence: Current therapy. *Am. J. Obstet. Gynecol.*, **79**, 545
Barter, R. H., Dusbabek, J. A., Riva, H. L. and Parks, J. (1958). Surgical closure of the incompetent cervix during pregnancy. *Am. J. Obstet. Gynecol.*, **75**, 511
Barter, R. H., Dusbabek, J. A., Tyndal, C. M. and Erkenbek, R. V. (1963). Further experiences with the Shirodkar operation. *Am. J. Obstet. Gynecol.*, **85**, 792
Bayer, H. (1977). Einige neue Gesichtspunkte bei der Prophylaxe und Therapie der drohenden. Fruhgeburt. *Zentralbl. Gynaekol.*, **99**, 547
Bergman, P. and Svennerund, S. (1957). Traction test for demonstrating incompetence of the internal os of the cervix. *Int. J. Fertil.*, **2**, 163
Brook, I., Feingold, M., Schwartz, A. and Zakut, H. (1981). Ullrasonography in the diagnosis of cervical incompetence in pregnancy – a new diagnostic approach. *Br. J. Obstet. Gynaecol.*, **88**, 640
Cousins, L. (1980). Cervical incompetence, 1980: A time for reappraisal. *Clin. Obstet. Gynecol.*, **23**, 467
Craig, C. J. T. (1973). Congenital anomalies of the uterus and foetal wastage. *S. Afr. Med. J.*, **47**, 2000
Danforth, D. W. and Buckingham, J. C. (1962).Cervical incompetence: A re-evaluation. *Postgrad. Med.*, **32**, 345
Dennerstein, G. J. (1971). Multiple pregnancy and cervical ligation with a case report of triplets. *Aust. NZ J. Obstet. Gynaecol.*, **2**, 51
Dumont, M. and Poizat, C. (1974). Etude d'un coefficient d'appréciation de la béance cervico-isthmique. A propos de 50 observations de béances traitées par cerclage. *J. Gynecol. Obst. Biol. Reprod.*, **3**, 981
Fisher, J. J. (1951). The effect of amputation of the cervix uteri upon subsequent parturition: preliminary report of 7 cases. *Am. J. Obstet. Gynecol.*, **62**, 644
Forster, F. M. (1967). Abortion and the incompetent cervix. *Med. J. Aust.*, **2**, 807
Gibbs, C. E. (1973). Diagnosis and treatment of uterine conditions that cause prematurity. *Clin. Obstet. Gynecol.*, **16**, 159
Gream, G. T. (1865). Dilation or division of the cervix uteri. *Lancet*, **1**, 381
Hefner, J. D., Patow, W. E. and Ludwig, J. M. (1961). A new surgical procedure for the correction of the incompetent cervix during pregnancy: The Wurm Procedure. *Obstet. Gynecol.*, **18**, 616
Heinonen, O. P., Slone, D., Monson, R. R., Hook, E. B. and Sahpiro, S. (1977). Cardiovascular birth defects and antenatal exposure to female sex hormones. *N. Engl. J. Med.*, **296**, 67
Hendrickx, A. G., Benirschke, K., Thompson, R. S., Ahern, J. K., Lucas, W. E. and Oi, R. (1979). The effects of prenatal diethylstilbestrol (DES) exposure on the genitalia of pubertal Macaca mulatta female offspring. *J. Reprod. Med.*, **22**, 233
Herbst, A. L. (ed.) (1978). *Intrauterine Exposure to Diethylstilbestrol in the Human: Proceedings of Symposium on DES, 1977 Annual Clinical Meeting of the ACOG.* (Washington: American College of Obstetricians and Gynecologists)
Hulka, J. F. *et al.* (1974). *Am. J. Obstet. Gynecol.*, **120**, 166
Javert, C. T. (1962). Further follow up on habitual abortion patients. *Am. J. Obstet. Gynecol.*, **84**, 1149

Jennings, C. L. (1972). Temporary submucosal cerclage for cervical incompetence: Report of 48 cases. *Am. J. Obstet. Gynecol.*, **113,** 1097

Johnstone, F. D., Beard, R. J., Boyd, I. E. and McCarthy, T. G. (1976). Cervical diameter after suction termination of pregnancy. *Br. Med. J.*, **1,** 68

Kaskarelis, D., Lolis, D., Papthanassiou, Z. and Michalas, S. (1976). Management of cervical incompetence with cerclage according to Shirodkar: A report on 110 cases. *Acta Eur. Fertil.*, **7,** 89

Kuhn, R. J. P. and Pepperell, R. J. (1977). Cervical ligation: a review of 242 pregnancies. *Aust. NZ. J. Obstet. Gynaecol.*, **17,** 79

Lash, A. F. (1960*a*). Fertility and reproduction following repair of the incompetent internal os of the cervix. *Fertil. Steril.*, **11,** 531

Lash, A. F. (1960*b*). Incompetent internal os of the cervix: diagnosis and treatment. *Am. J. Obstet. Gynecol.*, **79,** 552

Lash, A. F. and Lash, S. R. (1950). Habitual abortion: The incompetent internal os of the cervix. *Am. J. Obstet. Gynecol.*, **59,** 68

Lees, D. H. and Sutherst, J. R. (1974). The sequelae of cervical trasum. *Am. J. Obstet. Gynecol.*, **120,** 1050

McDonald, I. A. (1957). Suture of the cervix for inevitable miscarriage. *J. Obstet. Gynaecol. Br. Em.*, **64,** 346

McDonald, I. A. (1978). Incompetence of the cervix. *Aust. NZ J. Obstet. Gynaecol.*, **18,** 34

McDonald, I. A. (1980). Cervical cerclage. *Clin. Obstet. Gynaecol.*, **7,** 461

McLaren, H. C., Jordan, J. A. Glover, M. and Attwood, M. E. (1974). Pregnancy after cone biopsy of cervix. *J. Obstet. Gynaecol. Br. Commonw.*, **81,** 383

Moinian, M. and Andersch, B. (1982). Does cervix conization increase the risk of complications in subsequent pregnancy? *Acta Obstet. Gynecol. Scand.*, **61,** 101

Naver E. (1968). The incompetent cervix and its treatment in habitual abortion and premature labour. *Acta Obstet. Gynecol. Scand.*, **47,** 314

Nishijima, S. (1969). Antepartum cervical cerclage operations. *Am. J. Obstet. Gynecol.*, **104L,** 273

Nora, J. J., Nora, A. H., Blu, J., Ingram, J., Fountain, A., Peterson, M., Lortscher, R. H. and Kimberling, W. J. (1978). Exogenous progestogen and estrogen implicated in birth defects. *J. Am. Med. Assoc.*, **240,** 837

Novy, M. J. (1982). Transabdominal cervicoisthmic cerclage for the management of repetitive abortion and premature delivery. *Am. J. Obstet. Gynecol.*, **143, 44**

Olatunbosum, O. E. and Dyck, F. (1981). Cervical cerclage operation for a dilated cervix. *Obstet. Gynecol.*, **57,** 166

Orr, C. (1973). An aid to cervical cerclage. *Aust. NZ J. Obstet. Gynaecol.*, **13,** 114

Oster, S and Javert, C. T. (1966). Treatment of the incompetent cervix with the Hodge pessary. *Obstet. Gynecol.*, **28,** 206

Palmer, R. (1961). Eighty-one operations for repeated abortions due to incompetent isthmus. *Bull. Fed. Soc. Gynecol. Obstet. Fr.*, **13,** 328

Palmer, R. and Lacomme, M. (1948). La béance de l'orifice interne, cause d'avortements à repetition? Une observation de déchirure cervico-isthmique réparée chirurgicalement, avec gestation à terme consecutive. *Gynecol. Obstet.*, **47,** 905

Peterson, P. G. and Keifer, W. S. (1973). Diagnosis of an incompetent internal cervical os. *Am. J. Obstet. Gynecol.*, **116,** 498

Picot, H., Thompson, H. G. and Murphy, C. J. (1959). A consideration of the incompetent cervix. *Am. J. Obstet. Gynecol.*, **78,** 786

Ranney, B. (1963). Congenital cervical incompetence in primigravidas. *Am. J. Obstet. Gynecol.*, **86,** 52

Raphael, S. I., Thompson, H. G. and Murphy, C. S. (1958). Surgical treatment of the incompetent cervix in pregnancy. *Obstet. Gynecol.*, **12,** 269

Ritter, H. A. (1978). Surgical closure of the incompetent cervix: 15 years experience. *Int. J. Gynaecol. Obstet.*, **16,** 194

Robboy, M. S. (1973). The management of cervical incompetence. *Obstet. Gynecol.*, **41,** 108

Roddick, J. W., Buckingham, J. C. C. and Danforth, D. N. (1961). The muscular cervix: cause of incompetency in pregnancy. *Obstet. Gynecol.*, **17,** 562

Rorie, D. K. and Newton, M. (1967). Histological and chemical studies of the smooth muscle in the human cervix and uterus. *Am. J. Obstet. Gynecol.*, **99,** 466

Sarti, D. A., Sampke, W. F., Hobel, C. J. and Staisch, K. J. (1979). Ultrasonic visualization of a dilated cervix during pregnancy. *Radiology*, **130,** 417

Seppälä, M. and Vara, P. (1970). Cervical cerclage in the treatment of incompetent cervix. *Acta Obstet. Gynecol. Scand.*, **49,** 343

Sherman, A. I. (1966). Hormonal therapy for control of the incompetent os of pregnancy. *Obstet. Gynecol.*, **28,** 198

Shirodkar, V. N. (1955). A method of operative treatment for habitual abortions in the second trimester of pregnancy. *Antiseptic*, **52,** 299

Smith, S. G. and Seragg, W. H. (1969). Premature cervical dilatation and the McDonald cerclage. *Obstet. Gynecol.*, **33,** 535

Soihet, S. (1974). Surgical treatment in the incompetent internal os. In *Recent Advances in Human Reproduction*, p. 258. (Amsterdam: Excerpta Medica)

Strand, A. (1963). Isthmicocervical insufficiency as the cause of late abortion. *Nordisk Med.*, **69,** 103

Stromme, W. B. and Haywa, E. W. (1963). Intrauterine fetal death in the second trimester. *Am. J. Obstet. Gynecol.*, **85,** 223

Toaff, R. and Toaff, M. E. (1974). Diagnosis of impending late abortion. *Obstet. Gynecol.*, **43,** 756

Toaff, R. and Toaff, M. E. (1977). Cervical incompetence: diagnostic and therapeutic aspects. *Isr. J. Med. Sci.*, **13,** 39

Trythall, S. M. and Jeremias, R. C. (1961). Congenital inadequacy of the lower uterine segment as a cause of habitual abortion. *Int. J. Fertil.*, **6,** 67

Vitsky, M. (1961). Simple treatment of the incompetent os. *Am. J. Obstet. Gynecol.*, **81,** 1194

Vitsky, M. (1963). The incompetent cervical os and pessary. *Am. J. Obstet. Gynecol.*, **87,** 144

Vitsky, M. (1968). Pessary treatment of the incompetent cervical os. *Obstet. Gynecol.*, **31,** 732

Vogel, E. H. (1972). Electrocautery in the treatment of incompetent cervix. *Obstet. Gynecol.*, **39,** 27

Watkins, R. A. (1972). Transabdominal cervico-uterine suture. *Aust. NZ J. Obstet. Gynaecol.*, **12,** 62

Weingold, A. G., Palmer, J. I. and Stone, M. I. (1968). Cervical incompetence: A therapeutic enigma. *Fertil. Steril.*, **19,** 244

Youssef, A. F. (1958). The uterine isthmus and its sphincter mechanism. A radiographic study. *Am. J. Obstet. Gynecol.*, **75,** 1305

26
Management of the incompetent uterine cervix: a modified technique

B. COUTIFARIS and C. COUTIFARIS

It is well recognized that a significant percentage of second trimester habitual spontaneous abortions are due to incompetence of the internal os of the uterine cervix. This weakness of the internal cervical os appears to be due either to previous trauma (i.e. cervical laceration; multiple therapeutic abortions) or some congenital anatomic anomaly. The usual clinical presentation involves the slow, painless dilatation and effacement of the cervix with advancing gestational age and a sensation of lower abdominal pressure on the part of the patient. This slowly occurring series of events eventually leads to premature rupture of membranes and fetal wastage.

Cervical incompetence as a pathologic entity was first recognized in the early fifties (Lash and Lash, 1950) and several procedures for its correction have been described. The undisputed success of the cerclage operation during pregnancy as initially described by Shirodkar (1955) resulted in a flurry of modifications of the procedure around the world (McDonald, 1957; Barter *et al.*, 1958; Picot *et al.*, 1958; Stromme *et al.*, 1960). With the exception of the McDonald cerclage operation all other procedures involve extensive manipulation of the cervix and significant, usually bloody, surgical dissection of the cervical mucosa and bladder flap, thus increasing the risk of intraoperative and postoperative complications.

In the years since 1957, 551 cerclage operations were performed for the treatment of cervical incompetence according to the modified technique introduced and popularized in Greece by one of us (B.C.). The first successful case report in Greece was presented to the Hellenic Obstetrical Society in 1958 and, interestingly, involved an American woman residing in Greece who had experienced repeated second trimester fetal losses. The initial series of results of the procedure were reported in 1961 (Coutifaris and Theofanidis, 1961) and its effectiveness has withstood the test of time (Coutifaris *et al.*, 1972, 1982). The procedure is relatively simple and fast in its execution, involves no colpotomy or repulsion of the bladder, inflicts minimal (if any) damage to the cervix, has no significant blood loss and minimizes the danger of complications secondary to operative manipulations.

Of the total 551 cases, 319 were investigated, involving 264 pregnant women who complied with the experimental protocol and agreed to participate in the study. Fourty-five women had a cerclage placed during *two* consecutive pregnancies and five women underwent the procedure during *three* pregnancies. In the majority of the women the diagnosis of cervical incompetence was made in the non-gravid state by hysterosalpingography (129 patients), passage of a Hegar No. 8 dilator (79 patients), or by a characteristic obstetrical history (30 patients). In only 26 patients was the diagnosis made during an ongoing pregnancy with the recognition of premature cervical dilatation. It appears that most patients studied had experienced prior surgical manipulation of their cervix, with over half (146 patients) having undergone (often multiple) therapeutic abortions. Obvious uterine anatomic anomalies were evident in only eight women and no history of diethylstilbestrol exposure *in utero* was elicited in any of the patients. Forty of the 319 cerclage operations were emergency cases due to the unexpected premature cervical dilatation that occurred in these women who had no previous history suggestive of the condition of incompetent cervix or those who presented to the obstetrician for the first time at the time of diagnosis.

The surgical procedure is performed under general anesthesia and while the patient is in Trendelenberg in the dorsolithotomy position. The operative steps are graphically presented in Figure 26.1 (A–F). Over the years the suture material used for the ligature has changed: early on, silver wire or multiple strands of heavy silk suture were used, but at present, Mersilene is the suture material of choice. A large, atraumatic needle is employed for placement of the cerclage through the cervical submucosal tissue. Endocervical cultures are routinely obtained at the time of operation. The postoperative course involves bed rest in the hospital for 2 days and if complications do not arise the patient is discharged on the third postoperative day. Use of hormonal therapy (progesterone) or tocolytics is not routine, but is often employed when uterine irritability is observed following the surgical procedure. If no subsequent complications arise the cerclage is removed at term (37 weeks) or if active labor refractory to tocolytic therapy ensues. After its removal the ligature is always sent for culture since, more often than not, positive stitch cultures have been accompanied by negative endocervical cultures. If premature rupture of membranes occurs the mode of delivery (vaginal vs Cesarean section) is decided in consultation with the pediatricians to ensure minimal trauma to the premature infant. It should not be forgotten that these pregnant women have suffered multiple fetal losses in the past and thus are psychologically less prepared to face a possibly damaged baby. In such cases, oftentimes cesarean section has been chosen as the preferred mode of delivery.

Figure 26.2 shows the week of gestation the cerclage operation was performed in the 319 cases investigated, and Table 26.1 shows the results of the operation as compared to the outcome of a total of 829 pregnancies of the same patients prior to cerclage placement. Of significance is the decrease of second trimester spontaneous abortions from a rate of 62% to just 10% after cerclage placement, with a concomitant dramatic increase of term pregnancies (> 37 weeks) in these women from an 18% to an 82% overall rate. These results are further punctuated by the significant increase in viable neonates from a low 22% to an 85% rate after cerclage placement (Table 26.2). These

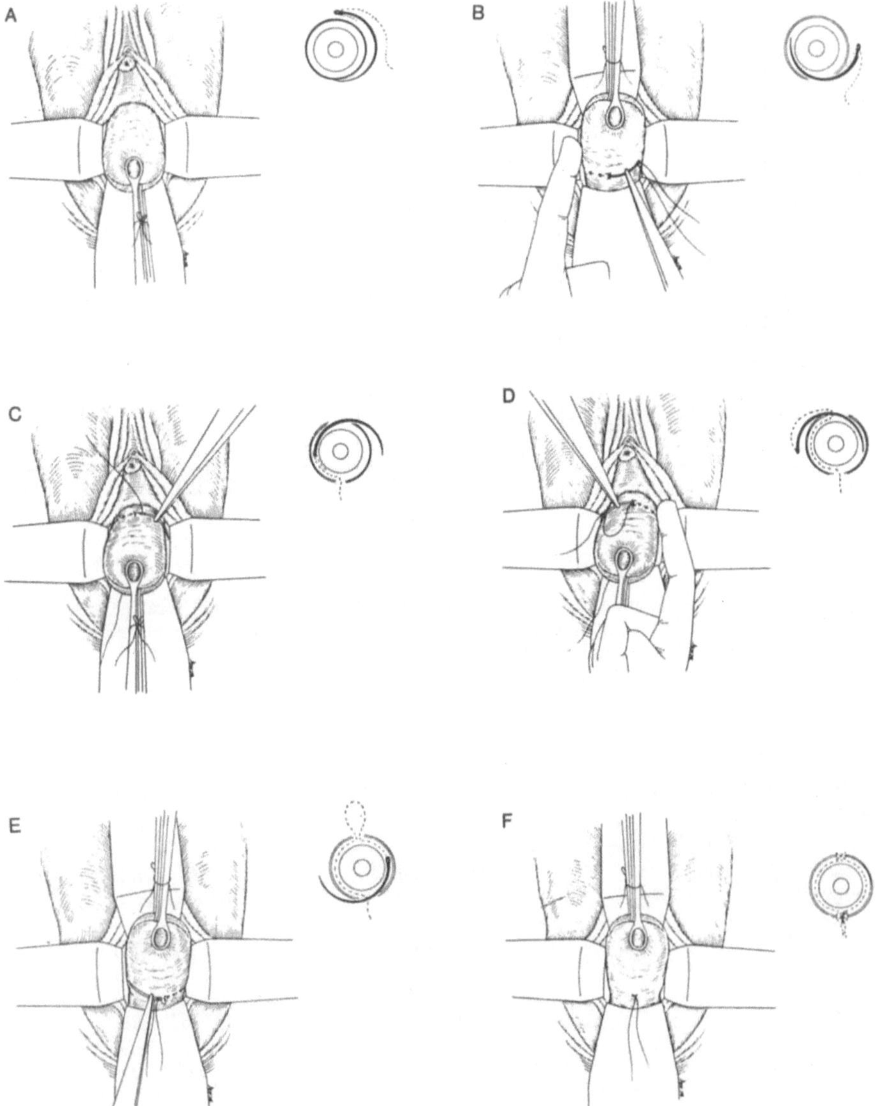

Figure 26.1 Schematic presentation of the technique for cervical cerclage. **A**, The anterior and posterior lips of the uterine cervix are grasped with two ring forceps. The forceps are held together with silk suture. **B**, Insertion of large, curved, atraumatic needle and suture at the level corresponding to the internal cervical os at the 6 o'clock position. Threading of the needle and suture through the submucosal tissue in a clockwise motion under the guidance of the index finger of the surgeon's other hand. **C**, Exit of needle at the 12 o'clock position. **D**, New insertion of the needle at the 12 o'clock position and threading of the needle and suture through the submucosal tissue in a clockwise motion. This is again achieved under control of the surgeon's index finger. **E**, Exit of the needle at the 6 o'clock position at the site of the primary insertion. **F**, Suture threads are apposed and tied together.

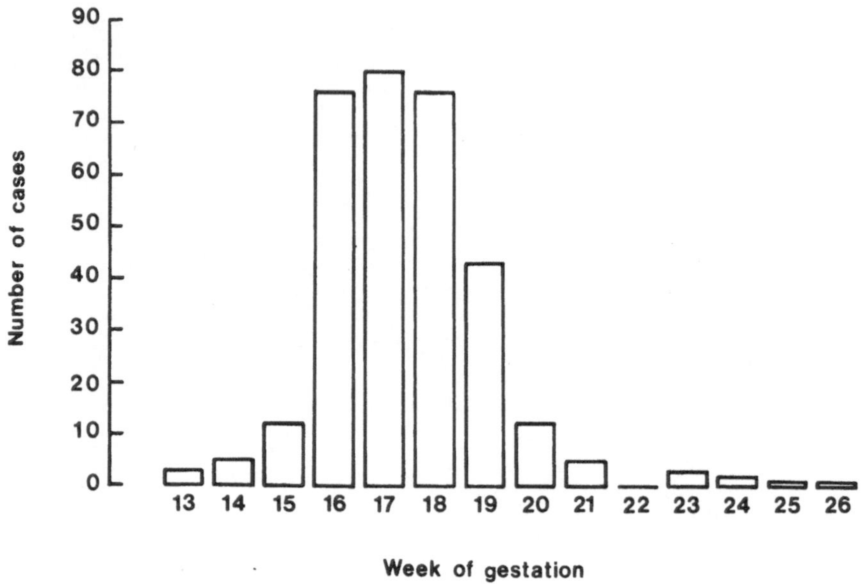

Figure 26.2 Schematic presentation of the number of cases of cervical cerclage performed during each week of gestation. (Total number of cerclages: 319; number of cerclages performed between the 16th and 18th week: 232).

Table 26.1 Duration of pregnancies in 264 women before and after placement of cervical cerclage

Duration of pregnancy (weeks)	*Before cerclage* *Pregnancies* (%)	*After cerclage* *Pregnancies* (%)
25	513 (62)	32 (10)
26–31	114 (14)	9 (3)
32–36	51 (6)	16 (5)
37	151 (18)	262 (82)
Total	829 100%	319 100%

Table 26.2 Fetal salvage rate before and after cervical cerclage placement

Neonates	*Before cerclage* *Babies* (%)	*After cerclage* *Babies* (%)
Non-viable	647 (78)	48 (15)
Viable	185 (22)	274 (85)

results compare favorably with the results from different types of cerclage procedures as reported by others (Seppälä and Vara, 1970; Lauersen and Fuchs, 1973; Hohlweg-Majert *et al.*, 1976; Fahmy, 1978; Goldstein, 1978). McDonald's initial report (1957) presented a 47% fetal salvage rate, but in his long series of 248 cases (McDonald, 1978) the success rate for term pregnancies was 94%.

The success rate for carrying pregnancies to term after emergency cerclage placement in women who presented with premature cervical dilatation and effacement with already visible (often bulging) membranes was only 57%. This is comparable to a 47% success rate reported by Fahmy (1978) in a series of similar emergency cases. It appears that cervical effacement with distension of the lower uterine segment might contribute to the failure of the cerclage to prevent the spontaneous abortions in these cases. This possibility is strengthened by the observation that in the present series the maximal success rate was observed when the cerclage was placed on the 16th week of gestation (90%) and it sharply decreased below 84% if the ligature was placed after the 19th week. In most cases performed after this gestational age, anatomic changes (effacement, lower uterine segment distension) were quite evident at the time of operation. These observations are in agreement with Robboy's study (1973) that showed a sharp decline in the success rate of the operation when this was performed on or after the 20th week of gestation.

Operative and postoperative complications in the present series of cases were rare (< 1%): there were two cases of rupture of membranes in the immediate postoperative period and there was one case of sepsis that became evident on the third postoperative day.

As to the question of the optimal gestational age for the placement of the cerclage, it appears that differing opinions are found in the literature. Hofmeister *et al.* (1968) and Cousins (1980) suggest that the cerclage be placed at 12–14 weeks of gestation; Occla and Lesinski (1967) and Hohlweg-Majert (1974) prefer the 14–16 week period and Stromme *et al.* (1961) advocate the 16–18 week period. The present results agree with the latter recommendation of 16–18 weeks and, at least for the present series, the 16th week was optimal producing a success rate for term pregnancy of 90%.

In summary, in this chapter, an attempt has been to present an alternative cervical cerclage technique that has been performed in Greece for over 25 years. Despite its simplicity and time efficiency, this technique has proven effective and just as successful as other commonly employed operative procedures for the management of the incompetent uterine cervix during pregnancy.

References

Barter, R. H., Dusbabek, J. A., Riva, H. L. and Parks, J. (1958). Surgical closure of the incompetent cervix during pregnancy. *Am. J. Obstet. Gynecol.*, **75**, 511

Cousins, L. (1980). Cervical incompetence 1980: A time for reappraisal. *Clin. Obstet. Gynecol.*, **23**, 467

Coutifaris, B., Chryssikopoulos, A. and Gnafakis, N. (1972). Current theories, results and treatment of cervical incompetence. Presented at *IIId European Conference on Fertility and Sterility*, Athens, Greece

Coutifaris, B., Chryssikopoulos, A., Vitoratos, N. and Kapatanakis, E. (1982). Cervical incompetence: Statistical results by Coutifaris' technique modified. Presented at *International Conference on Fertility and Sterility*, Honolulu, Hawaii

Coutifaris, B. and Theofanidis, K. (1961). Cervical incompetence. *Hellenic Obstet. Gynecol.*, **10**, 198

Fahmy, K. (1978). A close submucous cervical suture for the incompetent cervix. *Int. Surg.*, **63**, 77

Goldstein, D. P. (1978). Incompetent cervix in offspring to diethyl stilbestrol in utero. *Obstet. Gynecol.*, **52** (Suppl.), 73s

Hofmeister, F. J., Schwartz, W. R., Vondrak, B. F. and Martens, W. (1968). Suture reinforcement of the incompetent cervix. *Am. J. Obstet. Gynecol.*, **101**, 58

Hohlweg-Majert, P. (1974). Prophylaktische and Therapeutish zervixcerclage an der uni-frauenklinik Mannheim in der Jahren 1965–1973. *Geburtsh. Frauenheilk.*, **34**, 1047

Hohlweg-Majert, V. P., Taglieber, J. and Grumbtecht, C. (1976). Die zervix insuffizienz. *Fortschr. Med.*, **27**, 1443

Lash, A. F. and Lash, S. R. (1950). The incompetent internal os of the cervix. *Am. J. Obstet. Gynecol.*, **59**, 68

Lauersen, N. and Fuchs, F. (1973). Experience with Shirodkar's operation and postoperative alcohol treatment. *Acta Obstet. Gynecol. Scand.*, **52**, 77

McDonald, I. (1957). Suture of the cervix for inevitable miscarriage. *J. Obstet. Gynaecol. Br. Commonw.*, **64**, 346

McDonald, I. (1978). Incompetence of the cervix. *Aust. NZ J. Obstet. Gynaecol.*, **18**, 34

Occla, J. and Lesinski, J. (1967). Shirodkar's procedure in cervical incompetence. *Am. J. Obstet. Gynecol.*, **97**, 13

Picot, H., Thompson, H. C. and Murphy, C. J. (1958). Surgical treatment of the incompetent cervix in pregnancy. *Obstet. Gynecol.*, **12**, 269

Robboy, M. (1973). The management of cervical incompetence. *Obstet. Gynecol.*, **41**, 108

Seppälä, M. and Vara, P. (1970). Cervical cerclage in the treatment of incompetent cervix. A retrospective analysis of the indications and results of 164 operations. *Acta Obstet. Gynecol. Scand.*, **49**, 343

Shirodkar, U. N. (1955). A new method of operative treatment for habitual abortions in the second trimester of pregnancy. *Antiseptic*, **52**, 299

Stromme, W. B., Wagner, R. M. and Haywa, E. W. (1961). Incompetent cervix. *Minnesota Med.*, **49**, 393

Stromme, W. B., Wagner, R. M. and Reed, S. C. (1960). Surgical management of the incompetent cervix. *Obstet. Gynecol.*, **15**, 635

27
Immunological factors in spontaneous abortion

O. KANDIL, Z. EL-SHEIKHA, T. EL-MEKKAWI and M. MOUSA

The immunology of the materno-fetal relationship goes in a manner contravening the principles of transplantation immunity, i.e. the fetus receives passive immunity from its mother while developing its immune competence. The mother maintains her own abilities though not rejecting the trophoblast and placenta, which do not act as a complete tissue barrier and act in certain situations as a filter allowing the passage of potentially antigenic material between the mother and the fetus.

Antigenicity increases significantly during the second and third trimesters and continues to exert its effect during the postpartum period (Taylor *et al.*, 1976).

MATERNAL IMMUNE RESPONSE IN PREGNANCY

In normal pregnancy there is a maternal immune response to trophoblastic antigens that involves both cell-mediated and humoral factors (Hellestrom *et al.*, 1969; Youtananukorn and Matangkasombut, 1972; Maroni and Parrott, 1973; Kandil *et al.*, 1980). The fetus is known to inherit histocompatibility antigens from the father as well as from the mother. Thus, the fetus is antigenically foreign to the mother and may be considered as an allograft from the point of view of transplantation immunity (Han, 1974). Pregnancy has been considered as a very successful homotransplant. Various theories, including that of a physiological barrier between the mother and the fetus, anatomical separation of the fetus from the mother, antigenic immaturity of the fetus and immunological inertness of the mother, have been postulated (Nelson, 1965; Billingham, 1964; Anderson, 1971).

The maternal immunological unresponsiveness indicates depression of both the cell mediated and humoral immunity (Anderson, 1971; Kandil *et al.*, 1980, 1981). The mother is exposed to low doses of fetal and paternal antigens. This may occur at the placental interface or by trophoblastic deportation. Fetal lymphocytes cross the placenta in several species and are a potential source of histocompatibility antigens. Low grade antigenic exposure from the above sources either bypasses antigen processing mechanisms or provokes a weak humoral antibody response, but there is no true transplantation immunity. The efferent immune response mediated by these events may be either immunological tolerance or immunological enhancement.

In man, there is evidence for specific maternal, but not paternal, tolerance to skin grafts from offspring. The mixed lymphocytic reaction (MLR) between maternal and paternal or maternal and fetal lymphocytes is depressed compared with that between maternal cells and those from unrelated individuals (Jones, 1978).

EVIDENCE FOR ENHANCEMENT IN HUMAN PREGNANCY

The presence of factors in maternal serum which block cellular immunity directed against paternal and fetal lymphocytes was detected by Jenkins and Hancock (1972). Antibodies have been eluted from human placental homogenates, which could fulfil a blocking role (Bonneau *et al.*, 1973). *In vitro* cytotoxic action of maternal lymphocytes on trophoblast could be blocked by immunoglobulin fraction of the maternal serum (Taylor and Hancock, 1975). IgG is present in the placental villous stroma, particularly in vessel walls and the trophoblastic basement membrane (McCormick *et al.*, 1971). IgG obtained by acid elution of extensively washed human placental tissue homogenates was found to inhibit *in vitro* assays of lymphocyte reactivity (Faulk *et al.*, 1974). IgG is the main factor in the mechanism of non-rejection of the fetus by the mother. The blocking factors are important for the survival of the fetus in which the IgG is implicated (Rocklin *et al.*, 1976).

Immunological aspect of unexplained spontaneous abortion

In pregnancy, the lymphocyte reactivity to antigenic stimuli has revealed a weak cell-mediated response attributable wholly or partly to maternal serum factor or to a deficiency of responsive lymphocytes (Gatti, 1971; Kasakura, 1971; Purtilo *et al.*, 1972; Leikin, 1972; Smith *et al.*, 1972). There is a serum inhibitor factor whose nature or mode of action is not clearly understood. It was proposed that this inhibitory factor coats the leukocytes, rendering them poor responders to standard plasma (Kasakura and Jenkins, 1974). It is defined as a blocking factor present during pregnancy and may be relevant to the survival of fetal allograft (Yu *et al.*, 1975). Absence of this factor in maternal serum resulted in a high rate of spontaneous abortion in patients (Rocklin *et al.*, 1976).

Circulating antibody (blocking antibody) raised in response to paternal antigens provides protection against attack by maternal lymphocytes (Glass and Globus, 1978). Women with a history of habitual abortion lack appreciable levels of blocking factor found in the serum of normal multiparous women. Those with a history of recurrent abortion reject skin graft from their husbands in an accelerated fashion (Bardawil *et al.*, 1962). Fibrinoid and hyaline degeneration in villi of a majority of placentae resulted in spontaneous and habitual abortions (Gray, 1956, 1957). These could be attributed to the passage of placenta metabolic products to the mother's circulation stimulating antibody response. A portion of this antibody is absorbed by antigen in the maternal tissues and serum and the remaining free antibody reacts with the antigen-producing placental cells, thus leading to the specific pathological changes in the placenta.

The presence or absence of non-specific inhibitor normally present and known to exist in other immunological diseases had to be sought in spontaneous abortions. This non-specific inhibitor is part of the normal mechanisms regulating the immunological balance by blocking the pathogenicity of the antigen–antibody reaction, and indeed the absence of such an inhibitor has been demonstrated in the sera of the majority of spontaneous abortions. Using the macrophages migration inhibition test *in vitro*, it was found that women with recurrent abortion lacked a blocking factor present in the serum of multiparous women who had successful pregnancies (Rocklin *et al.*, 1978). It seems difficult to attribute abortion solely to immunologic factors, when up to 60% of conceptuses spontaneously aborted are chromosomally abnormal. It is possible that the presence of blocking factor is simply the result rather than the cause of successful pregnancies. The development of immunologic enhancement depends on such variables as the strength, dose and route of administration at the time of antigen exposure. Perhaps the blocking factor does not develop until there is a greater antigenic dose (large placenta) later in pregnancy. Despite these objections, if a blocking factor is found to be important in the prevention of abortion, this would open up new therapeutic possibilities by administering serum from women with successful pregnancies to women with recurrent pregnancy wastage.

The placenta and the attached fetus is a hybrid parasite with maternal and paternal components. Disturbances in the host–parasite balance may become under certain circumstances severe enough to bring about the expulsion of the conceptus. Habitual aborters manifest hypersensitivity to the paternal part of the placenta (Bardawil *et al.*, 1962). Since the mechanisms that allow a mother to tolerate her fetus are still puzzling, it is difficult to assess to what the failure of this normal relationship might be responsible for spontaneous abortions. The occurrence of such a rejection would require that the mother's body recognize the foreign antigens, produce antibodies and convey these agents to the fetus (Hancock *et al.*, 1968).

HISTOCOMPATIBILITY SYSTEMS IN SPONTANEOUS ABORTIONS

The fetus inherits histocompatibility antigens from the father, which probably is foreign to the mother. There is conflicting evidence in animals and humans concerning the influence of maternal–paternal tissue genetic disparity on favourable pregnancy outcome (Billington, 1964; Jenkins and Good, 1972; McLaren, 1975). Tissue genetic disparity in abortion has been measured by husband–wife MLRs (Halbrecht and Komlos, 1968). The percentage of transformed cells increased with higher number of abortions, suggesting that disparity may favour abortion and that repeated abortions may sensitize the women to paternal antigens. This situation is opposite to that found in term pregnancies (Anderson, 1971; Jenkins and Hancock, 1972), where increasing parity was associated with reduced maternal responsiveness to paternal antigens. Mixed lymphocyte reaction in a small group of reproductive partners gave highest reactivity in women with a history of habitual abortion and lowest in women with a history of recurrent hydatidiform mole (Takeuchi and Kanazawa, 1973). However, Kandil *et al.* (1983) reported depressed MLR in cases of habitual abortions.

The percentage of T-cells remained unaltered during the three trimesters of normal pregnancy. In patients with a previous history of spontaneous abortions the T-cells percentage was lower in the second and third trimester than in non-pregnant controls. The values did not differ statistically from corresponding values in those patients with no history of spontaneous abortion (normal pregnancy) (Garewal *et al.*, 1978). The phytohemagglutinin (PHA) induced transformation of lymphocytes was depressed in the second and third trimesters in patients with a normal pregnancy and in those with a previous history of spontaneous abortions. Thus, while the percentage of T-cells remained unaltered during pregnancy, their response to PHA falls in the second and third trimesters. Habitual aborters rejected skin grafts from their husbands earlier than grafts from unrelated males (Bardawil *et al.*, 1962), suggesting maternal sensitization to paternal strain antigens.

Couples with recurrent spontaneous abortions of karyotypically normal fetuses had a significantly depressed mitogenic response for mixed lymphocyte reaction when stimulated by unrelated donor lymphocytes. This hyperactivity was seen only when the fetus was karyotypically normal and was not seen when the fetus was karyotypically abnormal (Lauritsen *et al.*, 1976).

Habitual aborters may carry successfully to term following a change of husband, suggesting the possibility that immunological incompatibility of the original partner might have been responsible (Javert, 1962). Women with antisperm antibodies and otherwise unexplained infertility, who subsequently are liable to conceive, have a high incidence of spontaneous abortion, suggesting immunological incompatibility involving paternal antigens (Jones and Ing, 1974).

Significantly more male infants than expected were born to women who developed histocompatibility locus antigen (HLA) antibodies during their first full pregnancy. The male fetus stimulates a stronger HLA response than the female (Johansen and Festernstein, 1974). Lymphocytes reaction to paternal antigens was present both in women with three or more consecutive abortions and in normal nulliparous women.

Women with repeated idiopathic abortion had low level of IgG and increased level of IgM in their sera. The low concentration of trophoblastic antigen in early gestation will initiate a state of low zone tolerance. The antitrophoblastic antibodies in early gestation are of IgG group which act as a blocking factor against the activated T-lymphocytes. This blocking mechanism will protect trophoblast against lysis. The trophoblast develops gradually and starts to secrete materials which enhance leukocytic migration, initiating a process of immune repulsion (Gleicher *et al.*, 1979). This process is not inhibited by antibodies to estrogen or human chorionic gonadotropin, thus acting as a blocking factor in fetal graft enhancement. The growing trophoblast also secretes hormones, such as progesterone, estrogen and placental gonadotropin. At the same time the fetus starts to produce precursors of estrogen and corticosteroids; the latter participate in decreasing partially the immune patency of the mother. The increase in concentration of progesterone produces a local block of the myometrial activity, as it serves to stabilize phospholipase A_2 located in fetal membrane and decidua. A decrease in its release leads to prostaglandin production. IgM is known to be a complement fixing antibody and can cause lysis, trophoblastic injury and devitalization. This leads to decrease progesterone production which will lead to the destabilization of lysosomal phospholipidase A_2 located in fetal membranes and decidua, leading to the release of prostaglandins. At the same time the level of estrogen will increase to synthetize the uterine muscle. There is also no trophoblastic immune repulsion. All these factors help in initiating uterine contractions and abortion (Barden, 1977).

SERUM α2-GLOBULIN AND FETOPROTEIN IN SPONTANEOUS ABORTION

A protein specific band, in the α2-globulin, which ranged among the haptoglobulins is present in about 10% of the pregnant women studied. It is identified as the P.Z.P. Its importance and significance are not completely understood. Antibodies to α-fetoprotein can cause abortion in rabbits (Slade, 1973) and induced abortion in humans is associated with a sharp rise of α-fetoprotein. There is evidence that induced abortion may expose the mother to fetal antigens different in type from those which she is likely to experience as a consequence of term delivery. The abortion technique may provoke a greater passage of antigenic material into the maternal system or the mother's reactivity may be different. This is a subject which requires further study. Spontaneous abortion has been shown to be an extremely efficient method of

Table 27.1 The intensity of concentration of total immunoglobulins (Ig) and IgG in the decidua in cases of abortion

Concentration of immunoglobulins	*Light* +		*Moderate* ++		*Marked* +++		*Heavy* ++++	
	Total Ig	*IgG*	*Ig*	*IgG*	*Ig*	*IgG*	*Ig*	*IgG*
No. of cases with spontaneous abortion	10	16	17	11	5	3	–	–
No. of cases with induced abortion	–	–	3	5	6	8	5	1
No. of cases less than gravida 5 (G5)	8	10	8	7	2	1	1	–
No. of cases more than gravida 5 (G5)	2	6	13	10	8	9	4	1

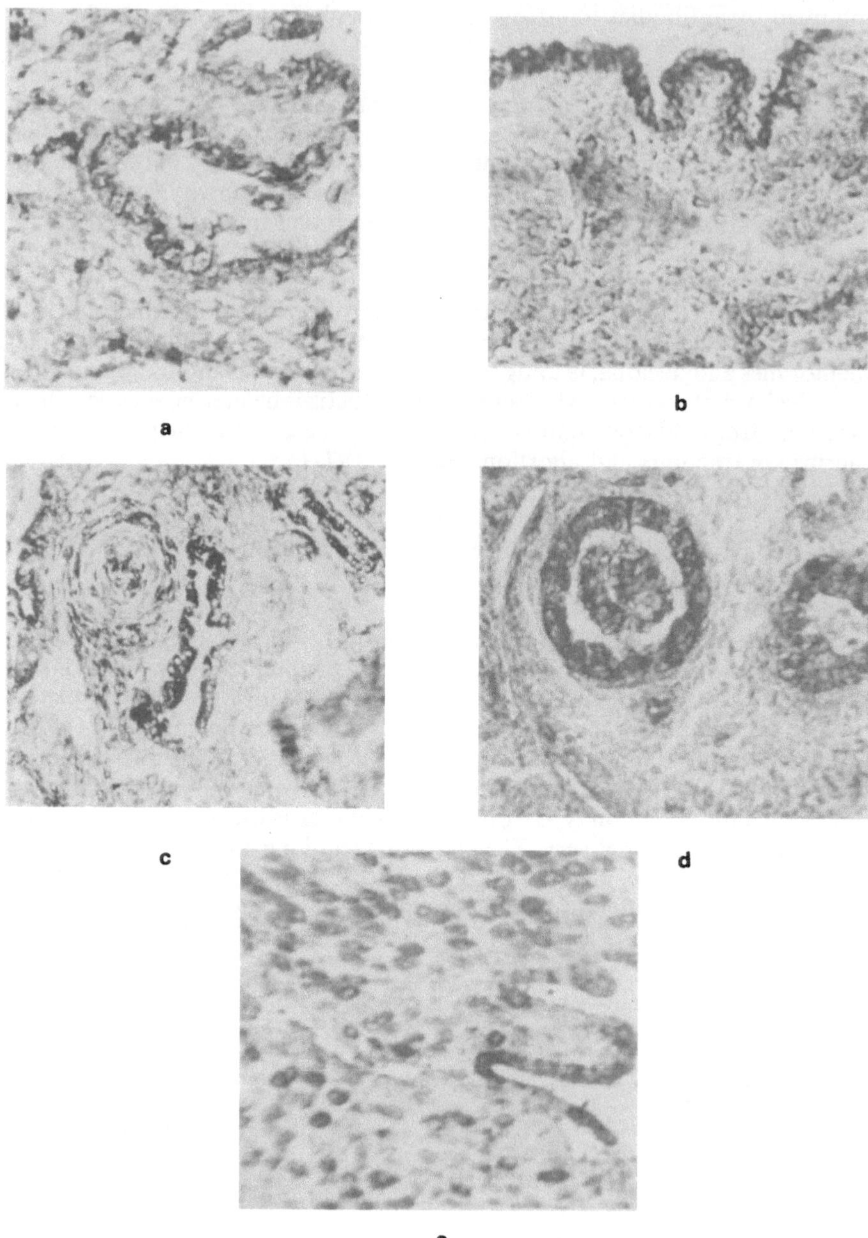

Figure 27.1 **a**, Decidua showing deposition of the stain (immunoglobulins). In a case of spontaneous abortion. (× 270). **b**, Deposition of the stain in the surface epithelium and stroma (spontaneous abortion). (× 270). **c**, Localization of immunoglobulins in the walls of blood vessels (spontaneous abortion). (× 150). **d**, Marked deposition of the stain (IgG) in the epithelium of the endometrial glands of a case of induced abortion. (× 270). **e**, Deposition of the stain (IgG) in the gland epithelium and in a large number of plasma cells in the decidua of a case of induced abortion. (× 270).

terminating a high percentage of pregnancies involving chromosomally abnormal fetuses (Austin, 1972). Although the evidence for an immunological factor in such abortions is absent, it is tempting to speculate that some failure by the abnormal fetus to organize its own immune defences may be operating.

DECIDUAL IMMUNOGLOBULINS IN SPONTANEOUS ABORTION

The decidua may play a protective role at the time of implantation. Immunological tolerance and enhancement has a major role in maternal immunological unresponsiveness. The immunoglobulins were localized in the decidua in cases of spontaneous and induced abortion in the first trimester, in which the latter was used as a control for normal pregnancy. (Kandil *et al.*, 1982).

Cases with spontaneous abortion had a lower concentration of blocking antibody, in particular IgG, compared to the cases with induced abortion. In the latter there was an evident higher concentration of total immunoglobulins and IgG (Table 27.1). These blocking immunoglobulins were found to be localized at different parts such as chorionic villi and walls of blood vessels as well as endometrial glands (Figure 27.1).

CONCLUDING REMARKS

High concentration of blocking antibody in the choriodecidual interface is essential for the survival of the fetus and its protection against the mother's immune system. Multiparous women with uninterrupted pregnancies have higher concentration of blocking antibody at the decidua. The higher the concentration of the blocking antibody at the decidua, the less the chance of having spontaneous abortion. There is no correlation between age and concentration of immunoglobulin G in the decidua of all cases studied. Immunoglobulins' concentration at the choriodecidual interface during second and third trimesters and at delivery should be further investigated.

References

Anderson, M. (1971). Transplantation, Nature's success. *Lancet*, **2**, 1077

Austin, C. R. (1972). In Austin, C. R. and Short, R. V. (eds.) *Reproduction in Mammals*. Vol. II, p. 134, (London: Cambridge University Press)

Bardawil, W. A., Mitchell, G. W., Mokeogh, R. P. and Morchant, D. J. (1962). Behaviour of skin homograft in human pregnancy. In habitual abortion. *Am. J. Obstet. Gynec.*, **15**, 1283

Barden, T. P. (1977). Labour. In Pitkin, R. M. and Scott, J. R. (eds.) *Yearbook of Obstetrics and Gynecology*, pp. 109–127. (Chicago: Year Book Medical)

Billingham, W. D. (1964). Transportation immunity of the maternal, fetal relationship. II. *N. Engl. J. Med.*, **270**, 720

Billington, W. D. (1964). Influence of immunological dissimilarity of mother and fetus on size of placenta in mice. *Nature (Lond.)*, **202**, 317

Bonneau, M., Latour, M., Revillard, J. P., Robert, M. and Traeger, J. (1973). Blocking antibodies eluted from human placenta. *Transplant. Proc.*, **3**, 582

Faulk, W. P., Jeannet, M. and Creighton, W. D. (1974). Immunological studies of the human placenta: Characterization of immunoglobulins on trophoblastic basement membranes. *J. Clin. Invest.*, **54**, 1011

Garewal, G., Sehgal, S. and Aikot, B. K. (1978). Cell-mediated immunity in pregnant patients with and without a previous history of spontaneous abortions. *Br. J. Obstet. Gynaecol.*, **83**, 221

Gatti, A. A. (1971). Serum inhibitor of lymphocyte responses. *Lancet*, **1**, 1351

Glass, R. H. and Globus, M. S. (1978). Habitual abortion. *Fertil. Steril.*, **29**, 257

Gleicher, N., Cohen, C. J., Kerengi, T. O. and Gusberg, S. B. (1979). *Am. J. Obstet. Gynecol.*, **133**, 386

Gray, J. D. (1956). The problem of spontaneous abortion. II. Changes in the placental villi. *Am. J. Obstet. Gynecol.*, **72**, 615

Gray, J. D. (1957). The problem of spontaneous abortion.

Halbrecht, I. and Kömlos, L. (1968). Lymphocyte transformation in mixed wife–husband leukocyte cultures in abortion and in hydatidiform stools. *J. Obstet. Gynecol.*, **31**, 173

Han, T. (1974). Inhibitory effect of human chorionic gonadotrophin on lymphocyte blastogenic response to mitogen, antigen and allogenic cells. *Clin. Exp. Immunol.*, **18**, 529

Hancock, J. L., McGovern, P. T. and Stamp, J. T. (1968). Failure of gestation of goat × sheep hybrids in goats and sheep. *J. Reprod. Fertil. Suppl.*, **3**, 92

Javert, C. T. (1962). Further follow-up of habitual abortion patients. *Am. J. Obstet. Gynecol.*, **84**, 1149

Jenkins, D. M. (1974). Lymphocyte transformation studies in normal and pathological pregnancy. *Proc. R. Soc. Med.*,

Jenkins, D. M. and Good, S. (1972). Mixed lymphocyte reaction and placentation. *Nature (New Biol.)* **240**, 211

Jenkins, D. M. and Hancock, K. W. (1972). Maternal unresponsiveness to paternal histocompatibility antigens in human pregnancy. *Transplantation*, **13**, 618

Jha, P., Talwar, G. P. and Hingorani, V. (1975). Depression of blast transformation of peripheral leukocyte by plasma from pregnant women. *Am. J. Obstet. Gynecol.*, **122**, 965

Johansen, K. and Festenstein, H. (1974). Possible relationships between maternal HL-A antibody formation and fetal sex. Evidence for a sex-linked histocompatibility system in man. *J. Obstet. Gynaecol. Br. Commonw.*, **81**, 781

Jones, W. P. (1978). Immunological aspects of pregnancy. In MacDonald, R. R. (ed.) *Scientific Basis of Obstetrics and Gynaecology*. 2nd edn., pp. 182–210. (Edinburgh and London: Churchill Livingstone)

Jones, W. R. and Ing, R. M. Y. (1974). Reproductive patterns in women with anti-sperm antibodies. In Centaro, A. and Corretti, N. (eds.) *Immunology in Obstetrics and Gynecology*, pp. 94–98. (Amsterdam: Excerpta Medica)

Kaliss, N. and Dagg, M. K. (1964). Immune response engendered in mice by multiparity. *Transplantation*, **2**, 416

Kandil, O., El-Nahas, H., El-Sheikha, Z., El-Mekkawi, T. and Aboul Fetouh, S. (1980). Plasma protein pattern and immunoglobulins in normal pregnancy and pre-eclamptic toxaemia. *J. Egypt. Soc. Obstet. Gynecol.*, **VI** (2) 45

Kandil, O., El-Nahas, H., El-Sheikha, Z. and El-Mekkawi, T. (1981). Lymphoblast transformation in normal pregnancy and pre-eclamptic toxaemia. *J. Egypt. Soc. Obstet. Gynecol.*, **VII** (1), 14

Kandil, O., El-Sheikha, Z., El-Mekkawi, T., Mousa, M. and El-Agizi, H. (1982). Presentation at the *International Symposium on Reproductive Health Care*, Maui, Hawaii, October

Kandil, O., Hefnawi, F., Eslam, M., Mahmoud, M., El-Mekkawi, T. (1983). Maternal immune response in cases of habitual abortion. (Under publication).

Kasakura, S. (1971). A factor in maternal plasma during pregnancy that suppress the reactivity of mixed leukocyte culture. *J. Immunol.*, **107**, 1296, 1301

Lauritsen, J. G., Kristensen, T. and Grummet, N. (1976). Depressed mixed lymphocyte culture reaction in mothers with recurrent spontaneous abortion. *Am. J. Obstet. Gynecol.*, **125**, 35

Leikin, S. (1972). Depressed maternal lymphocyte response to PHA in pregnancy. *Lancet*, **2**, 43

Maroni, E. S. and Parrott, D. M. V. (1973). Progressive increase in cell-mediated immunity against paternal transplantation antigens in parous mice after multiple pregnancies. *Clin. Exp. Immunol.*, **13**, 253

McCormick, J. N., Faulk, W. P., Fox, H. and Fudenberg, H. H. (1971). Immunohistological and elution studies of the human placenta. *J. Exp. Med.*, **133**, 1

McLaren, A. (1975). Antigenic disparity – does it affect placental size, implantation or populaton genetics? In Edwards, R. G. E., Howe, C. W. S. and Johnson, M. H. (eds.) *Immunobiology of Trophoblast*. pp. 255–276. (Cambridge: Cambridge University Press)

Nelson, J. M. (1965). Alterations in immune mechanisms in pregnancy. Their possible significance in collagen disease. *Clin. Obstet. Gynecol.*, **8**, 263

Purtilo, D. T., Haltgren, H. M. and Ynis, E. J. (1972). Depressed maternal lymphocyte response to PHA in human pregnancy. *Lancet*, **1**, 769

Rocklin, R. E., Kitzmiller, J. L., Carpenter, C. B., Garovoy, M. R. and David, J. R. (1976). Maternal–fetal relation. Absence of an immunologic blocking factor from the serum of women with chronic abortions

Rocklin, R. E., Kitzmiller, J. L. and Carpenter, C. B. (1978). Maternal–fetal relation: absence of an immunologic blocking factor from the serum of women with chronic abortions. In Pitkin, R. M. and Scott, J. R. (eds.) *Yearbook of Obstetrics and Gynecology 1978*, pp. 425, 441. (Chicago: Year Book Medical)

Slade, B. (1973). Antibodies to alpha-fetoprotein cause fetal mortality in rabbits. *Nature (Lond.)*, **246**, 493

Smith, C. A. (1959). *The Physiology of the Newborn Infant*, 3rd Edn. (Springfield: Thomas)

Smith, J. K., Casparg, E. A. and Field, E. J. (1972). Lymphocyte reactivity to antigen in pregnancy. *Am. J. Obstet. Gynecol.*, **113**, 602

Takeuchi, S. and Kanazawa, K. (1973). MLC tests in couples with histories of repeated hydatidiform moles and habitual abortion. In Centaro, A., Corretti, N. and Addison, G. M. (eds.), *1st International Congress on Immunology in Obstetrics and Gynecology* (International Congress Series, No. 281, Abstract No. 48), p. 19, (Amsterdam: Excerpta Medica)

Taylor, P. V. and Hancock, E. W. (1975). Antigenicity of trophoblast and some possible antigen-making effects during pregnancy. *Immunology*, **28**, 973

Youtananukorn, V. and Matangkasombut, P. (1972). Human maternal cell-mediated immune reaction to placental antigens. *Clin. Exp. Immunol.*, **17**, 349

Yu, V. Y. H., Walter, C. A., Mecleunan, I. C. M. and and Baum, J. D. (1975). Lymphocyte reactivity in pregnant women and newborn infants. *Br. Med. J.*, **1**, 428

28 Prevention of Rh immunization after spontaneous and induced abortion

L. G. KEITH, M. W. METHOD and G. S. BERGER

Immunologically immature until birth, the fetus can safely survive and thrive in the amniotic fluid, virtually sheltered from all outside menace, which would have to cross the placental barrier to gain access to the umbilical cord.

Protected by the trophoblastic tissue, one of the most sophisticated biologic defense systems, the fetal allograft resists maternal immunosuppressive hormones while accepting passage of maternal antibodies against infectious agents. The selectivity of the latter process, independent of antigenic specificity, is demonstrated by antibody–receptor reactions in which receptors bind the Fc portion of IgG only and not IgM. This system permits a true duality of effect (i.e., 'a cure that harms') – the same maternal antibodies that are meant to protect against infectious agents may also be noxious to the fetus, inducing antibody-mediated diseases ranging in severity from mild and temporary to grave and ultimately lethal.

A similar mechanism is responsible for the phenomenon of Rh immunization. An Rh-negative woman whose fetus is Rh-positive produces an antibody against Rh antigens that may cross the placental barrier and cause hemolytic anemia in the fetus.

MECHANISMS OF Rh IMMUNIZATION

The factors involved in the process of maternal Rh sensitization constitute a complex set of conditions, one or several of which act simultaneously to result in maternal Rh immunization. The logical construct of any cause-and-effect phenomenon may be simplistically represented as a linear sequence in which the cause *may* (only potentially) lead to effect. The favorable conditions needed to catalyze the process can be represented as oblique vectors of force that synergize the process of transformation of potentiality into reality. Thus, if the presence of an immunologically incompatible fetus is regarded as the cause, the favorable conditions leading to its effect (maternal sensitization) are the oblique vectors.

Several factors affect maternal sensitization to Rh antigen:

(1) spontaneous feto-maternal transfusions

(2) individual ability of Rh-negative women to react to the Rh antigen

(3) strength of the Rh antigen on the fetal erythrocyte

(4) ABO protection

(5) antepregnancy immunizations (e.g., transfusion of Rh incompatible blood)

(6) inadvertently induced feto-maternal transfusion (e.g., through induced abortion)

Feto-maternal transfusion

The maternal and fetal circulatory systems are separate entities. The barrier between them consists of three insulating layers, i.e., the endothelium of the fetal capillary, the connective tissue of the chorionic villus and the chorionic epithelium. The latter itself consists of two layers initially, namely the Langhans' cells on the inner side of the villus and the syncytium on the outer side. After the fourth month of pregnancy the Langhans layer of cells involutes and disappears.

In the advanced stages of pregnancy the barrier between the maternal and fetal blood circulation becomes increasingly irregular, particularly in places where the chorionic epithelium has disappeared, allowing the fetal capillary to come into direct contact with the intervillous spaces. The barrier thus is easily breached and only the pressure gradient between the fetal and maternal circulation determines the direction of blood flow between the two. The higher pressure present in the capillary as compared to that in the intervillous spaces explains why feto-maternal transfusion occurs more frequently than does maternofetal transfusion.

Detection of feto-maternal bleeding rests upon identification in the maternal circulation of fetal erythrocytes, based on their characteristic antigenic and chemical structure. The former can be ascertained by serologic analysis, the latter by differential elution (Kleihauer *et al.*, 1957) or the method in which an anti-Hb F serum is used.

Differences in chemical structure of hemoglobin, by virtue of being unequivocal, are the most useful in documenting the presence of fetal erythrocytes in maternal circulation. Fetal erythrocytes contain hemoglobin F (Hb F), which consists of two α and *two* γ polypeptide chains, while adult erythrocytes contain hemoglobin A (Hb A), which consists of two α and *two* β polypeptide chains.

Quantitation of feto-maternal bleeding can be achieved by identifcation of Hb F in maternal circulation. There are, however, a few factors that limit the accuracy of results. First, Hb F is known to decline gradually as pregnancy advances, i.e., from being the major fetal hemoglobin in the first 3 months to representing 60–75% of the fetal hemoglobin by the time of birth. Second,

Hb F also occurs in the erythrocytes of about 6% of all adults. Hb F production may be present in the adult in some cases of anaplastic anemia, leukemia, or even pregnancy. Thus, any interpretation of tests for fetal hemoglobin must take into account all these special considerations.

The differential elution (Kleihauer *et al.*, 1957) method entails bringing a thin blood smear after fixation into contact with a citric acid buffer of pH 3.3. Hb F remains in the cells in this buffer solution and clearly differentiates the fetal erythrocytes after the preparation has been stained and examined under the microscope. The test is, however, difficult both to perform and to interpret. Numerous modifications of it made since 1957 have not proved to be unanimously acceptable because of the delicate nature of the technique.

A more practical quantitative assay, the commercially available Fetaldex test, allows the adult hemoglobin to be eluted, while fetal hemoglobin remains intact within the erythrocytic membranes. The test allows measuring concentrations of fetal cells ranging from 0 to 1%. Below 0.2%, however, the KBB test appears to be more reliable (Keith *et al.*, 1978).

The more recent use of an enzyme immunoassay to detect feto-maternal bleeding is based on the identification of RH_0 (D)-positive cells in an Rh_0 (D)-negative milieu by use of an antiglobulin enzyme conjugate (Ness and Riley, 1982). The sensitivity of this test is of 0.2% or approximately 15 ml of whole blood, which makes it comparable with the KBB procedure.

Individual response of Rh-negative women to Rh antigen

The ability to produce antibodies to Rh_0(D) varies from individual to individual. Some women react to exposure to as little as 0.1 ml, while others fail to react even if massive antigenic onslaughts have resulted from transfusion of 1000 ml of Rh-positive blood, for instance.

Approximately 70% of Rh-negative individuals respond to antigenic stimulation of any magnitude by forming detectable anti-Rh antibodies (Pollack *et al.*, 1971*a*,*b*). Bowman found that if the amount of feto-maternal bleeding is less than 0.1 ml the incidence of demonstrable immunization is only 3% (Bowman, 1978).

The Rh-antigen on the fetal erythrocyte

Various antigens differ in terms of their capacity to elicit an antibody response in the mother. If the paternal genotype is *DcE* rather than *DCe*, the response elicited is stronger and the fetus will be more seriously affected. The D antigen, therefore, has a stronger effect in combination with E than with C.

ABO protection

When antibodies against the A or B antigen of the fetus are present in the maternal circulation, Rh immunization occurs less frequently than in ABO compatible pregnancies. The explanation is that in ABO incompatible pregnancies the fetal erythrocytes are eliminated more rapidly from the maternal circulation, which lessens their opportunity to incite an immunologic reaction. Nevertheless, ABO protection is not absolute and cannot be relied upon to protect against maternal immunization after abortion or delivery.

ABORTION AND Rh IMMUNIZATION

The risk of maternal immunization to the Rh_0 (D) antigen after spontaneous or induced abortion has been estimated in various studies to range from 5.5% (Queenan, 1970) to 10% (Judelsohn *et al.*, 1972). The risk of transplacental bleeding among patients with threatened abortion is more than twice as high as that among patients with incomplete abortions (Litwak *et al.*, 1970). All women undergoing spontaneous abortions (complete or incomplete) should receive Rh-immune globulin as prophylaxis (Queenan, 1970).

Any Rh-negative woman is at risk of developing immunization during and after spontaneous or induced abortion, which also entails risk for any future Rh-positive child she may bear.

Several conditions favor the development of maternal sensitization subsequent to abortion, as follows:

(1) *Rh incompatibility*. Since it is not routinely feasible to type the fetal blood at abortion, any abortus of an Rh-negative woman must be presumed to be Rh-positive unless the biologic father is known with certainty to be Rh-negative.

(2) *Feto-maternal bleeding*. The minimal quantity of Rh-positive erythrocytes capable of eliciting an antibody reaction in an Rh-negative individual has been estimated to vary from 0.1 to 1.25 ml.

(3) *Antibody–antigen reaction potential*. The antigen must have immunogenic capacity and the Rh-negative mother must be capable of responding with antibody production.

(4) *Prior obstetric history and length of gestation*. Feto-maternal bleeding occurs more frequently among women of low gravidity than among those with three or more pregnancies (Litwak *et al.*, 1970). The risk of Rh sensitization from abortion is proportional to the gestational age of the abortus, i.e., virtually inexistent at 1 month, 2% at 2 months, and up to 9% at 3 months and thereafter (Freda *et al.*, 1970).

Figure 28.1 plots differences in the incidence and magnitude of feto-maternal bleeding between first and second trimester abortions. The risk of sensitization depends upon a number of factors. Among these, the most important appear to be the duration of pregnancy and the manner of termination of pregnancy.

Postabortal anti-Rh prophylaxis

The standard dose of anti-Rh (D) immune globulin used in the United States contains 300 μg of immunoglobulin, which is capable of neutralizing 15 ml of

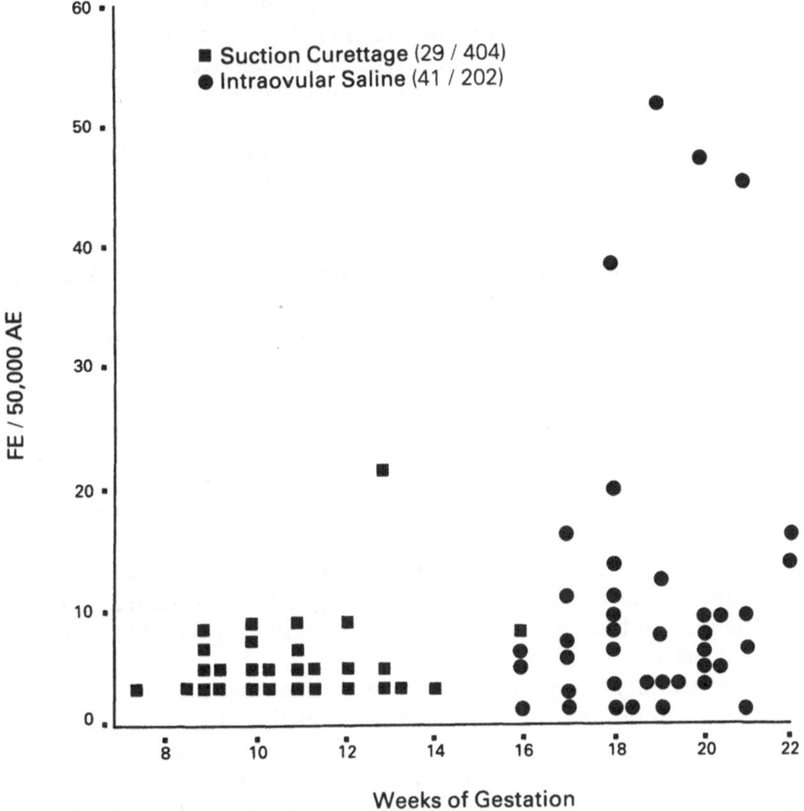

Figure 28.1 Incidence and magnitude of feto-maternal bleeding. (Courtesy of Dr William Peterson)

packed fetal red blood cells, vastly in excess of the entire quantity of fetal erythrocytes present in the fetal circulation in the first trimester of pregnancy. A 50 μg dose of Rh immune globulin can be used after first trimester abortions (WHO, 1971). This dose was deemed as sufficient for safe prophylaxis while reducing expense and conserving a valuable biologic commodity. This smaller dose has been in use in the USA since 1977, and has become accepted as efficacious, less costly, and more realistic in view of the risk (Keith and Bozorgi, 1977). Since 20 μg of anti-Rh immune globulin effectively suppresses the immunogenic potential of 1 ml of packed Rh-positive erythrocytes, 50 μg can be expected to protect against 2.5 ml of packed RBCs (5 ml of whole blood) – a volume that well exceeds that of the fetal circulation in the first trimester.

Various models and protocols have been proposed for postabortal immune prophylaxis. Blood type identification should be performed for all women about to undergo voluntary pregnancy termination or hospitalized with the diagnosis of threatened, imminent, incomplete or probably incomplete abortion. In women who are Rh-negative without antibodies, it is necessary to assume the fetal blood type is Rh-positive, unless the biologic father's blood type is known with certainty to be Rh-negative. Anti-Rh immune prophylactic therapy should be given to all suitable candidates. Those patients who refuse anti-Rh immune prophylaxis should be informed of the potential risk for the future. The manufacturer's advice regarding postabortal dosage (50 μg from a single vial) should be followed. This is preferable to splitting vials consisting of 300 μg of immunoglobulin in the interest of maintaining the sterility of the solution. Moreover, if attempts are made to get more than one dose from a single vial, inaccuracy is bound to occur due to retention of small amounts of fluid on the sides of the vial and the walls of the syringe.

MENSTRUAL REGULATION

Menstrual regulation refers to the procedure of vacuum aspiration of the uterus within 2 weeks of a missed period as a form of very early pregnancy termination. Prior to performing this procedure it may not be clear whether the patient is pregnant. Even after evacuating the uterine contents, a definite diagnosis may not be possible solely on the basis of gross inspection of the evacuated tissue.

The uncertainty of pregnancy at the time the menstrual regulation procedure prompts the question whether anti-Rh prophylaxis is indicated in these patients and, if so, whether prophylaxis should be given after confirmation of pregnancy by histopathologic examination.

Anti-Rh prophylaxis is definitely indicated before obtaining histopathologic confirmation of pregnancy in all Rh-negative women in view of the risks involved in the delays inherent in obtaining a histopathologic diagnosis, difficulties in locating patients a second time and ensuring compliance after patients leave the medical facility.

Even though some women undergoing menstrual extraction may in fact turn out not to have been pregnant, the safe policy is to treat all Rh-negative patients with a dose of 50 μg of anti-Rh immune globulin (human) at the time of menstrual extraction.

SECOND TRIMESTER ABORTION

In contrast to the almost unanimous consensus on the optimal sufficient dose of anti-Rh for prophylaxis in first trimester abortions, the optimal dosage for use after second trimester pregnancy termination is still a matter of speculation. It lies somewhere between the 50 μg dose, which is adequate for first trimester termination, and the 300 μg dose, which is required for use after full-term delivery. Nevertheless, the procedures used to induce abortion between the 12th and the 24th week of gestation unfortunately afford a maximal opportunity for transfer of fetal cells into the maternal circulation.

Amnio-infusion techniques, for example, often cause strong uterine contractions, increased intrauterine pressure, and occasional placental retention (which then necessitates manual removal or D & C). Late termination of pregnancy using some form of dilation and evacuation (D & E) may also lead to fragmentation of the placenta. The incidence of feto-maternal bleeding doubles between the 8th–10th week of gestation (21 %) and the 17th–20th week (41 %). The mean fetal red cell score similarly advances in the same period from 3 to 7 (Table 28.1). A proportionally increased incidence and volume of feto-maternal bleeding is seen as pregnancy advances (Figure 28.1).

Table 28.1 Incidence of feto-maternal hemorrhage, according to duration of gestation

Gestation (weeks)	*Cases* (*No.*)	*Positive* (%)	*Fetal red cell score* (*range*)
8–10	42	21	1–8
11–13	30	37	1–40
14–16	9	44	1–2
17–20	17	41	1–34

In a series of patients undergoing second trimester abortion, the relationship between the length of gestation and the magnitude of the feto-maternal bleeding at the time of induced abortion is continued. The fetal RBCs were detected and quantified by the Kleihauer–Betke–Braun test (Figure 28.2). Although the preponderance of bleedings involved was less than 5 ml of fetal cells, it is impossible, without performing a quantitation test, to predict accurately the precise dose required for each patient.

The D & E procedure is being increasingly used as a method of inducing abortion in the second trimester of pregnancy (Berger *et al.*, 1981). Many of these operations are performed as outpatient procedures in freestanding facilities that do not often have extensive laboratory capability. Such circumstances mandate the prudent recommendation that full prophylaxis (300 μg) be used after a second trimester abortion unless the exact dose required can be determined with accuracy by quantitation of the feto-maternal bleeding.

TIMING OF THERAPY

Timing of anti-Rh prophylaxis is as sensitively important as the dosage for obvious efficacy reasons. Standard procedures in the USA prescribe that anti-Rh prophylaxis be given within 72 hours of the potentially sensitizing event. The original human trials carried out at the Sing Sing Prison precluded the researchers' access to their subjects during weekends, which led to the incorporation of this time margin in further trials and eventually to its baseless acceptance as a meaningful threshold. Two serious misunderstandings resulting from this methodologic idiosyncrasy are that (1) some physicians do

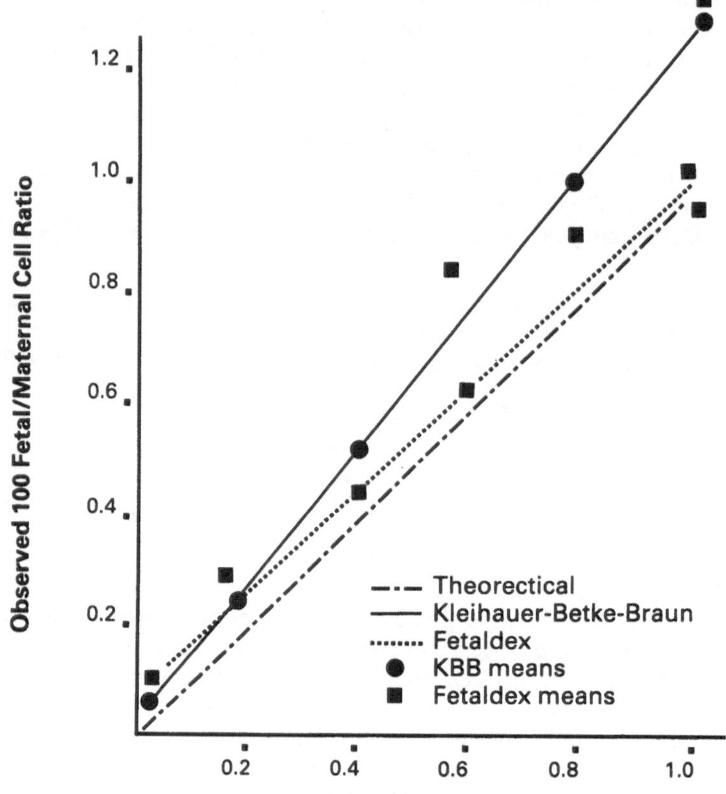

Figure 28.2 Kleihauer–Betke–Braun/Fetaldex cell ratio comparison.

not administer prophylaxis earlier than the 72nd hour and (2) others omit administering it altogether if this time limit has been exceeded.

Both concepts, arising from the same misinformation, are incorrect. Prophylaxis should be administered as soon after abortion or delivery as possible if the patient has any of the mandatory indications.

REMARKS

The nature of immunogenicity and the mode of inheritance of the Rh system are still largely unknown. Nevertheless, the means of providing prophylaxis against the unnecessary sensitization of Rh-negative women to the Rh-antigen are now widely available. Total and sustained prophylaxis can achieve the ultimate goal, i.e., that of virtually eliminating the risk of maternal sensitization and preventing the future occurrence of hemolytic disease in the newborn. Abortion represents a serious cause of maternal sensitization to Rh and that only appropriate prophylactic therapy can prevent such an occurrence.

The current standard recommendation for anti-Rh_0(D) immune prophylaxis after first trimester pregnancy termination is administration of 50 μg of immune globulin. The most appropriate dose should be administered after second trimester abortion. Considering the time and cost involved in determining the safe minimal amount in such cases, it is not unreasonable to advocate administration of 300 μg (standard 300 μg vial), although the amount may be in excess of the actual need.

Timing of therapy is not tied to any threshold of effectiveness; moreover, emphasis must be placed on the importance of administering prophylaxis as soon as possible after the spontaneous or induced abortion as after any potentially sensitizing event.

Continued collaborative efforts of physicians providing clinical services to patients, of blood bank laboratory staffs, and public health authorities who monitor hemolytic disease incidence rates and RhIg demand levels for large populations are necessary to eliminate this preventable cause of maternal sensitization and perinatal morbidity and mortality.

References

Berger, G. S., Brenner, W. E. and Keith, L. (1981). *Second Trimester Abortion: Perspective after a Decade of Experience*. (Littleton, MA.: Wright PSG)

Bowman, J. M. (1978). The management of Rh-isoimmunization. *Obstet. Gynecol.*, **52**, 1, 1

Freda, V. J., Gorman, J. G., Galen, R. S. and Treacy, N. (1970). The threat of Rh immunization from abortion. *Lancet*, **2**, 147

Judelsohn, R. G., Berger, G. S., Wallace, R. B. and Tiller, M. J. (1972). Rh immune globulin in induced abortion: Utilization in a high-risk population. *Am. J. Obstet. Gynecol.*, **114**, 1031

Keith, L. and Bozorgi, N. (1977). Small dose anti-Rh therapy after first trimester abortion. *Int. J. Gynaecol. Obstet.*, **15**, 235

Keith, L., Berger, G. S. and Edelman, D. (1978). Evaluation of Fetaldex: A new screening test for fetal erythrocytes in maternal circulation. *J. Reprod. Med.*, **20**, 109

Kleihauer, E., Braun, H. and Betke, K. (1957). Demonstration von fetalem Hämoglobin in den Erythocyten eines Blutausstrichs. *Klin. Wochenschr.*, **35**, 637

Litwak, O., Taswell, H., Banner, E. and Keith, L. (1970). Fetal erythrocytes in maternal circulation after spontaneous abortion. *J. Am. Med. Assoc.*, **214**, 531

Ness, P. M. and Riley, J. Z. (1982). The detection of feto-maternal hemorrhage by enzyme-linked antiglobulin test (ELAT). In Frigoletto, F. D., Jewett, J. F. and Konugres, A. A. (eds.) *Rh Hemolytic Disease: New Strategy for Eradication*, pp. 135–142. (Boston: G. K. Hall)

Pollack, W., Ascari, W. Q., Crispen, J. F., O'Connor, R. R., and Ho, T. (1971*a*). Studies on Rhesus prophylaxis. II. Rh immune prophylaxis after transfusion with Rh-positive blood. *Transfusion*, **11**, 340

Pollack, W., Ascari, W. Q., Kochesky, R. J., O'Connor, R. R., Ho, T. and Tripodi, T. (1971*b*). Studies in Rhesus prophylaxis. I. The relationship between dose of anti-Rh and the size of the antigenic stimulus. *Transfusion*, **11**, 333

Queenan, J. T. (1970). The role of Rh_0(D) immune globulin in induced abortions. *Clin. Obstet. Gynecol.*, **14**, 235

WHO (1971). Prevention of Rh sensitization: Report of a WHO Scientific Group. WHO Report 486. (Geneva: World Health Organization)

29
Molar pregnancy etiology

R. S. BERKOWITZ and D. P. GOLDSTEIN

Molar pregnancy has intrigued clinicians for several centuries due to its dramatic and varied patterns of presentation. Our knowledge of this unique complication of pregnancy has expanded enormously, particularly in the areas of pathology, cytogenetics, natural history, endocrinology and management. This chapter will review the natural history and management of molar pregnancy in light of these recent advances.

PRESENTING SIGNS AND SYMPTOMS

Vaginal bleeding

The most common presenting symptom in patients with molar pregnancy is irregular vaginal bleeding (Curry *et al.*, 1975). Vaginal bleeding develops in 97% of patients with molar gestation (Goldstein and Berkowitz, 1982). Molar tissues may separate from the uterine wall thereby disrupting maternal vascular channels and inducing bright-red vaginal bleeding. A large volume of retained blood may expand the endometrial cavity. When the intrauterine clots undergo oxidation and liquefaction, 'prune-juice'-like fluid may leak into the vagina. Molar vesicles may pass *per vagina* admixed with intrauterine clots. Because vaginal bleeding may be considerable and prolonged, 54% of patients with molar gestation present with anemia (hemoglobin level < 10 g).

Excessive uterine size

The uterus is excessively enlarged as compared to the gestational age in 51% of patients with molar pregnancy. The endometrial cavity may be expanded by both molar tissue and retained blood. The uterus may feel doughy on palpation and fill the entire abdominal cavity, reaching the xyphoid. Because uterine enlargement partially results from exuberant trophoblastic growth, excessive uterine size is generally associated with markedly elevated human chorionic gonadotropin (hCG) levels. While excessive uterine enlargement is one of the classic signs of hydatidiform mole, in fact half of the patients with molar pregnancy lack this clinical finding.

Toxemia

Pre-eclamptic toxemia is diagnosed in 27% of patients with molar pregnancy at the time of presentation (Goldstein and Berkowitz, 1982). Although pre-eclampsia is often associated with severe hypertension, proteinuria and clonus, eclamptic convulsions rarely develop. Toxemia occurs almost exclusively in patients with excessive uterine size and markedly elevated hCG titers. The uterus is large-for-dates in 81% of patients with molar pregnancy and toxemia (Curry *et al.*, 1975). When a patient develops toxemia early in pregnancy, the diagnosis of hydatidiform mole must be considered.

Hyperemesis gravidarum

Hyperemesis requiring antiemetic and/or intravenous therapy develops in 26% of patients with molar pregnancy (Goldstein *et al.*, 1979). Two percent of patients develop electrolyte disturbances and require hospitalization for intravenous fluids. Hyperemesis occurs primarily in patients with markedly elevated hCG levels and excessive uterine size. The etiology of hyperemesis in these patients has not been elucidated.

Hyperthyroidism

Clinically-evident hyperthyroidism is detected in 7% of patients with molar pregnancy at the time of diagnosis (Berkowitz and Goldstein, 1981*a*). These patients present with warm skin, tachycardia, tremor, fever and thyroid enlargement. The diagnosis of hyperthyroidism is confirmed by the detection of elevated serum levels of free thyroxine and triiodothyronine. Laboratory evidence of hyperthyroidism is commonly present in patients with molar pregnancy (Galton *et al.*, 1971). The hyperthyroid state promptly resolves in all patients following molar evacuation.

While a molar thyrotropin has been postulated to be the cause of hyperthyroidism, purified hCG has been shown to have intrinsic thyroid-stimulating activity (Kenimer *et al.*, 1975). Patients with molar gestations who develop hyperthyroidism generally have serum hCG levels exceeding 200 000 miu/ml. The high concentration of circulating hCG may bind to the thyroid follicular cells and induce marked thyroid stimulation. High levels of hCG may therefore be responsible for the development of hyperthyroidism in molar pregnancy.

Trophoblastic embolization

Two percent of patients with molar pregnancy develop trophoblastic embolization to the pulmonary vasculature and present with the acute onset of tachypnea, tachycardia, chest pain and cough (Kohorn *et al.*, 1978). After molar evacuation, patients may experience severe respiratory distress in the recovery room due to trophoblastic embolization. Auscultation of the chest may reveal bilateral rales and chest roentgenogram may demonstrate diffuse pulmonary infiltrates. Arterial blood gases may show hypoxia, hypocarbia and respiratory alkalosis. Because of an acute increase in the pulmonary vascular resistance, the electrocardiogram may indicate right-sided heart strain. The signs and symptoms of respiratory distress generally resolve with supportive care with supplemental oxygen within 72 hours. Anticoagulation is usually not indicated in the treatment of trophoblastic embolization.

Theca lutein ovarian cysts

About half of the patients with molar gestation have prominent theca lutein cysts. Ovarian enlargement occurs almost exclusively in patients with markedly elevated hCG levels and results from ovarian hyperstimulation. The formation of theca lutein cysts may also be related to increased serum levels of prolactin (Osathanondh *et al.*, 1981). The cysts are usually multilocular and contain serosanguineous or amber-colored fluid. Because these patients often have excessively enlarged uteri, the theca lutein cysts may be difficult to palpate. However, the presence of theca lutein cysts can be accurately detected by ultrasonography. Following molar evacuation, theca lutein cysts normally regress spontaneously within 2–4 months (Scheer and Goldstein, 1973).

Patients with prominent theca lutein cysts may have symptoms of marked pelvic pressure or fullness. After molar evacuation, prominent theca lutein cysts may be decompressed by laparoscopic aspiration to relieve symptoms of pelvic pressure and to reduce the risk of cystic torsion or rupture. If a patient with theca lutein cysts develops acute pelvic pain, laparoscopy should be performed to assess possible cystic torsion or rupture (Berkowitz *et al.*, 1980). Laparoscopic manipulation may successfully manage small cystic rupture or incomplete ovarian torsion. However, if the ovary is infarcted due to torsion and vascular compromise, oophorectomy is mandatory.

DIAGNOSIS OF MOLAR PREGNANCY

HCG

HCG is a predictable and constant secretory product of the trophoblastic cell. Like the other glycoprotein hormones (FSH, LH and TSH), hCG is composed of two polypeptide chains attached to a carbohydrate moiety. There is considerable cross-reactivity between LH and hCG in several immunologic and biologic assays because they share indistinguishable α-chains. The β-subunit of the four glycoprotein hormones is biochemically unique and confers immunologic and biologic specificity (Goldstein, 1976). A highly specific and sensitive radioimmunoassay (RIA) was developed for hCG based upon the immunologic properties of the β-subunit structure (Vaitukaitis *et al.*, 1972). Because the β-subunit RIA is specific for hCG and has a sensitivity of 5 miu/ml, it is the most reliable assay for the management of patients with gestational trophoblastic tumors. The β-subunit RIA is particularly useful in quantitating low levels of hCG to prevent interference from physiologic levels of LH.

Patients with molar pregnancy may have markedly elevated hCG levels.

When there is exuberant trophoblastic growth, the hCG measurement may far exceed the normal hCG level of a singleton pregnancy of the same gestational age. However, in about half of the patients with an hydatidiform mole, the endometrial cavity is not excessively expanded by trophoblastic growth. The hCG levels in these patients may actually be lower than the values seen in normal pregnancies of the same gestational age. Furthermore, the physician must consider the possibility of multiple gestation when a patient presents with markedly elevated hCG levels, excessive uterine size and vaginal bleeding. Therefore, the measurement of hCG should not be used as a sole criterion for the diagnosis of molar pregnancy.

Ultrasonography

Ultrasonography has been demonstrated to be a sensitive and reliable non-invasive technique in the diagnosis of molar pregnancy (Kobayashi, 1976). The diffuse hydatidiform swelling of molar chorionic villi gives rise to a characteristic vesicular pattern on ultrasound. If a normal gestation is present, the gestational sac should be identified from the 6th to the 10th week. The fetal cranium should be predictably detected by ultrasonography after the 14th week of gestation. The following conditions may infrequently be confused with an hydatidiform mole on ultrasound: (1) early intrauterine pregnancy with coexisting uterine leiomyomas, (2) normal pregnancy between 10 and 13 weeks of gestation, (3) tangential section of a normal placenta, (4) missed abortion and (5) intrauterine clotted blood. However, ultrasonography is remarkably accurate in diagnosing molar gestation when it is performed and interpreted by a skilled and experienced individual.

CLASSICAL vs PARTIAL MOLAR PREGNANCY

Pathologic and chromosomal features

Hydatidiform mole may be categorized as either a classical (complete) mole or partial mole on the basis of gross morphology, histopathology and karyotype.

Classical moles have no identifiable embryonic or fetal tissues and generalized hydatidiform swelling of the villi. The molar chorionic villi are diffusely enveloped by hyperplastic and atypical trophoblast. The genesis of complete molar pregnancy has been elucidated by recent cytogenetic studies. Complete moles generally have a 46,XX karyotype and the molar chromosomes are derived entirely from paternal origin (Kajii and Ohama, 1977). Complete moles appear to develop from an ovum which has been fertilized by an haploid sperm which then duplicates its own chromosomes after meiosis (Yamashita *et al.*, 1979). The ovum nucleus may be either absent or inactivated. While most complete moles have a 46,XX karyotype, about 3–13% of hydatidiform moles have a 46,XY constitution (Pattillo *et al.*, 1981). The molar chromosomes in a 46,XY mole also appear to be derived entirely from paternal origin (Surti *et al.*, 1979).

In contrast, partial moles are characterized by the following pathologic features: (1) identifiable fetal or embryonic tissues, (2) varying-sized chorionic villi with foci of hydropic swelling and cavitation, (3) foci of trophoblastic hyperplasia with or without atypia, (4) marked villous scalloping and (5) prominent stromal trophoblastic inclusions (Szulman and Surti, 1978*b*). Partial moles generally have a triploid karyotype (Szulman and Surti, 1978*a*). When whole fetuses are identified with partial moles, these fetuses have stigmata of triploidy, including growth retardation and multiple congenital anomalies.

Clinical features of partial molar pregnancy

Limited information is available concerning the clinical features of partial molar pregnancy (Berkowitz *et al.*, 1979). We therefore reviewed our experience with partial molar pregnancy in 33 patients at the New England Trophoblastic Disease Center (NETDC). Prior to endometrial curettage, 85% of these patients were diagnosed as having incomplete or missed abortion. The diagnosis of partial mole was only considered after histologic review of the curettage specimens. Patients with partial moles usually lack the clinical features that are characteristic of complete molar pregnancy. At presentation, only 15% of patients with partial moles have excessive uterine enlargement and/or pre-eclampsia. Only one patient with a partial mole developed persistent gestational trophoblastic neoplasia (GTN) and required chemotherapy to achieve remission. Therefore, partial moles have a limited (3%) potential for the development of persistent GTN.

HIGH-RISK vs LOW-RISK MOLAR PREGNANCY

Following evacuation of a complete molar pregnancy, local uterine invasion occurs in 15% of patients and metastasis develops in 4% of patients (Berkowitz and Goldstein, 1981*a*).

Certain factors can be identified in molar pregnancy that predispose to the development of persistent GTN (Goldstein *et al.*, 1981). At the time of presentation, 41% of patients have the following signs of marked trophoblastic growth: hCG level >100 000 miu/ml, uterine size > gestational age, and theca lutein cysts >6 cm in diameter (Table 29.1). Following molar evacu-

Table 29.1 Sequelae of low- and high-risk molar pregnancy (New England Trophoblastic Disease Center, July 1965–June 1979)*

Outcome	*Low-risk*	*High-risk*
Normal involution	96.0%	60.2%
Non-metastatic trophoblastic disease	3.4%	31.0%
Metastatic trophoblastic disease	0.6%	8.8%

* 506 patients had low-risk and 352 patients had high-risk molar pregnancy; all patients underwent evacuation with no prophylactic chemotherapy

ation, 31% of these patients develop local uterine invasion and 8.8% develop metastases. The risk for persistent GTN is greatly reduced in the patients who do not present with signs of exuberant trophoblastic growth. After molar evacuation only 3.4% of these patients develop local uterine invasion and 0.6% develop metastases. Therefore, molar pregnancies with excessive uterine enlargement and markedly elevated hCG levels are at increased risk for developing persistent GTN.

Women older than 40 with molar gestations also have a greater incidence of developing persistent GTN (Tow, 1966). In a study conducted in Singapore, 37% of patients with molar pregnancy older than 40 developed persistent GTN. Hydatidiform moles in older women are frequently aneuploid and this may be related to their increased potential for local invasion and metastasis (Tsuji *et al.*, 1981).

TREATMENT

Molar evacuation

After diagnosing a molar pregnancy, the patient is thoroughly examined for the presence of associated medical problems including marked anemia, pre-eclampsia and hyperthyroidism. The patient is first stabilized and then a decision must be made regarding the most appropriate method of evacuation.

Suction evacuation is the preferred technique regardless of uterine size in patients who desire to preserve fertility (Goldstein *et al.*, 1981). An oxytocin infusion is started in the operating room at the time of anesthesia induction. A rigid 12 mm cannula is preferred because this size enables rapid evacuation and prompt involution of the uterus. If the uterus is larger than 14 weeks' size, one hand is placed on top of the fundus and the uterus is massaged to stimulate uterine contraction and to reduce the risk of perforation. When suction evacuation is thought to be complete, a sharp curettage using a large Reynold's curet is performed to remove any residual molar tissue. The curettings from suction and sharp curettage are submitted separately for pathologic review.

Prophylactic chemotherapy

The use of prophylactic chemotherapy at the time of molar evacuation is controversial (Goldstein, 1974). The controversy primarily concerns the wisdom of exposing all patients to potentially toxic treatment when only about 19% are at risk for developing persistent GTN.

Prophylactic chemotherapy with actinomycin-D has been employed at the time of molar evacuation at the NETDC. Local uterine invasion subsequently developed in only 4% of patients and no patient developed metastases. Furthermore, all patients treated with prophylactic chemotherapy, who developed local uterine invasion, subsequently achieved remission after only one additional course of chemotherapy. Prophylactic chemotherapy therefore not only prevents metastatic disease but also reduces the incidence and morbidity of non-metastatic trophoblastic disease. Prophylactic chemotherapy may be particularly helpful in the management of high-risk molar pregnancy, especially when hormonal follow-up is unavailable or unreliable.

HORMONAL FOLLOW-UP

After molar evacuation, patients are carefully followed with weekly β-subunit hCG levels until they are normal for 3 consecutive weeks and then monthly levels until they are normal for 6 consecutive months. Patients are encouraged to use effective contraception during the entire interval of gonadotropin follow-up. Patients are counseled regarding the relative risks and benefits of different methods of contraception.

The incidence of postmolar trophoblastic disease has been reported to be increased in patients who used oral contraceptives before gonadotropin remission (Stone *et al.*, 1976). Their data indicate that persistent GTN develops in 25 % of patients using oral contraceptives and in 9.3 % of patients using barrier methods after molar evacuation. However, data from the NETDC indicate that oral contraceptives do not increase the risk of postmolar trophoblastic tumors (Berkowitz *et al.*, 1981). Postmolar trophoblastic disease developed in 18.9 % of patients using oral contraceptives and 14.3 % of patients using barrier methods. The mean hCG regression time was also not influenced by the contraceptive method. Therefore, oral contraceptives do not appear to increase the risk of postmolar trophoblastic disease and may be safely prescribed after molar evacuation during the entire interval of gonadotropin monitoring.

SUBSEQUENT PREGNANCIES

Patients with molar pregnancies can anticipate normal reproduction in the future (Pastorfide and Goldstein, 1973). Subsequent pregnancies have no increase in the incidence of congenital anomalies, prematurity, ectopics or stillbirths (Table 29.2) (Berkowitz and Goldstein, 1981*b*). First trimester

Table 29.2 Subsequent pregnancies in patients with molar pregnancy (New England Trophoblastic Disease Center)*

Outcome	%
Term delivery	65.3
Premature delivery	9.7
Stillbirth	0.5
Spontaneous abortion	
1st trimester	18.7
2nd trimester	1.3
Therapeutic abortion	2.6
Ectopic	0.8
Repeat molar pregnancy	1.1
Congenital anomalies	5.0

* Based upon 783 subsequent pregnancies

spontaneous abortion occurs in 18.7% of their later pregnancies. Because these patients undergo careful clinical scrutiny and hCG monitoring, their incidence of spontaneous abortion is most likely consistent with the general population.

However, when a patient has had a molar pregnancy, any future gestation is at increased risk for developing trophoblastic neoplasia (Federschneider *et al.*, 1980). Nine patients (1:150) have had at least two consecutive molar pregnancies at the NETDC. The later molar pregnancies are characterized by worsening histology and increased risk of postmolar trophoblastic disease. Patients with repetitive molar pregnancies also have a limited capacity to sustain a normal gestation. Only one patient has had a normal subsequent term pregnancy after two prior molar gestations.

It is our recommendation that ultrasonography should therefore be performed in the first trimester of subsequent pregnancies to confirm normal gestational development. The placentas or products of conception from later pregnancies should undergo thorough pathologic review. Furthermore, hCG should be measured 6 weeks after the completion of any future conception to exclude occult trophoblastic neoplasia.

References

Berkowitz, R. S., Goldstein, D. P., Marean, A. R. and Bernstein, M. R. (1979). Proliferative sequelae after evacuation of partial hydatidiform mole. *Lancet*, **2**, 804

Berkowitz, R. S., Goldstein, D. P. and Bernstein, M. R. (1980). Laparoscopy in the management of gestational trophoblastic neoplasms. *J. Reprod. Med.*, **24**, 261

Berkowitz, R. S. and Goldstein, D. P. (1981*a*). Pathogenesis of gestational trophoblastic neoplasms. *Pathobiol. Annu.*, **11**, 391

Berkowitz, R. S. and Goldstein, D. P. (1981*b*). Pregnancy outcome after molar gestation. Contemp. *OB/GYN*, **18**, 69

Berkowitz, R. S., Goldstein, D. P., Marean, A. R. and Bernstein, M. R. (1981). Oral contraceptives and post molar trophoblastic disease. *Obstet. Gynecol.*, **58**, 474

Curry, S. L., Hammond, C. B., Tyrey, L., Creasman, W. T. and Parker, R. T. (1975). Hydatidiform mole: Diagnosis, management and long-term follow-up of 347 patients. *Am. J. Obstet. Gynecol.*, **45**, 1

Federschneider, J. M., Goldstein, D. P., Berkowitz, R. S., Marean, A. R. and Bernstein, M. R. (1980). The natural history of recurrent molar pregnancy. *Obstet. Gynecol.*, **55**, 457

Galton, V. A., Ingbar, S. H., Jimenez-Fonseca, J. and Hershman, J. (1971). Alterations in thyroid hormone economy in patients with hydatidiform mole. *J. Clin. Invest.*, **50**, 1345

Goldstein, D. P. (1974). Prevention of gestational trophoblastic disease by use of actinomycin-D in molar pregnancies. *Obstet. Gynecol.*, **43**, 475

Goldstein, D. P. (1976). Chorionic gonadotropin. *Cancer*, **38**, 453

Goldstein, D. P., Berkowitz, R. S. and Cohen, S. M. (1979). The current management of molar pregnancy. *Curr. Probl. Obstet. Gynecol.*, **3**, 1

Goldstein, D. P., Berkowitz, R. S. and Bernstein, M. R. (1981). Management of molar pregnancy. *J. Reprod. Med.*, **26**, 208

Goldstein, D. P. and Berkowitz, R. S. (1982). *Gestational Trophoblastic Neoplasms – Clinical Principles of Diagnosis and Management*, pp. 1–301. (Philadelphia: Saunders)

Kajii, T. and Ohama, K. (1977). Androgenetic origin of hydatidiform mole. *Nature (Lond.)*, **268**, 633

Kenimer, J. G., Hershman, J. M. and Higgins, H. P. (1975). The thyrotropin in hydatidiform moles is human chorionic gonadotropin. *J. Clin. Endocrinol. Metab.*, **40**, 482

Kobayashi, M. (1976). Use of diagnostic ultrasound in trophoblastic neoplasms and ovarian tumors. *Cancer*, **38**, 441

Kohorn, E. I., McGinn, R. C., Gee, B. L., Goldstein, D. P. and Osathanondh, R. (1978). Pulmonary embolization of trophoblastic tissue in molar pregnancy. *Obstet. Gynecol.*, **51,** 165

Osathanondh. R., Berkowitz, R., deCholnoky, C., Goldstein, D. P., Tyson, J. E. and Smith, B. (1981). Endocrine factor for theca lutein cyst in gestational trophoblastic neoplasia. *Placenta, Suppl.*, **3,** 270

Pastorfide, G. B. and Goldstein, D. P. (1973). Pregnancy after hydatidiform mole. *Obstet. Gynecol.*, **42,** 67

Pattillo, R. A., Sasaki, S., Katayama, K. P., Roesler, M. and Mattingly, R. F. (1981). Genesis of 46,XY hydatidiform mole. *Am. J. Obstet. Gynecol.*, **141,** 104

Scheer, K. I. and Goldstein, D. P. (1973). Use of ultrasonography to follow regression of theca lutein cysts. *Radiology*, **108,** 673

Stone, M., Dent, J., Kardana, A. and Bagshawe, K. D. (1976). Relationship of oral contraception to development of trophoblastic tumour after evacuation of a hydatidiform mole. *Br. J. Obstet. Gynaecol.*, **83,** 913

Surti, U., Szulman, A. E. and O'Brien, S. (1979). Complete (classic) hydatidiform mole with 46,XY karyotype of paternal origin. *Hum. Genet.*, **51,** 153

Szulman, A. E. and Surti, U. (1978*a*). The syndromes of hydatidiform mole: I. Cytogenetic and morphologic correlations. *Am. J. Obstet. Gynecol.*, **131,** 665

Szulman, A. E. and Surti, U. (1978*b*). The syndromes of hydatidiform mole: II. Morphologic evolution of the complete and partial mole. *Am. J. Obstet. Gynecol.*, **132,** 20

Tow, W. S. H. (1966). The influence of the primary treatment of hydatidiform mole on its subsequent course. *J. Obstet. Gynaecol. Br. Commonw.*, **73,** 545

Tsuji, K., Yagi, S. and Nakano, R. (1981). Increased risk of malignant transformation of hydatidiform moles in older gravidas: A cytogenetic study. *Obstet. Gynecol.*, **58,** 351

Vaitukaitis, J. L., Braunstein, G. D. and Ross, G. T. (1972). A radioimmunoassay which specifically measures human chorionic gonadotropin in the presence of human luteinizing hormone. *Am. J. Obstet. Gynecol.*, **113,** 751

Yamashita, K., Wake, N., Araki, T., Ichinoe, K. and Makoto, K. (1979). Human lymphocyte antigen expression in hydatidiform mole: Androgenesis following fertilization by a haploid sperm. *Am. J. Obstet. Gynecol.*, **135,** 597

30
Epilogue

E.S.E. HAFEZ

REPRODUCTIVE PARAMETERS

Various reproductive parameters are extremely variable for the purpose of planning obstetric and neonatal care facilities and personnel training and for making informed decisions concerning the practice of family planning, obstetrics, pediatrics and neonatology; e.g. fertility rate, birth rate, abortion (spontaneous and induced) rate, maternal and fetal mortality (CDC, 1980; Grebenik and Hill, 1974; IPPF, 1971; Moore-Cavor, 1974; Tietze, 1983; WHO, 1970; Population Reports, 1980; Hodgson, 1981; Berger *et al.*, 1981). However, there are apparent controversies and uncertainty with some of the parameters and definitions (Tables 30.1, 30.2). It is generally assumed that the gestational age is an estimate of fetal age in completed weeks, calculated from the first day of the last normal menstrual period (LMP). Radiological techniques, conventional B-scanning and linear real-time diagnostic ultrasonography (Tables 30.3 and 30.4) have been used extensively to measure fetal circumferance, fetal crown–rump length (CRL), fetal biparietal deamenter (BPD) and gestational sac volume at different gestational ages (Meudt and Hinselmann, 1975; Robinson, 1975; Reinold, 1976; Adam *et al.*, 1979: Robinson *et al.*, 1979). However, ultrasonographical evaluation of fetal measurements as a function of gestational age is subject to racial differences.

Various clinical and physiological parameters should be considered in the evaluation of gestational age; e.g. the duration of amenorrhea, gestational age as judged by ultrasonography, clinical examination, the results of pregnancy tests and the onset of fetal movements. The duration of amenorrhea refers to the interval in days from the first day of a normal menstruation. The regularity or irregularity (as well as the use of contraceptives) have to be considered in the computation. Thus, the gestational age should be calculated from the day of temperature elevation on a basal body temperature chart. The ultrasound fetal age is evaluated according to the crown–rump length (SD 0.5 week) or fetal biparietal diameter (SD 2 weeks). The duration of pregnancy can be estimated utilizing clinical, internal and/or external examination.

According to the Committee on Terminology of the American College of Obstetricians and Gynecologists, 'abortion is the expulsion or extraction of

Table 30.1 Some definitions related to pregnancy, spontaneous abortion in relation to reproductive health*†

Term	*Definition*
Abortion induced	Expulsion or extraction from a pregnant woman of intrauterine components of conception up to 500 g of fetal weight or approximately 20–24 weeks of gestational age. It is still controversial whether the stage of conception is calculated from LMP or from fertilization or conception Voluntary termination of intrauterine pregnancy Molar and ectopic pregnancies are excluded
Abortion failed	Failure of induced abortion with subsequent continuation of pregnancy
Abortion habitual	Repeated, usually three or more consecutive spontaneous abortions; etiology is often uncertain
Abortion inevitable	Bleeding and/or myometrial contraction associated with rupture of amniotic membranes, during the 20 weeks of gestation; dilation of the cervix, prior to expulsion of the products of conception; spontaneous abortion cannot be normally prevented after the onset of cervical dilatation
Abortion infected	Abortion associated with uterine microbiological contaminant
Abortion missed	Fetal death 20 weeks from LMP (*see below*), without expulsion of products of conception; vaginal discharge and arrested fetus, common in diabetic patients
Abortion septic	Abortion associated with passage of microbiological contaminants into the bloodstream
Abortion spontaneous	Abortion resulting from genetic defect, maternal disease, accidental injury, or known or unknown cause excluding wastage induced
Abortion threatened	Intrauterine bleeding affecting intact pregnancy before 20 weeks of gestation without expulsion of products of conception, and without cervical dilation
Abortus	(Plural abortus or abortuses, never aborti.) Expelled or extracted fetus or stillborn infant with gestation of less than 20 weeks from LMP Hydramniotic sac, without any fetal tissues
Blastocyst	A hollow embryonic structure resulting from the accumulation of blastocelic fluid within the expanding morula, found in uterus from day 3 to 7 of gestation
Conception	Confusing term: Not recommended term whereas others refer to the onset of fertilization of the egg in the tube
Conception product of	All structures developing from the blastocyst, including the fetus and the placental membranes and fluid
Death fetal	Termination of fetal viability to the complete expulsion or extraction of a product of conception, irrespective of the duration of pregnancy Fetal death at less than 20 weeks from LMP corresponds to spontaneous abortion; fetal death at more than 20 weeks corresponds to 'stillbirth' (*see below*) In certain European countries, the term 'fetal death' is used only after the 28th week

Table 30.1 (*Contd.*)

Term	*Definition*
Death maternal	The death of any pregnant woman or within 6 weeks of abortion (irrespective of duration and location of pregnancy) or due to complications of parturition and puerperium Maternal death due to complications or chain of events initiated by abortion; or aggravation of an unrelated condition due to abortion
Embryo	The conceptus from the time of implantation to the 2-, 4-, 8-, 16-blastomeres, morula, blastocyst and implanted blastocyst until completed organogenesis, later is a fetus
Fertilization	Penetration of the ovum by the spermatozoon and completed by the fusion of the female and male chromosomes with subsequent formation of male and female pronuclei and expulsion of the second polar body, syngamy leading to cleavage to two blastomeres
Fetus	Unborn offspring from completed organogenesis, end of 8 weeks, until the completion of pregnancy
Fetus excessive size	Larger than the corresponding gestation stage; birth weight over 4500 g
Gestational age (menstrual weeks of gestation)	Fetal age in completed weeks, calculated from the first day of the last normal or calculated menstrual period (LMP), assuming a 28-day cycle Gestational age is expressed in completed weeks; whereas developmental age (fetal age), calculated from the time of implantation of blastocyst
Gestation (pregnancy; gravidity)	The period from implantation of the blastocyst in the endometrium until the termination of pregnancy
Implantation	The blastocyst adheres to, penetrates and establishes nutritional support from maternal tissues, normally the endometrium
Infant Low birth weight	Live newborn with birth weight of 2500 g or less
Infant Mature	Live newborn completed 38 weeks of gestation, with birth weight over 2500 g
Infant Mortality rate	Death during the first year after birth. Infant mortality rate is inversely related to age. 70 % of infants die before 4 weeks of birth, and over 50 % before 1 week of life
Infant Postmature	Prolonged gestation beyond 42 weeks associated with (1) excessive fetal size, (2) diminished placental integrity for sufficient exchange and (3) cutaneous metabolic changes in the newborn
Infant Preterm	Live birth before 37 weeks of gestation
Life signs of	Cardiovascular activity; breathing, heartbeat, pulsation of umbilical cord, movement of involuntary muscles
Live birth	Complete expulsion of extraction of product placental membrane from the mother, irrespective of gestation length, attachment of umbilical cord and of placenta. Evidence of life in newborn, e.g. heartbeat, pulsation of umbilical cord, and definite movements of involuntary muscles

Table 30.1 (*Contd.*)

Term	*Definition*
LMP	Last menstrual period; date of first day of the last normal or calculated menstrual period
Menstrual regulation (menstrual extraction)	Very early evacuation of the uterine contents of a woman (usually 42–49 days from LMP) with suspected pregnancy and before definite pregnancy diagnosis
Morula	A 16-, 32- or 64-blastomere embryo resulting from cleavage of zygote, usually found in fallopian tube or uterus
Neonatal interval	First 4 weeks of life, this interval may be divided into 3 periods. Neonatal period I: less than 24 h after birth. Neonatal period II: less than 7 days of life. Neonatal period III: 1–4 weeks after birth
Parity	Live or dead births (weighing 500 g or more) after the 20th week of gestation, as calculated from LMP A multiple birth is considered as a single parous episode
Pregnancy	The period from implantation of the blastocyst until the expulsion or extraction of the fetus and placental membranes
Pregnancy duration of	Duration of pregnancy, calculated as number menstrual weeks, from LMP, corresponding to a term delivery at 40 weeks Prefer to calculate from the estimated date of fertilization, i.e., 2 weeks after LMP
Pregnancy extrauterine (ectopic)	A pregnancy outside of the uterine cavity, including abdominal, ovarian, intestinal, intramural, cervical and tubal implantation
Pregnancy intrauterine	Implantation of blastocyst and pregnancy within the uterine cavity
Pregnancy molar	Gestational trophoblastic irregular mass of ingrowth and organization of remnants after abortion
Pregnancy prolonged	Prolonged gestation beyond 2 SD (from mean and with a duration of 42½ weeks (297 days) Restricted placental exchange of fetus may cause increased intrauterine death
Stillbirth	Expulsion or extraction of a fetus weighing more than 500 g at more than 20 weeks from LMP
Viability	Neonatal period associated with independent extrauterine life of fetus or infant Alive fetus or infant is not necessarily viable; whereas a non-viable fetus shows transient signs of life at delivery
Zygote	Fertilized ovum, after the penetration of spermatozoa into zona pellucida and the vitellus, with subsequent formation of the male and female pronuclei at syngamy, until the completion of the first cleavage and formation of 2-blastomere egg.

* Thanks are due to all those who kindly reviewed this table and provided valuable critical remarks: G. S. Berger, J. Danezis, T. N. Evans, T. Eskes, U. Gethman, K. Green, A. A. Haspels, H. M. Hasson, J. Lauritzen, Y. Manabe, M. Thiery, W. A. A. van Os and B. Viel.

† (Data from Adam *et al.*, 1979; Berger *et al.*, 1981; Cook and Senanayake, 1978; CDC, 1980; Grebenik and Hill, 1974; Hughes, 1975; IPPF, 1971; Kleinman, 1971; Meudt and Hinselmann, 1975; Moore-Cavar, 1974; Pernoll, 1980; Population Reports, 1980; Robinson, 1975; Robinson *et al.*, 1979; Tietze, 1981; WHO, 1970, 1977, 1978)

Table 30.2 Morphological and pathological characteristics of empty chorionics during postimplantation stage

Syndrome	*Characteristics*
Presence of spot(s)	Sparse and irregular distribution of chorionic villi
Hydropic swollen villi	Increased syncytial and cytotrophoblastic proliferation Avascular and lyalinized stroma
Anomalies of amnion	With or without amniotic cyst
Hydatidiform mole	
Slender atrophic villi	

(Nishimura and Shiota, 1984)

Table 30.3 Clinical uses of ultrasonography

Indication in early pregnancy	(1) assessment of pregnancy well-being: (a) threatened abortion (b) lack of uterine growth (c) recurrent abortion (d) negative pregnancy tests (2) estimation of gestational age: (a) for continuation of pregnancy (b) for termination of pregnancy (3) suspected multiple gestation (4) suspected ectopic pregnancy (5) suspected molar pregnancy (6) suspected gynecological tumor associated with pregnancy (7) gynecologic scanning – pregnancy not suspected (8) gestational sac/placenta localization (prior to genetic amniocentesis)
Indication for referral of patients for biparietal diameter measurements	(1) diabetes mellitus (2) premature rupture of membranes (3) late pregnancy bleeding (4) uncertain dates (5) small-for-dates (6) large-for-dates (7) multiple gestation (8) Rh incompatibility
Complicated early gestations Final diagnosis	(1) normal, single gestation (2) arrested pregnancy (3) multiple gestation (4) pregnancy with uterine fibroids (5) ectopic pregnancy (6) pregnancy with ovarian cysts (7) molar pregnancy

(Adam *et al.*, 1979; Duff, 1979*a,b*; Meudt and Hinselmann, 1975; Robinson, 1975; Robinson *et al.*, 1979, after adaptation from Martin; Stocker, 19xx)

the placenta or membranes, without an identifiable fetus or with a live-born infant or a stillborn infant weighing less than 500 g'.

In most countries of Western Europe, including the Netherlands, the following terms are used:

Table 30.4 Ultrasonographic characteristics and early pregnancy and certain types of spontaneous abortion

Parameters	*Gestational age* (weeks*)	*Ultrasonic characteristics*
Normal gestation sac	$5\frac{1}{2}$	Bright, luminous and completely closed ring of equal thickness (Ring echo)
	7–8	Fetal heart
	9	Loss of regular ring shape (configuration ovoid)†
	11	Club shape
	12	Filling entire uterine cavity
Normal embryo	6	Profuse and dense fetal echoes**
	10	Constant dense echoes
Missed abortion		A common phenomenon
		A fetus is clearly apparent and measured by sonar within the gestation sac but no fetal heart movements
		Loss of definition of gestational sac, fragmentation of sac, or a break in the sac
		Absence of fetal echo from 9 weeks onward
		Absence of fetal head from 12 weeks onward and failure of growth of sac or fetal head for 1–2 weeks
		An error in maturity can be mistaken for arrested progress of pregnancy (ultrasonic examination is useful in differentiating these two conditions)
Hydatidiform mole		Uterus is filled with echoes of similar size and amplitude, but without a gestation sac or fetus
		Speckling at high insonation which disappears very rapidly at only very slightly less insonation; empty uterus.
		If the fetus is present, the echoes are different and are still obtainable at an insonation setting at which molar tissue fails to produce visible echoes
		Enlarged uterus, 'snow-storm' pattern or multiple echoes.
		Typical molar pattern appears within uterine cavity, mole is often well delineated from myometrium presence of hydatidiform mole
		Condition most likely to cause diagnostic confusion is early normal pregnancy with a bulky decidua, but incomplete abortion and

Table 30.4 (*Contd.*)

Parameters	*Gestational age (weeks*)*	*Ultrasonic characteristics*
		uterine fibroid may be confused with hydatidiform mole
Type of abortion		
Blighted ovum (anembryonic pregnancy)		A gestation sac is defined, but is not demonstrated to contain a fetus, either by sonar or by subsequent examination of the aborted products of conception
Ectopic pregnancy		Normal or bulky empty uterus with a gestational sac outside the cavity, or adjacent mass

(Data from Mendt and Hinselmann, 1975; Robinson, 1975).

abortion – 1–16 weeks from LMP
immature (partus immaturus) – 16–28 weeks from LMP
premature (partus prematurus) – 28–37 weeks from LMP
at term (partus at term) – 37–42 weeks from LMP
partus serophius – 42 weeks from LMP

This terminology is based on certain physiological concepts: e.g. the uterus grows due to estrogen as a sphere until the 16th week. At later stages, the gestational sac which is surrounded by chorionic villi develops the final placental disc. Uterine distension occurs primarily after the 16th week. From the neonatal stand point, the 28th week is of special significance since survival is minimal outside the uterus. From the perinatal viewpoint, three parameters should be considered: the duration of amenorrhea, birth weight and percentiles.

Birth weight

The birth weights of infants preceding a spontaneous fetal loss are lower than for babies preceding a live birth. In women who experienced repetitive early fetal loss, the birth weight declines in subsequent pregnancies. There is a tendency for mothers to repeat preterm births, low weight births, and small-for-gestational age (SGA) births.

Among mothers whose first births were late abortions (less than 28 weeks of gestation), the risk of a late abortion the second time seems to be higher than in mothers who delivered their first infant at term (39–41 weeks of gestation). The risk of preterm birth increases among mothers whose first birth is also preterm compared to mothers whose first birth was delivered at term. The rate of perinatal survival is associated with this tendency to repeat similar gestational ages in subsequent deliveries. SGA birth is usually associated with congenital anomalies. Major malformations are more common among births to mothers with only a single SGA birth compared to births of mothers who had three successive SGA deliveries (Abstracts of Reproductive Health Care Symposium, Maui, 1982).

PHYSIOLOGICAL MECHANISMS OF SPONTANEOUS ABORTION

Spontaneous abortion may be associated with environmental pollutants, maternal anatomical anomalies, drugs, nutritional deficiencies, radiation, immunologic disorders, cytogenetic anomalies, smoking and alcohol consumption. Immunological mechanisms involved in spontaneous abortion may be associated with the presence of blocking antibodies in response to parental antigens, parental blood group incompatability or HLA incompatability (Elias and Simpson, 1980).

Various chromosomal anomalies are associated with spontaneous abortion. Structural chromosomal rearrangements such as balanced translocations in couples lead to increased risk of recurrent fetal loss. Little is known about the effects of chromosomal variants, polymorphism, increased chromosomal breakage and chromosome aneuploidy in parents with a history of recurrent abortion. Several chromosomal abnormalities in repeated abortions may be due to sporadic errors in mieiosis and mitosis within the sperm or oocyte prior to or following fertilization. Common abnormalities in abortuses include monosomy 45X polyploidy and various trisomies. Further chromosome studies on larger numbers of couples with habitual abortion and a detailed account of their environmental exposures are needed to evaluate the role environmental conditions play in human fetal loss.

Cervical incompetency, associated with increased repeated and painless midtrimester abortion, can be corrected by several techniques: Shirodkar (intrafascial closure), Lash (hernia repair), Page (scarification), Benson and Durfee (intraabdominal cerclage), and McDonald (pursestring suture). Ultrasonography is employed to measure the internal os during pregnancy to diagnose cervical insufficiency, and to assess surgical techniques in the management. Combined vaginal cerclage and trachelorraphy are used for cervical tears and incompetent internal os, whereas the transabdominal approach for cervical cerclage is used in severe cases after failure of transvaginal route.

Several methods have been utilized for the management of missed abortion in the second trimester. Priming of the uterus with synthetic estrogen for 5 days is followed by i.v. drip administration of prostaglandin $F_{2\alpha}$. 15(S)-15-methyl-PGF_2 (15-me-PGF_2) is used for terminating missed abortion. Pretreatment with extra-ovular PG-gel decreases the amount of 15-me-PGF_2 required to elicit expulsion of the dead ovum and decrease the incidence of complications and side-effects. The treatment–abortion interval, however, is reduced.

DIAGNOSTIC TECHNIQUES

Diagnostic tests used to assess threatened abortion must be easy, fast, inexpensive, accurate and reliable, with high diagnostic specificity (prediction of abortion), sensitivity (prediction of successful outcome), and with minimal day-to-day analytical and diurnal variation. The half-life of the parameter should be short (minutes or hours) so that acute deterioration in the physiological integrity of the conceptus is rapidly reflected. The levels of placental hormones may remain unaltered for some time after fetal death or be normal in anembryonic gestations. Gross and microscopic examination of the placenta is essential to obtaining a complete evaluation of mechanisms of perinatal morbidity and mortality.

The Appendix contains a summary of some recent studies reported on the etiology, physiology, physiopathology, diagnosis, evaluation and management of spontaneous abortion.

References

Adam, A. H., Robinson, H. P. and Dunlop, C. (1979). A comparison of crown–rump length measurements using a real-time scanner in an antenatal clinic and conventional B-scanner. *Br. J. Obstet. Gynaecol.*, **86**, 521

Berger, G. S., Brenner, W. E. and Keith, L. G. (eds.) (1981). *Second Trimester Abortion: Perspectives after a Decade of Experience*. (Littleton, MA: Wright PSG)

Cook, R. J. and Senanayake, P. (eds.) (1978). *The Human Problem of Abortion. Medical and Legal Dimensions*. International Planned Parenthood Federation, Bellagio, Italy

CDC (1980). *Abortion Surveillance 1978*. (Atlanta, GA: Center for Disease Control)

Duff, G. B. (1979*a*). Routine fetal maturity estimation by ultrasound. *Aust. NZ, J. Obstet. Gynaecol.*, **19**, 77

Duff, G. B. (1979*b*). A comparison of early fetal growth curves, *Aust. NZ, J. Obstet. Gynaecol.*, **19**, 80

Elias, S. and Simpson, J. L. (1980). Evaluation and clinical management of patients at apparent increased risk for spontaneous abortions. In Porter, I. H. and Hook, E. B. (eds.) *Human Embryonic and Fetal Death*, pp. 331–349. (New York: Academic Press)

Grebenik, E. and Hill, A. (1974). International demographic terminology: fertility, family planning and nuptiability. *International Union for the Scientific Study of Population Papers*, No. 4, p. 53

Hodgson, J. E. (ed.) (1981). *Abortion and Sterilization: Medical and Social Aspects*. (New York: Grune & Stratton)

Hughes, E. C. (ed.) (1975). *Obstetrics-Gynecologic Terminology with Section on Neonatology and Glossary of Congenital Anomalies*. (Philadelphia: Davis)

IPPF (International Planned Parenthood Federation) (1971). *Abortion: Classification and Techniques*, p. 27. (London: IPPF).

Kleinman, R. L. (1971). *Abortion: Classification and Techniques*, p. 7. (London: International) Planned Parenthood Federation)

Meudt, R. O. and Hinselmann, M. (1975). *Ultrasonoscopic Differential Diagnosis in Obstetrics and Gynecology*. (New York: Springer)

Moore-Cavar, E. C. (1974). *International Inventory of Information on Induced Abortion*, p. 654. (New York; Columbia University International Institute for the Study of Human Reproduction)

Nishimura, H. and Shiota, K. (1984). Early embryonic death – pathology and associated factors, This volume, Chapter 8

Pernoll, M. L. (1980). Maternal and perinatal statistics, In Benson, R. C. (ed.) *Current Obstetric and Gynecologic Diagnosis and Treatment*, 3rd Edn. (Los Altos, CA: Lange)

Population Reports (1980). Series F, Number 7. *Pregnancy Complications of Abortion in*

Developing Countries. Population Information Program, The Johns Hopkins University, Hampton House, 624 North Broadway, Baltimore, MD

Reinold, E. (1976). *Ultrasonics in Early Pregnancy. Diagnostic Scanning and Fetal Motor Activity*. (Basel: Karger)

Robinson, H. P. (1975). The diagnosis of early pregnancy failure by sonar. *Br. J. Obstet. Gynaecol.*, **82**, 849

Robinson, H. P., Sweet, E. M. and Adam, A. H. (1979). The accuracy of radiological estimates of gestational age using early fetal crown–rump length measurements by ultrasound as a basis for comparison. *Br. J. Obstet. Gynaecol.*, **86**, 525

Tietze, C. (1979). *Induced abortion*. 3rd Edn, p. 108. (A Population Council Fact Book) New York: Population Council)

Tietze, C. (1983). *Induced Abortion*. 4th Edn. (A Population Council Fact Book) (New York: Population Council)

WHO (World Health Organization) (1970). Spontaneous and induced abortion: report of a WHO Scientific Group. *WHO Tech. Rep.*, **461**, 51

World Health Organization (WHO) (1977). *Manual of the international statistical classification of diseases, injuries and causes of death, International Classification of Diseases*, Vol. 1. (Geneva: WHO)

World Health Organization (WHO) (1978). Induced abortion. *WHO Tech Rep. Ser.*

Appendix
Summary of some studies related to etiology, physiology, diagnosis, evaluation and management of spontaneous abortion

Concepts	*Parameters studied*	*References*
Adverse effects	Psychiatric sequelae	Cavenar *et al.* (1978)
	Epileptiform convulsion	Kaplan (1978)
	Hormonal changes	Murashko (1978)
Blood	α-Fetoprotein (AFP)	Lidbjork *et al.* (1977)
	Hemostasis	Talaat *et al.* (1976)
	Serum folic level	Dutta (1977)
	Hormonal changes	Murashko (1978)
	Plasma hormone	Miyakawa *et al.* (1977)
Chemically induced	Sugar substitutes	Kline *et al.* (1978*a*)
	Around a smelter	Nordstrom *et al.* (1978)
	Partial resorption and retardation of fetal growth/barbital sodim	Champakamalini *et al.* (1977)
	Anesthetic practice and pregnancy	Knill-Jones *et al.* (1975)
	Hospital laboratory	Strandberg *et al.* (1978)
Classification	Spontaneous abortion	Rushton (1978)
Complications	Fetal abnormality	Gardiner *et al.* (1978)
	Adrenal necrosis	Young *et al.* (1977)
	Chromosomal abnormalities	Alberman *et al.* (1977)
Diagnosis	Prognostic value of pregnancy/zone protein	Damber *et al.* (1978)
	Progesterone values and cornification index/vaginal smears	El-Maraghy *et al.* (1978)
	Ultrasonography	Smith *et al.* (1978)
	Echoscopy	Bal *et al.* (1978)
	Serum hCG analysis	Clasen *et al.* (1977)
	Vaginal cytologic	Busch (1978)

Concepts	*Parameters studied*	*References*
	Echographic study	Saavedra *et al.* (1977)
	Ultrasound	Schillinger *et al.* (1978)
Drug therapy	Fever index	Ledger *et al.* (1977)
	Amoxicillin and ampicillin	Lopez Ortiz *et al.* (1978)
Epidemic, abortion	Surveillance	Kline *et al.* (1977)
	Primary sex ratio	Creasy (1977)
	Preterm delivery	Keirse *et al.* (1978)
	Laparoscopic sterilization	Quan *et al.* (1977)
	Contraceptive practice	Rushwan *et al.* (1977)
	Cytophotometric DNA measurements	Gehring *et al.* (1977)
Etiology	Cigarette smoking	Kline *et al.* (1978*b*)
	Chromosome abnormalities	Worton (1977)
	Central nervous system abnormalities	Bell *et al.* (1978)
	Ectopic pregnancies IUD	Sivin (1978)
	Toxoplasma antibodies	Lolis *et al.* (1978)
	Autoimmune hemolytic anaemia	Jain *et al.* (1977)
	Virus	Suffin *et al.* (1977)
	Bicornuate uterus	McArdle (1978*a*)
	Mechanism	Amino *et al.* (1978)
	Immunobiological mechanism	Breshnihan *et al.* (1977)
	α-Fetoprotein screening	Gordon *et al.* (1978)
	Migraine	Wainscott *et al.* (1978)
	Viral hepatitis	Theile (1977)
	Pathogenetic factors	Kozhevnikov (1977)
	Septic abortion and IUDs	Sparks *et al.* (1978*a,b*)
	Complications	Nemec *et al.* (1978)
Familial and genetic	Monosomy	Kuliev *et al.* (1977)
	Reciprocal translocation	Fried *et al.* (1977)
	Cytogenetics	Kajii *et al.* (1978)
	Anencephaly or spina bifida	James (1978)
	α-1-Antitrypsin	Aarskog *et al.* (1978)
	Sex ratio	Bear (1978)
	Large Y chromosome	Nielsen (1978)
	Genetic aspects	Lauritsen (1977)
	Acrocentric trisomies	Niikawa *et al.* (1977)
	HLA markers	Couillin *et al.* (1977)
Immunology	B and T lymphocytes	Sulovic *et al.* (1977)

Concepts	*Parameters studied*	*References*
Metabolism	Placental proteins	Pogorelova (1978)
	Oxidative metabolism	Kampo *et al.* (1978)
Methods	Karmans	Vasilev (1978)
	Blood coagulation	During *et al.* (1977)
Microbiology occurrence	Epizootiology	Islamov *et al.* (1978)
Missed abortion	Fetus papylaceus in twin pregnancy	Livnat *et al.* (1978)
	Management and fetal death *in utero*	Kamarawy *et al.* (1977)
	Extra-amniotic injection	Kerekes *et al.* (1977)
	Induction of labor	Paladini *et al.* (1977)
Mortality	Lethality	Sol'skii *et al.* (1978)
Occurrence	Autosomal recessive disorder	Kate (1978)
	Fetal wastage and chromosome anomalies	King *et al.* (1977)
	Terathanasi	Warkany (1978)
	Down's syndrome	Cernay *et al.* (1977)
	Inborn developmental defects	Gencik *et al.* (1978)
Physiopathology	Hypophyseal-ovarian relationship	Kononova *et al.* (1977)
	Amniotic fluid embolism	Lees *et al.* (1977)
Psychology	Narcissim and abortion	Ruiz-Mateos Jimenez de Tejada (1977)
Radiography	Radiographic studies	Kirchoff *et al.* (1977)
Septic abortion	Heparin	Schwarz (1978)
	Hemostatic disorders	Sanches Avalos *et al.* (1977)
Therapeutic abortion	Outpatient	Moller *et al.* (1978*a*)
	General and local anesthesia	Moller *et al.* (1978*b*)
	Catecholamines	Brenner *et al.* (1978)
	Septate uterus	McArdle (1978*b*)
	Paracervical block	McKenzie *et al.* (1978)
	Vasopressin analogue	Akerlund *et al.* (1978)
	Intra-amniotic prostaglandin $F_{2\alpha}$	Ward *et al.* (1978)
	Infanticide	Humphries (1978)
	Return of ovarian function	Lahteenmaki *et al.* (1978)
	Computerized screening	Hunton (1977)
	Laparoscopic sterilization	Weil (1978)
	Psychiatric indications	Dilling *et al.* (1978)

Concepts	*Parameters studied*	*References*
Threatened abortion	Extra-amniotic prostaglandin	Arshat (1977)
	Hormonal profile	Jovanovic *et al.* (1978)
	Hormonic colpocytotest	Teleman *et al.* (1977)
Urine	Fromino-glutamic acid	Friedman *et al.* (1977)

References

Aarskog, D. *et al.* (1978). Alpha-1-antitrypsin (Pi)-types in recurrent miscarriages. *Clin. Genet.*, **13,** 81

Akerlund, M. *et al.* (1978). Myometrial response to a long acting vasopressin analogue in early pregnancy. *Br. J. Obstet. Gynaecol.*, **85,** 525

Alberman, E. D. *et al.* (1977). Frequency of chromosomal abnormalities in miscarriages and perinatal deaths. *J. Med. Genet.*, **14,** 313

Amino, N. *et al.* (1978). Mechanism for spontaneous abortion in S.L.E. (Letter) *Lancet,* **1,** 447

Arshat, H. (1977). Extra-amniotic prostaglandin E2 and intravenous oxytocin in termination of mid-trimester pregnancy and the management of missed abortion and hydatiform mole. *Med. J. Malaysia,* **31,** 220

Bal, H. *et al.* (1978). Echoscopy as an aid in management planning in threatened abortion. *Ned. Tijdslar. Geneskl.*, **122,** 83

Bell, J. E. *et al.* (1978). Central nervous system abnormalities: contrasting patterns in early and late pregnancy. *Clin. Genet.*, **13,** 387

Brenner, W. E. *et al.* (1978). Catecholamines during therapeutic abortion induced with intra-amniotic Prostaglandin F2 alpha. *Am. J. Obstet. Gynecol.*, **130,** 178

Breshnihan, B. *et al.* (1977). Immunobiological mechanism for spontaneous abortion in systemic lupus erythematosus. *Lancet,* **2,** 1205

Busch, W. (1978). Prediction of spontaneous abortion by vaginal cytologic smears. (Author's transl.) **100,** 23

Cavenar, J. O. *et al.* (1978). Psychiatric sequelae of therapeutic abortions. *N.C. Med. J.*, **39,** 101

Cernay, J. *et al.* (1977). Morbidity and abortions in mothers of children with Down's Syndrome. *Bratisl. Lek. Listy,* **68,** 559

Champakamalini, A. V. *et al.* (1977). Abortion, partial resorption and retardation of foetal growth in rats chronically treated with barbital sodium during pregnancy. *Indian J. Exp. Biol.*, **15,** 346

Clasen, C. *et al.* (1977). The prognostic value of serum hCG analysis with the aid of an hCG-receptor assay in patients with imminent abortion (proceedings). *Arch. Gynaekol.*, **224,** 89

Couillin, P. *et al.* (1977). HLA markers in parents of triploid conceptuses. *Pathol. Biol. (Paris)*, **25,** 647

Creasy, M. R. (1977). The primary sex ratio of man. (Letter) *Ann. Hum. Biol.*, **4,** 390

Damber, M. G. *et al.* (1978). Prognostic value of the pregnancy zone protein during early pregnancy in spontaneous abortion. *Obstet. Gynecol.*, **51,** 677

Dilling, H. *et al.* (1978). Psychiatric indications for pregnancy interruption. *Internist (Berlin)*, **19,** 315

During, R. *et al.* (1977). Blood coagulation studies of therapeutic abortion induced by 15-methyl-prostaglandin F2 alpha. *Zentralbl. Gynaekol.*, **99,** 1361

Dutta, G. P. (1977). Serum folic level in abortion. *J. Indiana Med. Assoc.*, **69,** 149

El-Maraghy, M. A. *et al.* (1978). The prognostic value in threatened abortion of plasma progesterone values and the cornification index of vaginal smears. *Br. J. Obstet. Gynaecol.*, **85,** 533

Fried, K. *et al.* (1977). Familial balanced reciprocal translocation ascertained because of multiple abortions in a carrier. *Hum. Hered.*, **25,** 362

Friedman, S. *et al.* (1977). Fromino-glutamic acid (Figulu) excretion and abortion. *Panminerva Med.*, **19**, 271
Gardiner, A. *et al.* (1978). Spontaneous abortion and fetal abnormality in subsequent pregnancy. *Br. Med. J.*, **1**, 1016
Gehring, H. *et al.* (1977). 2-BR-alpha-ergocryptine (Pariodel) in primary and secondary lactation suppression following child-birth or abortion. *Praxis*, **66**, 985
Gencik, A. *et al.* (1978). Analysis of spontaneous abortiveness, child mortality, and of inborn developmental defects in two population series from Horna Nitra. (Author's transl.) *Bratisl. Lek. Listy*, **69**, 678
Gordon, Y. B. *et al.* (1978). Fetal wastage as a result of an alpha fetoprotein screening programe.
Humphries, S. V. (1978). The problems of therapeutic abortion and infanticide. *Cent. Afr. J. Med.*, 2411
Hunton, R. B. (1977). Computerized screening for medical, psychiatric and social problems: review of the technique and results in 1296 consecutive applications for therapeutic abortions. In Coblentz, A. M.
Islamov, R. Z. *et al.* (1978). Epizootiology of enzootic (viral) abortion in sheep. *Veterinariia*, 57
Jain, S. *et al.* (1977). Autoimmune hemolytic anaemia and foetal loss. *J. Assoc. Physicians India*, **25**, 765
James, W. H. (1978). Birth ranks of spontaneous abortions in sibships of children affected by anencephaly or spina bifida. *Br. Med. J.*, **1, 72**
Jovanovic, L. *et al.* (1978). Hormonal profile as a prognostic index of early threatened abortion. *Am. J. Obstet. Gynecol.*, **130**, 274
Kajii, T. *et al.* (1978). Cytogenetics of aborters and abortuses. *Am. J. Obstet. Gynecol.*, **131**, 33
Kamarawy, H. *et al.* (1977). Management of missed abortion and fetal death in utero. *Prostaglandins*, **14**, 583
Kampo, M. A. *et al.* (1978). Oxidative metabolism of the placenta in miscarriage. *Pediatr. Akush. Ginekol.*, 43
Kaplan, E. S. (1978). A generalized epileptiform convulsion after intra-amniotic prostaglandin with intravenous oxytocin infusion, a case report. *Afr. Med. J.*, **53**, 17
Kate, L. P. (1978). On estimating the actual rate of foetal loss in families with an autosomal recessive disorder and Wolfs data on PKU ten. *Ann. Hum. Genet.*, **41**, 463
Keirse, M. J. *et al.* (1978). Risk of pre-term delivery in patients with previous pre-term delivery and/or abortion. *Br. J. Obstet. Gynaecol.*, **85**, 81
Kerekes, L. *et al.* (1977). Termination of mid-term spontaneous and missed abortions by extra-amniotic injection of a single prostaglandin F2 alpha dose. *Ther. Hung.*, **25**, 102
King, C. R. *et al.* (1977). Fetal wastage and chromosome anomalies in offspring of patients with Turner Syndrome. (Letter) *Lancet*, **2**, 928
Kirchoff, H. *et al.* (1977). Value of radiographic studies on the cervix uteri and internal uterine orifice with reference to irregular pregnancies (abortus-premature labor). *Zentralbl. Gynaekol.*, **99**, 1159
Kline, J. *et al.* (1977). Surveillance of spontaneous abortion. Power in environmental monitoring. *Am. J. Epidemiol.*, **106**, 345
Kline, J. *et al.* (1978*a*). Spontaneous abortion and the use of sugar substitutes (saccharin). *Am. J. Obstet. Gynecol.*, **130**, 708
Kline, J. *et al.* (1978*b*). Cigarette smoking and spontaneous abortion. *Br. Med. J.*, **1**, 259, 4
Knill-Jones, R. P. *et al.* (1975). Anesthetic practice and pregnancy. Controlled survey of male anaesthetists in the United Kingdom. *Lancet*, **2**, 807
Kononova, E. S. *et al.* (1977). Characteristics of the hypophyseal-ovarian relationship in miscarriage. *Akush. Ginekol., (Mosk.)*, **37**
Kozhevnikov, V. N. (1977). Pathogenetic factors in miscarriage and prolonged pregnancy. *Akush. Ginekol.*, 40
Kuliev, A. M. *et al.* (1977). Monosomy 21 in a human spontaneous abortus. Morphogenetic disturbances and phenotype at the cellular level. *Hum. Genet.*, **38**, 137
Kunze, W. P. (1978). Cytophotometric DNA measurements in abortion. *Pathol. Res. Pract.*, **162**, 253
Lahteenmaki, P. *et al.* (1978). Return of ovarian function after abortion. *Clin. Endocrinol.*, **8**, 123
Lauritsen, J. G. (1977). Genetic aspects of spontaneous abortion. *Dan. Med. Bull.*, **24**, 169
Ledger, W. J. *et al.* (1977). A fever index evaluation of chloramphenicol or clindamyclin in patients with serious pelvic infections. *Obstet. Gynecol.*, **50**, 523

Lees, D. E. *et al.* (1977). Probable amniotic fluid embolism during curettage for a missed abortion; a case report. *Anesth. Analg.*, **56**, 739
Lidbjork, G. *et al.* (1977). Alpha-fetoprotein (AFP) levels in maternal serum in 115 patients with spontaneous abortion. *Acta Obstet. Gynecol. Scand.*, 50
Livnat, E. J. *et al.* (1978). Fetus papylaceus in twin pregnancy. *Obstet. Gynecol.*, **51**, (1 Suppl.), 41
Lolis, D. *et al.* (1978). Toxoplasma antibodies and spontaneous abortion. *Int. J. Gynaecol. Obstet.*, **15**, 299
Lopez Ortiz, E. *et al.* (1978). Value of amoxicillin and ampicillin in the treatment of septic abortion (double blind and random comparative studies). *Ginecol. Obstet.*, **43**, 123
McArdle, C. R. (1978*a*). Pregnancy in a bicornuate uterus. *JCU*, **6**, 185
McArdle, C. R. (1978*b*). Failed abortion in a septate uterus. *Am. J. Obstet. Gynecol.*, **131**, 910
McKenzie, R. *et al.* (1978). A safer method for paracervical block in therapeutic abortions. *Am. J. Obstet. Gynecol.*, **130**, 317
Miyakawa, I. *et al.* (1977). Plasma hormone profile of threatened abortion and its prognosis. *Int. J. Gynaecol. Obstet.*, **15**, 12
Moller, B. R. *et al.* (1978*a*). Therapeutic abortion in an out patient clinic. A prospective investigation of complications and patient acceptability. *Acta. Obstet. Gynecol. Scand.*, **57**, 41
Moller, B. R. *et al.* (1978*b*). Effect of general and local anaesthesia on blood loss during and after therapeutic abortion. *Acta. Obstet. Gynecol. Scand.*, **57**, 133
Murashko, L. E. (1978). Hormonal changes in artificial abortion in the 7th and 8th weeks of pregnancy. *Sov. Med.*, 75
Nemic, D. K. *et al.* (1978). Medical abortion complications. An epidemiologic study at a mid-Missouri clinic. *Obstet. Gynecol.*, **51**, 433
Nielsen, J. (1978). Large Y chromosome (Yq +) and increased risk of abortion. *Clin. Genet.*, **13**, 415
Niikawa, N. *et al.* (1977). Origin of acrocentric trisomies in spontaneous abortuses. *Hum. Genet.*, **40**, 73
Nordstom, S. *et al.* (1978). Occupational and environmental risks in and around a smelter in northern Sweden, III. Frequencies of spontaneous abortion. *Hereditas*, **88**, 51
Paladini, A. *et al.* (1977). Induction of labor in missed abortion, fetal death and vesicular mole, using PGF2 alpha by extra-amniotic intracavitary administration. *Minerva Ginecol.*, **29**, 931
Pogorelova, T. N. (1978). Physiocochemical properties of placental proteins, in physiological and interrupted pregnancy. *Akush. Ginekol. (Mosk.)*, 27
Quan, A. *et al.* (1977). Laparoscopic sterilization after spontaneous abortion. *Int. J. Gynaecol. Obstet.*, **15**, 258
Ruiz-Mateos Jimenez de Tejada, A. M. (1977). Narcissism and abortion. *Actas Luso. Esp. Neurol. Psiquiatr.*, **5**, 241
Rushton, D. I. (1978). Simplified classification of spontaneous abortions. *Med. Genet.*, **15**, 1
Rushwan, H. *et al.* (1977). Contraceptive practice after women have undergone spontaneous abortion in Indonesia and Sudan. *Int. J. Gynaecol. Obstet.*, **15**, 241
Saavedra, J. A. *et al.* (1977). Echographic study in early pregnancy. I. Parameter of uterus. *Zentralbl. Gynaekol.*, **99**, 1421
Sanches Avalos, J. C. *et al.* (1977). Hemostatic disorders in acute renal failure post-abortion. Study of 60 cases. *Medicina (B Aires)*, **37**, (*Suppl.* 2), 70
Schillinger, H. *et al.* (1978). Ultrasound and semiquantitative chorionic gonadotropin secretin in the diagnosis of abortiona. *Zentralbl. Gynaekol.*, **100**, 76
Schwarz, R. (1978). Experiences with the preventive use of heparin in septic abortion. *Zentralbl. Gynaekol.*, **100**, 486
Sivin, I. (1978). Ectopic pregnancies, IUDs and abortion. *Contraception*, **12**, 575
Smith, C. *et al.* (1978). Ultrasonography in threatened abortion. *Obstet. Gynecol.*, **51**, 173
Sol'skii, IaP *et al.* (1978). Lethality in abortions and the ways for its further decrease.
Sparks, R. A. *et al.* (1978*a*). Septic abortion and IUDs. *Br. Med. J.*, 6114, 719.
Sparks, R. A. *et al.* (1978*b*). Mid-trimester septic abortion and Escherichia coli septicaemia in copper IUCD users. *Br. Med. J.*, **1**, 481
Strandberg, M. *et al.* (1978). Spontaneous abortions among women in hospital laboratory. (Letter) *Lancet*, **1**, 384
Suffin, S. C. *et al.* (1977). Vesicular stomatitis virus causes abortion and neonatal death in ferrets. *J. Clin. Microbiol.*, **6**, 437

Sulovic, V. *et al.* (1977). Population of B and T lymphocytes and lymphocyte blast transformation test in spontaneous and missed abortions in the first trimester of pregnancy. In B. Boettcher (ed.) *Immunological Influence on Human Fertility.* (New York: Academic Press)

Talaat, M. *et al.* (1976). Hemostasis in the Egyptian female in abortion, with a case report. *J. Egypt Med. Assoc.*, 59-98-105

Teleman, G. *et al.* (1977). Hormonic colpocytotest in diagnosis and therapy of some spontaneous abortion. *Rev. Med. Chir. Soc. Med. Nat. Iasi,* **81,** 499

Theile, U. (1977). Rate of abortions and abnormalities following viral hepatitis. *Med. Klin.*, **72,** 1554

Vasilev, D. (1978). Early artificial termination of pregnancy by Karmans method. *Akosh. Ginekol. (Sofiia)*, **17,** 98

Wainscott, G. *et al.* (1978). The outcome of pregnancy in women suffering from migraine. *Postgrad. Med. J.*, **54,** 98

Ward, H. *et al.* (1978). Plasma non-esterified fatty acids, cortisol and glucose in maternal blood during abortion induced with intra-amniotic prostaglandin F2alpha. *Br. J. Obstet. Gynaecol.*, **85,** 344

Warkany, J. (1978). Terathanasia. *Teratology*, **17,** 187

Weil, A. (1978). Laparoscopic sterilization with therapeutic abortion versus sterilization or abortion alone. **52,** 79

Worton, R. G. (1977). Chromosome abnormalities; a major cause of birth defects, stillbirth and spontaneous abortion. *Can. Med. Assoc. J.*, **117,** 849, 51

Young, R. H. *et al.* (1977). Adrenal necrosis following abortion. *Ir. J. Med. Sci.*, **146,** 340

Index